T0292632

Lecture Notes in Computational Science and Engineering

111

Editors:

More information about this series at http://www.springer.com/series/3527

Aslak Tveito • Glenn T. Lines

Computing Characterizations of Drugs for Ion Channels and Receptors Using Markov Models

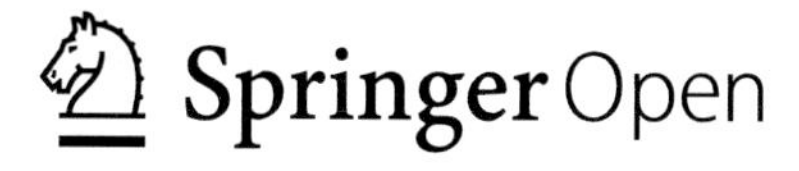

Aslak Tveito
Center for Biomedical Computing
Simula Research Laboratory
Lysaker, Norway

Glenn T. Lines
Center for Biomedical Computing
Simula Research Laboratory
Lysaker, Norway

ISSN 1439-7358 ISSN 2197-7100 (electronic)
Lecture Notes in Computational Science and Engineering
ISBN 978-3-319-30029-0 ISBN 978-3-319-30030-6 (eBook)
DOI 10.1007/978-3-319-30030-6

Library of Congress Control Number: 2016937425

Mathematics Subject Classification (2010): 34F05, 60J20, 60J28, 62M05, 80A30, 92C45

Printed on acid-free paper

This Springer imprint is published by Springer Nature
The registered company is Springer International Publishing AG Switzerland

Preface

The summer of 2013 was very good; we found a series of papers published by Gregory D. Smith and his coauthors. We spent several weeks trying to understand the paper [35], which introduces and carefully studies a stochastic model of calcium release from internal stores in cells. Then we found a whole series of papers [36, 57, 102, 103], and the results more or less kept us busy for months. The beauty of the theory presented in these papers is that they introduce a systematic way of analyzing models that are of great importance for understanding essential physiological processes.

So what is this theory about? It has been fairly well known for a while that stochastic models are useful in studying the release of calcium ions from internal storage in living cells. Some authors even argue that this process *is* stochastic. That is debatable, but it is quite clear that stochastic models are well suited to study such processes. Stochastic models are also very well suited to study the change of the transmembrane potential resulting from the flow of ions through channels in the cell membrane. Both these processes are of fundamental importance in understanding the function of excitable cells. In both applications, ions flow from one domain to another according to electrochemical gradients, depending on whether the channel is in a conducting or nonconducting mode. The state of the channel is described by a Markov model, which is a wonderful tool used to systematically represent how an ion channel or a receptor opens or closes based on the surrounding conditions. In this context, the contribution of the papers listed above is to present a systematic way of analyzing the stochastic models in terms of formulating deterministic differential equations describing the probability density distributions of the states of the Markov models.

As pointed out in the papers by Smith et al., this approach is not really new; the authors cite a number of earlier papers and we have been quite influenced by the paper of Nykamp and Tranchina [63] because of its elegant way of developing the deterministic differential equation describing the probability density functions of the states involved in the stochastic process. The key observation is that we can study stochastic release in two fundamentally different ways: (1) We can run a number of simulations using a stochastic model. Because of the stochastic state of the channel, the results will differ, but we can gather numerous results and summarize them in terms of histograms describing the probability density functions of being in a given state. (2) We can find a deterministic partial differential equation modeling the probability density functions and obtain the distributions by solving this system numerically. By increasing the number of simulations in (1) and by refining the numerical discretization in (1) and (2), we observe that the results of the two methods converge to the same distributions. Therefore, we have a very powerful tool for analyzing the stochastic models: We can simply solve deterministic partial differential equations to find the probability density functions. In some simple cases, the deterministic partial differential equations can be studied analytically and no numerical solution is needed. The relation between the stochastic simulation and the solution of the deterministic partial differential equations will be studied repeatedly in these notes.

More recently, we found the book by Bressloff [6] to be an astonishing source of material concerning stochastic processes in cells. It will clearly become a standard reference in the field together with its companion volume [7]. The theory of stochastic processes is also introduced in a most readable manner by Jacobs [39], and elements of the theory are covered in the monumental work of Keener and Sneyd [43, 44].

One reason for our enthusiasm in finding the papers listed above is that, for a while, we have been trying to understand how to theoretically devise suitable drugs for mutations affecting both ion channels and receptors. It has been clear for some time that the effect of mutations on ion channels and various receptors can be successfully modeled using Markov models to describe the state of the channel. A comprehensive review is presented by Rudy [74] (see also Rudy and Silva [75]). Clancy and Rudy and their coauthors (e.g., [16]) have also shown how to use Markov models to describe the function of various drugs aimed at repairing the function of mutated channels or receptors. This is very useful, since it allows simulation based on stochastic models and the models can also be interpreted as continuous representations for whole cell simulations. However, analysis of the Markov models is taken to a new level by the introduction of probability density functions defined in terms of deterministic partial differential equations.

Our approach has been as follows: Let the properties of the drug be free parameters and use a setup based on Markov models to find the best possible drugs. This problem is much easier to approach using the results of Smith et al. because it amounts to understanding how the solution of the extended system of partial differential equations (including the effect of the drug) behaves as a function of the parameters characterizing the drug. Typically, we will end up comparing the solutions of three systems of partial differential equations: (1) a system modeling the dynamics of healthy (wild type) cells, (2) a system modeling the dynamics of non-healthy (mutant) cells, and (3) a system modeling the dynamics of non-healthy cells with a drug added to repair the effect of the mutation. *The problem we would like to address is how to adjust the parameters describing the drug such that the solution of (3) is as close to the solution of (1) as possible.* This turns out to be much easier using a deterministic system of partial differential equations describing the probability density functions than using stochastic simulations.

We have decided to present our results in the form of lecture notes. There are several reasons for this choice. First, we strongly believe that the theory described above is very useful, and we want to help make it as comprehensible as possible. That is more or less impossible to do in scientific papers because their focus must be on new results and not on careful derivations of established insights. A second reason is that the problem of understanding cell physiology and how drugs affect their function is inherently multidisciplinary, and we therefore write these notes in such a way that we hope readers who are not primarily applied mathematicians can understand. We also hope to give applied mathematicians glimpses of interesting problems of great importance.

As mentioned above, these notes aim to explain known theory that we think can be useful to researchers working on a mathematical understanding of living cells. There are also new results. We show in some detail how to derive formulas describing the optimal properties of theoretical drugs. Most of the results are stated for rather simple models, but it is quite clear that the methods can be extended to more intricate cases.

The million dollar question when you read these notes is, of course, can these drugs actually be created? Do they exist? We do not know. We know that Markov models have been used to successfully represent the actions of drugs, but is it possible to go the other way and first compute what properties the drug should have and then create it? We have found no clear answers in the literature or through discussions with colleagues, so we decided to just formulate these ideas as precisely as possible in the hopes that someone will find them useful. We have tried to carefully underline in the notes that we are discussing *theoretical drugs*, and we state in many places that this work is about possible drugs.

Acknowledgments

It is pleasure to thank Dr Martin Peters at Springer for a very fruitful collaboration through many years.

We would also like to thank the six reviewers of these notes. One reviewer wrote an unusually comprehensive and encouraging report counting seven pages; we spent two months working on his or her comments and it was clearly worth the effort. We have never experienced a referee report of equal depth and usefulness and we deeply appreciate the reviewer's labor.

These lecture notes were largely written during visits to the University of California, San Diego, and the authors are grateful for the hospitality of the Department of Bioengineering and the Department of Computer Science and Engineering.

Finally, we would like to thank Karoline Horgmo Jæger, who read the entire document twice and found numerous small (and actually some not so small) errors.

Her efforts are highly appreciated. We would also like to thank Achim Schroll for helpful discussions regarding the hyperbolic problems encountered in this text.

This work was supported by a Centre of Excellence grant from the Norwegian Research Council to the Center for Biomedical Computing at Simula Research Laboratory.

Lysaker, Norway Aslak Tveito
Lysaker, Norway Glenn T. Lines
October 2015

Contents

Chapter 1
Background: Problem and Methods

Drugs are generally devised to alter the function of cells in a favorable manner. The actions of drugs can in some cases be represented by mathematical models often phrased in terms of differential equations. Our aim in these notes is to study such models and show how the effect of drugs can be optimized. More precisely, drugs are represented in terms of a set of parameters and we show how optimal drugs can be characterized by tuning the parameters. Our approach is to consider models of a healthy cell and a non-healthy cell and a model of a non-healthy cell to which a drug has been applied. The problem we are trying to resolve is how to tweak the parameters of the drug such that the drugged non-healthy cell behaves as similarly to the healthy cell as possible.

We will use this approach to address two processes of immense importance in physiology: (1) voltage-gated ion channels and (2) calcium release from storage structures inside the cell. We will also study combinations of these processes occurring in a space in which the release through voltage-gated ion channels interacts with calcium release from the internal storage structures.

Both processes can be affected by disease and by mutations. In these notes we will concentrate on wild type (healthy) cells and mutant cells. We will assume that the behavior of the wild type cell can be described in terms of Markov models and that a Markov model can represent the effects of the mutation.

1.1 Action Potentials

Suppose a group of engineers were given the task of developing a pump weighing about 300 g that is supposed to work uninterruptedly and basically without maintenance for about 80 years, pump about 7,000 l of blood every day, and beat every second. The group would—and should—agree that the task is impossible but,

A. Tveito, G.T. Lines, *Computing Characterizations of Drugs for Ion Channels and Receptors Using Markov Models*, Lecture Notes in Computational Science and Engineering 111, DOI 10.1007/978-3-319-30030-6_1

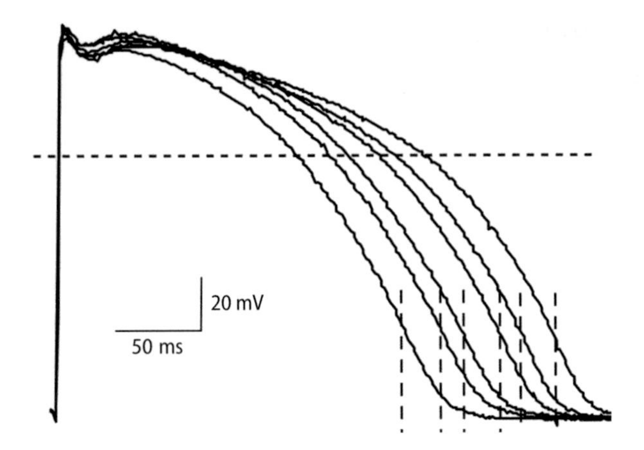

Fig. 1.1 Action potentials obtained by measurements taken from Jost et al. [40]

under pressure from their employer, they would probably agree that the mechanism would have to be extremely simple. Fortunately for us all, the pump has already been developed by evolution, but it is very far from being simple; it is an extremely complex piece of machinery, so complex that how it works is still not completely understood. For an intriguing illustration of this, the reader is encouraged to consult the fascinating joint paper by Lakatta and DiFrancesco [47] in which they debate the following fundamental question: How is the heartbeat initiated? It is remarkable that such a basic question is still open. Two plausible and completely different mechanisms are discussed, with supporting experimental data and mathematical models for both. The interested reader can also consult Li et al. [50] for an introduction to this discussion.

Even if the exact mechanism for initiating the heartbeat is still under debate, it is completely clear that every normal heartbeat is initiated in the sinoatrial node. From that node, an electrochemical wave spreads throughout the cardiac muscle. With every beat, billions of cardiac cells undergo an action potential that is a characteristic temporal change of the transmembrane potential of the cell V, defined by

$$V = V_i - V_e,$$

where V_i and V_e are the intracellular and extracellular electrical potentials, respectively.

In Fig. 1.1 we show an action potential obtained by measurements. The recordings are taken from the paper by Jost et al. [40]. Mathematical models have been used to represent action potentials ever since the groundbreaking paper by Hodgkin and Huxley [33] from 1952. The first models of cardiac cells were developed by Noble [61, 62] in 1960–1962. In Fig. 1.2 an action potential is presented based on the mathematical model of ventricular cardiac cells developed by Grandi et al. [29].

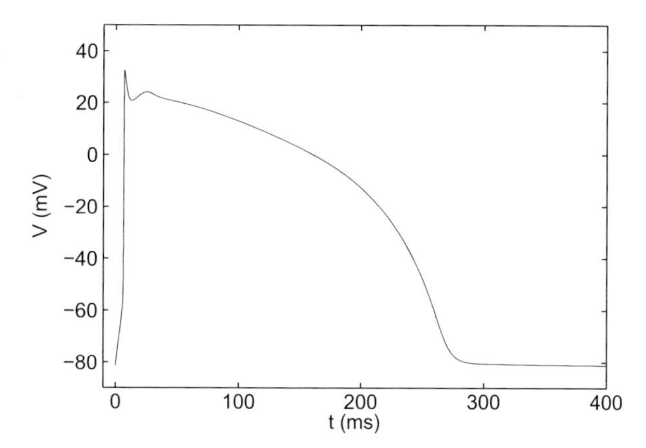

Fig. 1.2 Action potential computed using the model of Grandi et al. [29]

When an electrical wave of the increased transmembrane potential approaches a cell, the cell's transmembrane potential is elevated above a critical value. This elevation leads to the opening of sodium channels, resulting in a huge influx of sodium ions into the cell. This rapid process dramatically increases the transmembrane potential and is referred to as the upstroke of the action potential. When the transmembrane potential increases, voltage-gated calcium channels in the cell membrane open and calcium ions flow into the cell because of the huge difference in concentrations; the extracellular concentration of calcium ions is much greater than the intracellular (cytosolic) concentration when the cell is at rest. The increased concentration of calcium ions within the cell triggers the opening of channels to internal stores and a great deal more calcium floods into the cytosol. The increased level of calcium in the cytosol leads to the cell's contraction, which is basically the main goal of the whole operation. Then everything returns to the resting state: Calcium is pumped out of the cell and into internal stores—every cell prepares for a new wave.

Even if this process is amazingly stable and versatile and a masterpiece by any standard in the universe, it is not infallible. It can be harmed by disease, by the side effects of drugs, and by mutations. In these lecture notes, we shall focus on the effect of mutations and search for theoretical drugs that can, in principle, repair the effect of dangerous mutations. The study of mutations affecting cardiac cells is a huge field and we will simply look at prototypical models that capture the characteristic effects of well-known mutations. Our main objective is to present methods for computing characterizations of optimal theoretical drugs using prototypical models of ion release.

Most of these lecture notes will be focused on what happens in single ion channels. However, in the final chapter we will return to the action potential of the whole cell.

1.2 Markov Models

The cell membrane is densely populated with ion channels that can open and close to control the flow of ions across the cell membrane. In Fig. 1.3, we show the recordings of a single channel and we note the frequent transitions between the open and closed states and how the frequency changes with the transmembrane potential. It is commonly believed that the state of a single channel is adequately modeled using a stochastic approach. Actually, it is common to claim that the process is stochastic. It is hard, if not impossible, to prove that something is stochastic, but for modeling purposes it suffices to state that a stochastic approach leads to reasonable models of the gating dynamics.

A Markov model in its simplest form is usually written as the chemical reaction scheme

$$C \underset{k_{co}}{\overset{k_{oc}}{\leftrightarrows}} O, \tag{1.1}$$

where k_{oc} and k_{co} are reaction rates that may depend on the transmembrane potential. We will return to the interpretation of this notation many times, but let us just roughly describe what it means. Suppose at a given time t that the gate is open so the channel is in state O and suppose that Δt is a very short time interval. Then (1.1) states that the probability that the channel changes state from open to closed is given by $k_{oc}\Delta t$. Similarly, if the channel is closed (C), the probability for a change to the open state is given by $k_{co}\Delta t$.

More formally, we let $S = S(t)$ denote a random variable representing the state of the channel at time t, so $S \in \{O, C\}$. Then the transition rates k_{oc} and k_{co} give the probability of changing state during a small time interval Δt :

$$k_{oc}\Delta t = \text{Prob}\,[S(t + \Delta t) = C \mid S(t) = O(t)]$$

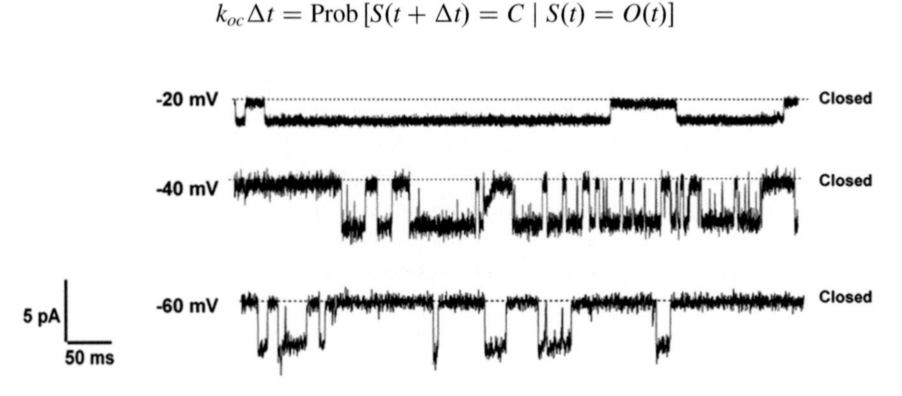

Fig. 1.3 Single-channel recording of a sodium current (from Shaya et al. [81]). The levels of the current indicate whether the channel is closed (as indicated in the figure) or open. The probability that the channel is open is low at −60 mV, higher at −40 mV, and even higher at −20 mV

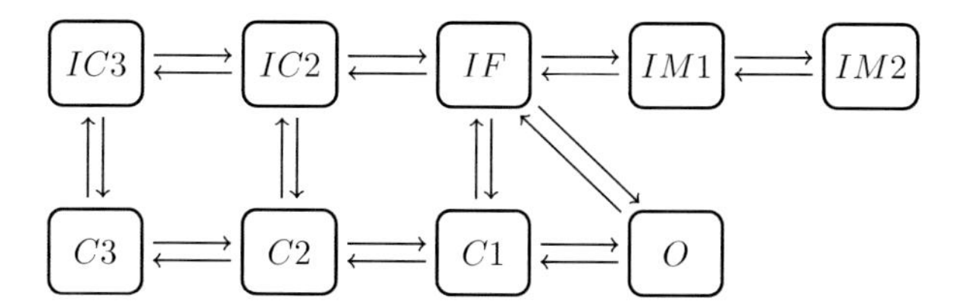

Fig. 1.4 The sodium channel model of Clancy et al. [15]; O is the open state, C1, C2 and C3 are the closed states, while the rest of the states represent different kinds of inactivation

and

$$k_{co}\Delta t = \text{Prob}\left[S(t + \Delta t) = O \mid S(t) = C(t)\right],$$

respectively. With this notation, we easily see that we can play with the properties of the channels by changing the values of the parameters k_{oc} and k_{oc}. We also see that we can make the reaction scheme dependent on the transmembrane potential V (mV) by allowing the reaction terms to depend on V.

The case of just one closed and one open state is particularly simple but it is still the base model and it is frequently used in modeling ion channels. However, much more intricate models have been derived and one is shown in Fig. 1.4. It represents a Markov model with one open state, three closed states, and five inactivated[1] states.

The popularity of these models stems from the fact that it is possible to adjust the parameters involved to obtain a model that reflects data quite well. However, it should also be mentioned that models can be so complex that it is virtually impossible to uniquely determine all the parameters involved. In these notes, we shall confine ourselves to relatively simple Markov models but the methods we describe can be applied, at least in principle, to Markov models of higher complexity.

1.2.1 *The Master Equation*

From the Markov model written on the form (1.1), we can derive an equation giving the evolution of the probability of the two states, open (O) and closed (C). Let $o = o(t)$ be the probability that the channel is in the open (O) state at time t and let $c = c(t)$ denote the probability that the channel is closed (C). We assume that the probabilities o and c are known at time t and then use the Markov model (1.1) to compute the probabilities at time $t + \Delta t$. Here Δt is assumed to be so small that the

[1] Inactivated states are discussed in Chap. 11.

channel changes state at most once during the time step from t to $t + \Delta t$. Then the scheme (1.1) states that the open probability at time $t + \Delta t$ is given by

$$o(t + \Delta t) = \text{Prob}\,[(S(t) = C) \text{ and } (C \to O \text{ during } \Delta t)] \tag{1.2}$$

$$+ \text{Prob}\,[(S(t) = O) \text{ and not}(O \to C \text{ during } \Delta t)] \tag{1.3}$$

$$= c(t) \cdot (\Delta t k_{co}) + o(t) \cdot (1 - \Delta t k_{oc}) \tag{1.4}$$

so

$$o(t + \Delta t) = o(t) + \Delta t(k_{co}c(t) - k_{oc}o(t)).$$

From this equation, we obtain

$$\frac{o(t + \Delta t) - o(t)}{\Delta t} = k_{co}c(t) - k_{oc}o(t),$$

and, therefore, by passing to the limit $\Delta t \to 0$, we get the differential equation

$$o'(t) = k_{co}c(t) - k_{oc}o(t). \tag{1.5}$$

Similarly, we find that the probability of being in the closed state evolves according to

$$c'(t) = k_{oc}o(t) - k_{co}c(t). \tag{1.6}$$

Since we are dealing with probabilities, it is reasonable to assume that the initial conditions add up to one (the channel is either open or closed) and therefore, by adding the equations above, we find that

$$o(t) + c(t) = 1$$

for all time. Hence the variable c in (1.5) can be replaced by $1 - o$ and the system (1.5,1.6) can be written as a scalar equation of the form

$$o'(t) = (k_{co} + k_{oc}) \left(\frac{k_{co}}{k_{co} + k_{oc}} - o\,(t) \right). \tag{1.7}$$

Here we see that

$$o = \frac{k_{co}}{k_{co} + k_{oc}}$$

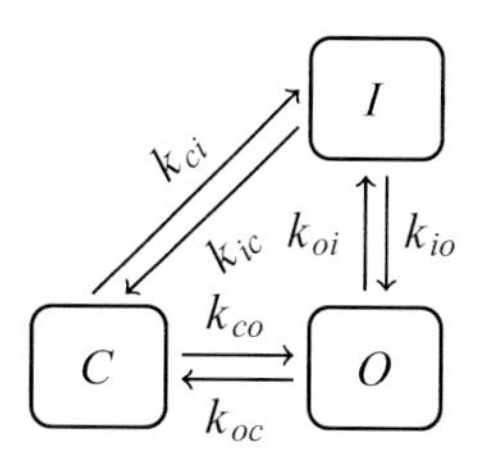

Fig. 1.5 Markov model including three possible states: open (O), closed (C), and inactivated (I)

is a stable equilibrium solution. Furthermore, if we know that the channel is closed initially, that is, $o(0) = 0$, we get the solution

$$o(t) = \frac{k_{co}}{k_{co} + k_{oc}} \left(1 - e^{-(k_{co}+k_{oc})t}\right)$$

and we notice that the equilibrium is reached more quickly as the sum of the rates $k_{co} + k_{oc}$ increases.

1.2.2 The Master Equation of a Three-State Model

The development of the master equation for the two-state model above can be carried out for any Markov model. For instance, if we consider the three-state Markov model shown in Fig. 1.5, we realize that the probabilities of the open (O), closed (C), and inactivated (I) states are governed by the following system of ordinary differential equations:

$$\begin{aligned} o' &= k_{io}i + k_{co}c - (k_{oi} + k_{oc})\, o, \\ c' &= k_{oc}o + k_{ic}i - (k_{co} + k_{ci})\, c, \\ i' &= k_{oi}o + k_{ci}c - (k_{io} + k_{ic})\, i, \end{aligned} \tag{1.8}$$

Since

$$i = 1 - (o + c)\,, \tag{1.9}$$

we have the following 2×2 system:

$$o' = k_{io} + (k_{co} - k_{io})\, c - (k_{oi} + k_{oc} + k_{io})\, o, \tag{1.10}$$

$$c' = k_{ic} + (k_{oc} - k_{ic})\, o - (k_{co} + k_{ci} + k_{ic})\, c. \tag{1.11}$$

We will now show, using a numerical computation, that the solution of the system (1.10,1.11) coincides with the average result of Monte Carlo simulations using the Markov model shown in Fig. 1.5 as the number of Monte Carlo runs goes to infinity.

1.2.3 Monte Carlo Simulations Based on the Markov Model

Before we compare the two computational schemes, let us briefly describe how the Monte Carlo simulation can be implemented. We choose a small timestep Δt and we assume that the state at time $t = t_n = n\Delta t$, where n is a non-negative integer, is either O, C, or I. For simplicity, we describe how the computation proceeds in the case of the channel being in the open (O) state at time $t = t_n$. In order to decide the state at time $t_{n+1} = t_n + \Delta t$, we divide the unit interval into three non-overlapping parts: $A_c = [0, k_{oc}\Delta t)$, $A_i = [k_{oc}\Delta t, k_{oc}\Delta t + k_{oi}\Delta t)$, $A_o = [k_{oc}\Delta t + k_{oi}\Delta t, 1]$. Then, at time $t_{n+1} = t_n + \Delta t$, we can update the state of the channel based on a random number r_n in the unit interval drawn from a uniform distribution. Specifically, if $r_n \in A_o$, the channel remains open; if $r_n \in A_c$, the state of the channel changes from open to closed; and, finally, if $r_n \in A_i$, the state of the channel changes from open to inactivated.

Similar steps are straightforward to devise for the case of the channel being in the closed or inactivated states at time $t = t_n$.

1.2.4 Comparison of Monte Carlo Simulations and Solutions of the Master Equation

In Fig. 1.6 we compare the probabilities computed by solving the master equation (1.10,1.11) (red lines) and by Monte Carlo simulations using the Markov model as described above. In the simulations we have used the initial conditions $o(0) = i(0) = 0$ and $c(0) = 1$ and the rates used in the computations are given in Table 1.1. As the number of Monte Carlo simulations increases, we see that the average approaches the solution of the continuous master equation. In these computations the master equation was solved using the function ODE15s in Matlab.

1.2.5 Equilibrium Probabilities

The equilibrium state of the reaction shown in Fig. 1.5 is characterized by the equations

$$\begin{aligned} k_{co}c &= k_{oc}o, \\ k_{oi}o &= k_{io}i, \\ k_{ic}i &= k_{ci}c, \end{aligned} \tag{1.12}$$

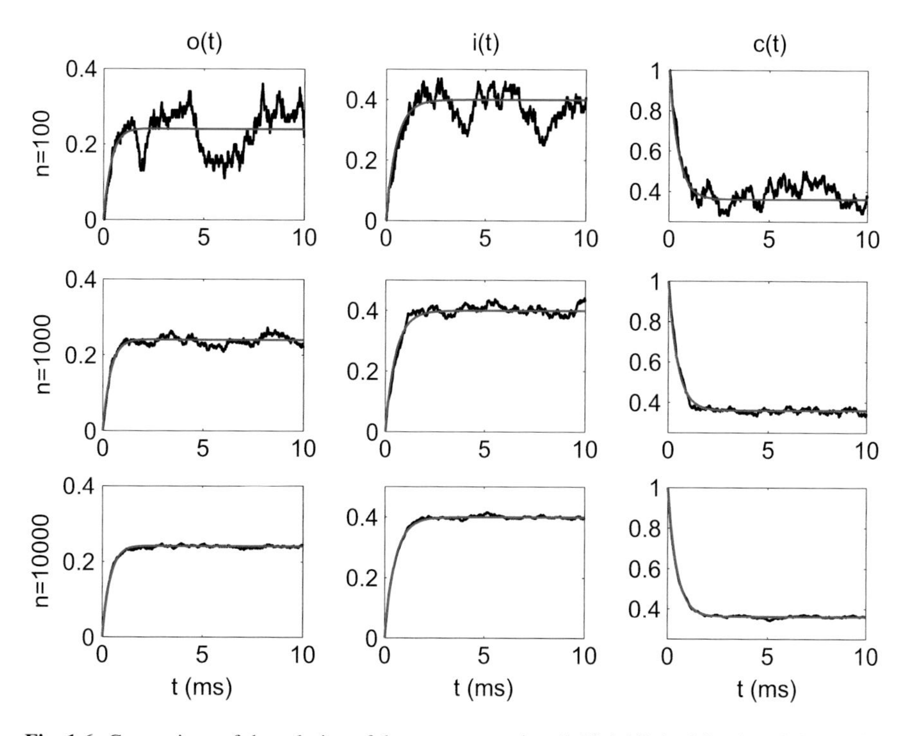

Fig. 1.6 Comparison of the solution of the master equation (1.10,1.11) (*red lines*) and the results of Monte Carlo simulations based on the Markov model given in Fig. 1.5. The time step used in the Monte-Carlo simulations was $\Delta t = 0.01$ ms in all the panels and the simulations were run for 10 ms. The number of Monte Carlo simulations increases from 100 (*top*) to 10,000 (*bottom*)

Table 1.1 Rates (in 1/ms) of the Markov model given in Fig. 1.5 used in the computations presented in Fig. 1.6

k_{oi}	k_{io}	k_{co}	k_{oc}	k_{ic}	k_{ci}
0.5	0.3	0.6	0.9	0.72	0.8

where o, c, and i denote the probabilities of the channel being open, closed, or inactivated, respectively. It follows that

$$c = \frac{k_{oc}}{k_{co}} o$$

and

$$i = \frac{k_{oi}}{k_{io}} o.$$

By using the fact that $o + c + i = 1$, we obtain

$$\left(1 + \frac{k_{oc}}{k_{co}} + \frac{k_{oi}}{k_{io}}\right) o = 1$$

and therefore

$$o = \frac{1}{1 + \frac{k_{oc}}{k_{co}} + \frac{k_{oi}}{k_{io}}},$$

$$c = \frac{\frac{k_{oc}}{k_{co}}}{1 + \frac{k_{oc}}{k_{co}} + \frac{k_{oi}}{k_{io}}},$$

$$i = \frac{\frac{k_{oi}}{k_{io}}}{1 + \frac{k_{oc}}{k_{co}} + \frac{k_{oi}}{k_{io}}}.$$

For the particular rates given in Table 1.1, we get the following equilibrium probabilities: $o = 0.24$, $c = 0.36$, and $i = 0.4$.

1.2.6 Detailed Balance

In order to compute the equilibrium solution of (1.8) above, we assumed that each of the sub-transitions of the diagram given in Fig. 1.5 was in equilibrium. More precisely, we assumed that

$$k_{co}c = k_{oc}o, \; k_{oi}o = k_{io}i, \; \text{and } k_{ic}i = k_{ci}c.$$

These three relations yield

$$k_{co}k_{oi}k_{ic} = k_{ci}k_{io}k_{oc}. \tag{1.13}$$

This relation is referred to as the condition of *detailed balance*. In these notes, we will always assume that Markov models satisfy this condition. More generally, the product of the rates in a loop (e.g. the I-O-C loop of Fig. 1.5) in the clockwise direction equals the product of the rates in the counterclockwise direction. Under this assumption, the equilibrium solution can always be computed by the method indicated above. We will use the same technique many times in these notes.

1.3 The Master Equation and the Equilibrium Solution

We have seen that the Markov model written in the form

$$C \underset{k_{co}}{\overset{k_{oc}}{\leftrightarrows}} O \tag{1.14}$$

leads to a master equation of the form

$$o'(t) = k_{co}c(t) - k_{oc}o(t), \tag{1.15}$$

$$c'(t) = k_{oc}o(t) - k_{co}c(t). \tag{1.16}$$

Since $o + c = 1$, we can reduce the system to the scalar equation,

$$o'(t) = (k_{co} + k_{oc}) \left(\frac{k_{co}}{k_{co} + k_{oc}} - o(t) \right)$$

and we readily see that the equilibrium solution is given by

$$o = \frac{k_{co}}{k_{co} + k_{oc}}.$$

Exactly the same steps can be followed for the three-state Markov model illustrated in Fig. 1.5. The associated Markov model reads

$$o' = k_{io}i + k_{co}c - (k_{oi} + k_{oc})\, o$$
$$c' = k_{oc}o + k_{ic}i - (k_{co} + k_{ci})\, c$$
$$i' = k_{oi}o + k_{ci}c - (k_{io} + k_{ic})\, i$$

and since

$$i = 1 - (o + c) \tag{1.17}$$

we arrive at the following 2×2 system:

$$o' = k_{io} + (k_{co} - k_{io})\, c - (k_{oi} + k_{oc} + k_{io})\, o,$$
$$c' = k_{ic} + (k_{oc} - k_{ic})\, o - (k_{co} + k_{ci} + k_{ic})\, c.$$

The equilibrium solution is now defined by a 2×2 linear system of equations of the form

$$Bq = b, \tag{1.18}$$

where

$$B = \begin{pmatrix} k_{oi} + k_{oc} + k_{io} & k_{io} - k_{co} \\ k_{ic} - k_{oc} & k_{co} + k_{ci} + k_{ic} \end{pmatrix}, \ q = \begin{pmatrix} o \\ c \end{pmatrix}, \text{ and } b = \begin{pmatrix} k_{io} \\ k_{ic} \end{pmatrix}.$$

By solving this linear system and using (1.17), we find (as above) that

$$o = K^{-1}, \ c = \frac{k_{oc}}{k_{co}} K^{-1}, \ i = \frac{k_{oi}}{k_{io}} K^{-1},$$

where

$$K = 1 + \frac{k_{oc}}{k_{co}} + \frac{k_{oi}}{k_{io}}.$$

1.3.1 Linear Algebra Approach to Finding the Equilibrium Solution

Calculations to find the equilibrium solution will be done repeatedly in these notes. We will always use the special structure of the Markov model to derive the equilibrium solution, but it also worth noting that this can be done by solving a linear system. The master equation associated with a Markov model of the form (1.14) or of the form given in Fig. 1.4 can always be written in the form

$$p' = Ap,$$

where p is a vector containing the probabilities of occupying the different states of the Markov model. Since the sum of the probabilities adds up to one, the number of unknowns can be reduced by one and the system takes the form

$$q' = b - Bq.$$

Therefore, the equilibrium solution can be found by solving the linear system (1.18).

Instead of reducing the number of unknowns, we can also address the problem more directly by computing the eigenvector associated the eigenvalue $\lambda = 0$. For instance, using Matlab we can put $z = \text{null}(A)$ and then define

$$p = \frac{z}{\sum_i z_i}$$

where z_i denote the components of the vector z.

1.4 Stochastic Simulations and Probability Density Functions

Given the Markov model, defining a stochastic differential equation describing changes of the transmembrane potential due to the opening and closing of the channel is quite straightforward. Additionally, based on the stochastic differential equation, we will derive deterministic differential equations describing the probability density functions of the states involved in the Markov model. We thus have two ways to analyze models of ion channels: We can either run numerous Monte Carlo simulations using the stochastic differential equation or solve the deterministic differential equations defining the probability density functions. Both these methods will be used throughout the notes. Although one method is the average of the other, we will see that both provide distinct insights useful to understanding the mechanisms under consideration.

1.5 Markov Models of Calcium Release

The contraction of the heart is a collective and very well-coordinated effort achieved in a collaboration involving billions of cells. For each of these cells, the contraction depends on the release of a massive amount of calcium from internal storage. The release takes place in many thousands of release units within each cell and the state of the release process is believed to be adequately modeled using Markov models.

We will study this release in several steps and we start by assuming that the only varying concentration is in the dyad and that the reaction rates of the Markov model vary only with this single concentration. This case will be studied in great detail and we will explain how drugs can be theoretically constructed to repair mutations affecting the release mechanism. The analysis is based on a scalar stochastic differential equation representing the concentration of calcium in the dyad. The properties of this model will be analyzed using Monte Carlo simulations. Furthermore, we will derive a system of deterministic partial differential equations describing the probability density function of the states of the Markov model.

It is more common to divide the calcium concentration into two values—not only one—which leads to 2×2 stochastic differential equations to be analyzed. This model will also be analyzed using Monte Carlo simulations and by a 2D deterministic system of partial differential equations representing the probability density functions of the states of the Markov model.

Next, we shall couple the calcium concentration to the voltage-gated release of calcium through so-called L-type calcium channels. This model will allow us to study optimal drugs, combining the effect on calcium release and L-type channels. The balance of these mechanisms rules the calcium-induced calcium release that is at the crux of cardiac contraction. The calcium-induced calcium release model is stated in terms of a 2×2 model of stochastic equations where the transmembrane potential V is included as a parameter in the model. The associated model for the probability density functions is given by a 2D system of partial differential equations where the transmembrane potential is again included as a parameter.

1.6 Markov Models of Ion Channels

After analysis of the calcium release we move on to study voltage-gated ion channels. We will immediately see that in mathematical terms the problem is very similar to the calcium release problem. For the ion channel case, however, the stochastic equation is one-dimensional and so is the associated deterministic partial differential equation. The basic Markov model is still based on the open and closed states, but we will also see that an inactivated state plays a central role. Optimal theoretical drugs will be derived and we will observe that they work nicely.

1.7 Mutations Described by Markov Models

A trademark of mutations affecting ion channels and calcium release mechanisms is that they change the open probability and possibly also the mean open time and other characteristics of the channels involved. We will show below that the equilibrium open probability of the channel described by the Markov model of the form (1.1) is given by

$$o = \frac{k_{co}}{k_{co} + k_{oc}}$$

and the mean open time is given by

$$\tau_o = \frac{1}{k_{oc}}.$$

The concept of mean open time will be discussed in Chap. 13 and the formula $\tau_o = 1/k_{oc}$ will be derived in that chapter. Given these formulas, it is straightforward to see that the effect of mutations affecting the open probability or the mean open time can be modeled by changing the parameters of the Markov model. In these notes we shall focus on rather simple changes in the model but, again, the techniques can be generalized to more intricate cases.

Two examples of the effect of mutations are given in Figs. 1.7 and 1.8. Figure 1.7 shows recordings of the open and closed states for the wild type and the V2475F mutation of the ryanodine receptor (RyR). The graphs in Fig. 1.8 show similar results for the voltage-gated sodium channel when the wild type recordings are compared with recordings from a mutant (ΔKPQ) channel.

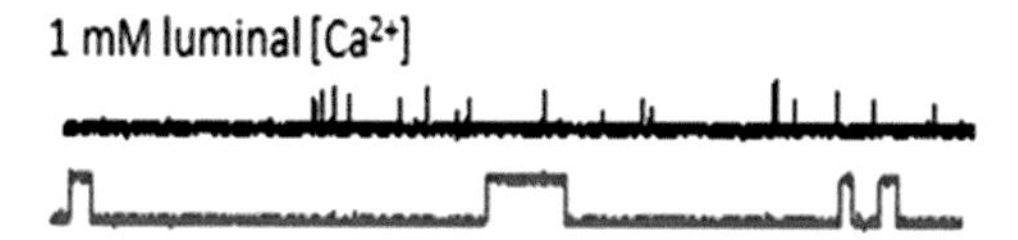

Fig. 1.7 Single-channel recordings of wild type (*black*) and mutant (*red*) cardiac RyR channels. The open probability and the mean open time are significantly increased for the mutant (V2475F) case. The graphs are from Figure 3 of Loaiza et al. [52]

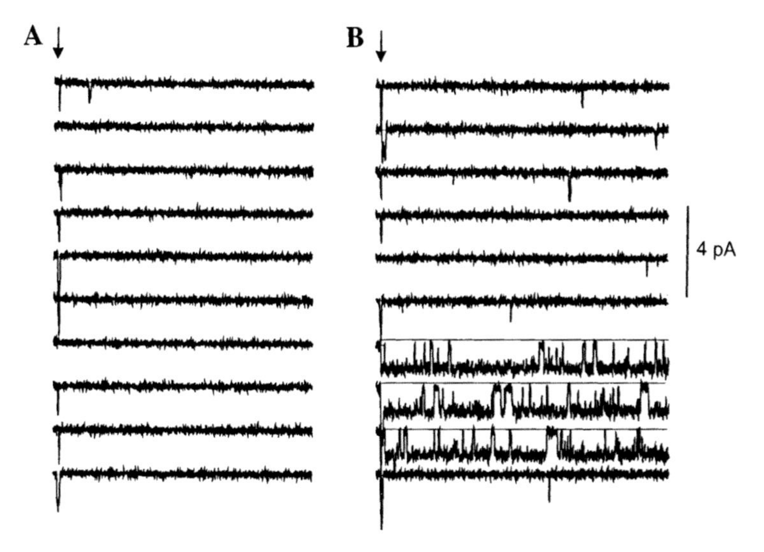

Fig. 1.8 Sodium current recordings taken from Figure 4 of Chandra et al. [13]: A represents the wild type and B represents the ΔKPQ mutant. The recordings are based on 200-ms depolarizing pulses from −100 to −40 mV

1.8 The Problem and Steps Toward Solutions

Assume that experimental data on wild type cells can be used to identify the parameters of a Markov model faithfully describing the stochastic properties of the wild type channel and that experimental data on mutant cells can be used to establish a Markov model of similar structure representing the stochastic properties of the mutant channel. Furthermore, we assume that the Markov model of the mutant can be extended to account for the effect of a theoretical drug. *The problem is then to compute the reaction rates of the drug such that, after the drug is applied, the mutant channel behaves as similarly to the wild type channel as possible.* The essence of these notes is to show how to solve this problem mathematically; we show how to compute an optimal theoretical drug. To clarify what we mean by an optimal theoretical drug, we will give a few examples that will be discussed later and then we will briefly discuss the concept of a theoretical drug more generally.

1.8.1 Markov Models for Drugs: Open State and Closed State Blockers

By using the notation of chemical reactions introduced above, we can explain the problem in a bit more detail. The reaction scheme for an open state blocker can be illustrated as follows:

$$C \underset{k_{co}}{\overset{k_{oc}}{\leftrightarrows}} O \underset{k_{ob}}{\overset{k_{bo}}{\leftrightarrows}} B. \tag{1.19}$$

For theoretical purposes, this drug is well defined, provided that we know the values of the parameters k_{ob} and k_{bo}. We will often assume that these parameters are constants. As mentioned above, one example of a problem we want to overcome is mutations leading to an increased open probability; so either the release mechanism is too prone to releasing calcium from internal storage or the ion channels are too prone to allowing current to flow through the cell membrane.

Since the problem involves too high of an open probability, it seems reasonable to try to fix the open probability by extending the reaction scheme and directly affecting this state, as illustrated in the reaction scheme above. By allowing the probability to be moved from O to B, the open probability will be reduced and thus the goal will be achieved. This reasoning seems impeccable and it seems much less intuitive to use a closed state drug of the form

$$B \underset{k_{bc}}{\overset{k_{cb}}{\leftrightarrows}} C \underset{k_{co}}{\overset{k_{oc}}{\leftrightarrows}} O. \tag{1.20}$$

We will see, however, that both open and closed state blockers may be optimal, depending on the nature of the mutation.

1.8.2 Closed to Open Mutations (CO-Mutations)

We have seen that for a Markov model written in the form

$$C \underset{k_{co}}{\overset{k_{oc}}{\leftrightarrows}} O, \tag{1.21}$$

the equilibrium open probability is given by

$$o = \frac{k_{co}}{k_{co} + k_{oc}} = \frac{1}{1 + \frac{k_{oc}}{k_{co}}}$$

and the mean open time is given by

$$\tau_o = \frac{1}{k_{oc}}.$$

A mutation leading to an increased open probability can be represented by a Markov model written in the form

$$C \underset{\mu k_{co}}{\overset{k_{oc}}{\leftrightarrows}} O, \tag{1.22}$$

where $\mu \geq 1$ will be referred to as the *mutation severity index* and we always use the convention that $\mu = 1$ refers to the wild type case. At this point, it is useful to recall the interpretation of a scheme of this form. In particular, it is useful to note that the probability of going from the closed state (C) to the open state (O) during a time step Δt is now given by $\mu \Delta t k_{co}$, compared to $\Delta t k_{co}$ for the wild type channel. It is pretty clear that increasing the mutation severity index will increase the probability of being in the open state and this is also reflected by the equilibrium open probability given by

$$o_\mu = \frac{1}{1 + \frac{k_{oc}}{\mu k_{co}}},$$

which clearly increases as a function of the mutation severity index μ. It is also interesting to observe that, for this mutation, the mean open time is unchanged. We will refer to a mutation of this form as a CO-mutation and we will show repeatedly that, for CO-mutations, closed state blockers are theoretically optimal.

1.8.3 Open to Closed Mutations (OC-Mutations)

Another way to introduce a mutation that increases the open probability is to decrease the rate from open to closed. This can be written as follows:

$$C \underset{k_{co}}{\overset{k_{oc}/\mu}{\leftrightarrows}} O, \tag{1.23}$$

where, again, $\mu \geq 1$ is the mutation severity index and $\mu = 1$ represents the wild type. The probability of leaving the open state is now reduced and this will lead to an increased open probability. In particular, the equilibrium open probability is again given by

$$o_\mu = \frac{1}{1 + \frac{k_{oc}}{\mu k_{co}}},$$

as above, but now the mean open time changes; it is given by

$$\tau_o = \frac{\mu}{k_{oc}}$$

and thus increases with the mutation severity index.

We will refer to a mutation of this form as an OC-mutation and we will show that, for such mutations, open state blockers are theoretically optimal.

1.9 Theoretical Drugs

The concept of a theoretical drug is essential in these notes. Basically, we will *refer to a theoretical drug*[2] *as a purely mathematical construction* that may or may not have a viable pharmaceutical counterpart. A mental image of how the drug may work is given in Fig. 1.9; the figure is taken from Starmer [87]. With no drug involved, the channel can take on two conformational states: the open state (O), when ions can flow freely through the channel, and the closed state (C), when there is no flow of ions through the channel. An open blocker can change the open state such that there is no flow through the channel. The reaction scheme of the situation described in the figure is given by

$$C \underset{k_{co}}{\overset{k_{oc}}{\leftrightarrows}} O \underset{k_{ob}}{\overset{k_{bo}}{\leftrightarrows}} B. \tag{1.24}$$

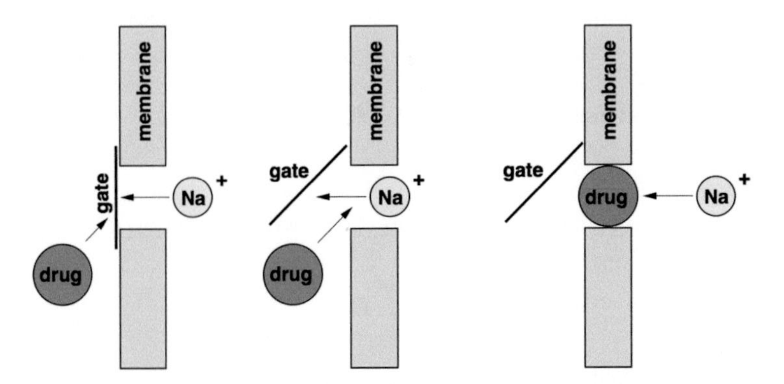

Fig. 1.9 Illustration of a blocker associated with the open state. In the leftmost case the channel is closed and no ions can pass through it. In the center case, the channel is open and ions may flow freely. In the rightmost case the channel is blocked by the drug and no ions can pass through it. The figure is taken from Starmer [87]

[2]We also use the terms *mathematical drug, numerical drug*, and so forth interchangeably with *theoretical drug*.

where we again note that the properties of the theoretical drug are solely given by the values of the rates k_{ob} and k_{bo}.

This way of describing the effect of a drug has been used for many years, see e.g. Hille [31] or Hondeghem and Katzung [34]. Our use of this notation is clearly motivated by the paper of Clancy et al. [16]. In these papers, an existing drug is characterized using a scheme of the form (1.24). That is, data obtained from experiments using a particular drug are used to characterize the rates k_{bo} and k_{ob} referred to, respectively, as the on and off rates of the drug. As mentioned above, we often view the rates as free parameters that can be optimized in order to create the best possible theoretical drug in the sense that the channel should work as much like the healthy case as possible. This way of describing a theoretically optimal drug was introduced in [99] and clearly motivated by the drug vector approach discussed in [97].

1.10 Results

Many of the models, methods, and results described in these notes are well known in the literature. All the Markov models are taken from the literature and so are the stochastic differential equations and the models describing the probability density approach. Compared to earlier published models, we will often derive simplified models, but the ideas behind them are basically the same as those used by many authors. Concerning the modeling of mutations, we aim to consistently model the effect of mutations as simply as possible and preferably only by changing a single parameter: the mutation severity index.

The novel part of these notes is that we attempt to systematically describe how to compute characterizations of drugs that are optimal in a specific sense and we do so for a number of applications. We almost exclusively address so-called gain-of-function mutations. For such mutations, the open probability of the channel or receptor is too large, which can lead to severe difficulties for the cell and, ultimately, for large collections of such cells.

1.11 Other Possible Applications

The focus in this text will be on how to compute characterizations of optimal theoretical drugs defined in terms of parameters describing the associated Markov model. The methods can, however, also be used to compare existing drugs. If Markov models are developed for two drugs, the associated probability density functions can be computed and thus a comparison of the quality of the two drugs can be computed. This approach will rely heavily on accurate representations of the function of a drug in terms of a Markov model, which is a problem beyond the scope of the present notes.

1.12 Disclaimer

These notes are written to explain in some detail how we can compute characterizations of theoretical drugs in terms of Markov models. However, we specifically avoid discussing whether it is possible to realize a certain drug given the characterization in terms of a Markov model, simply because we do not know and have been unable to find any reasonable answer to this in the literature. The applicability of our results therefore remains uncertain.

1.13 Notes

1. Several excellent introductions to Markov models of the stochastic behavior of receptors and ion channels are available (e.g., [39, 42, 79, 85]). In particular we recommend the recently published book by Bressloff [6] (see also [7]). Bressloff [6] provides a broad introduction to stochastic processes in cells and covers most of the models covered in the present text and much more. It is an excellent text that will become a standard reference in the field.
2. A comprehensive mathematical analysis of the stochastic properties of single ion channels using Markov models was initiated by Colquhoun and Hawkes (e.g., [19–21]).
3. Insight into the electrophysiology of excitable cells was fundamentally enhanced by the development of the patch clamp technique of Sakmann and Neher (see, e.g., [77, 78]). The authors received the Nobel Prize in Physiology or Medicine in 1991 for their work on single ion channels. The patch clamp technique is used to generate measurements of the form illustrated in Fig. 1.3. These data are used to determine the Markov model and are therefore of fundamental importance. As mentioned below, however, the problem of finding the Markov model based on experimental data is still an active research problem.
4. The models studied in these notes address the flow of ions through various types of channels. An excellent introduction to ion channels is given in the book by Hille [32].
5. Our discussion is focused on mechanisms of the heart but, at the level of single channels, these mechanisms are similar to channel-based mechanisms of the brain or, more specifically, the mechanisms of neurons. There are several excellent introductions to neuroscience (e.g., [22, 23, 38, 90]).
6. Given the Markov model, we have seen that it is pretty straightforward to compute what state the channel is in as a stochastic function of time. We have also seen that we can solve the master equation and find the average behavior of the channel when the rates are independent of the surroundings. Furthermore, we will show how to compute probability density functions for each state when the rates depend on the transmembrane potential. Such simulations are forward

problems: Given the model, compute the solution. The inverse problem in this setting is quite a bit harder; the problem is to compute the rates (i.e., the values of k_{oc}, k_{co} etc.) of the Markov model in order for the stochastic behavior of the model to match the measurements of the channel. The analysis of the inverse problem was started by Colquhoun and Hawkes [19], beginning in 1977, and their findings are summarized by Sakmann and Neher [78] (see also [17]). More recently the problem has been addressed in a series of papers by Sachs and his co-authors; see [59, 68, 69]. Their methods are available in the open-source QuB software package. Furthermore, Markov chain Monte Carlo (MCMC) has been used in a series of papers by Siekmann, Sneyd and his co-authors [27, 82–84]. Interestingly, their analysis shows that certain Markov models cannot be identified using standard data. The MCMC method was used for inversion of single ion channel data more than 15 years ago by Ball et al [1], and Rosales and co-authors, see [72, 73].

7. For whole cell data, the problem of identifying the parameters of Markov models is carefully studied by Fink and Noble [24].
8. The terms *CO-mutation*, *OC-mutation*, and *mutation severity index* are not standard and introduced here for convenience.
9. A thorough discussion of the principle of detailed balance can be found in the paper by Colquhoun et al. [18]. The validity of the principle for given data can be tested as shown by Song and Magleby [86] and Ullah et al. [101] (suppl. material). There are examples of Markov models that do not satisfy the principle of detailed balance (see, e.g., [6], p. 208).
10. The numerical method for handling the Markov model described on page 8 is not particularly efficient. For the case of constant rates in the Markov model, considerable acceleration can be achieved by using the method of Gillespie [26]. The Gillespie method is particularly useful for simulations involving many channels (see, e.g., [85]).
11. For comprehensive introductions to modeling the cardiac action potential, we refer to the recent overview by Rudy [74] and to Rudy and Silva [75]. For the action potential shown in Fig. 1.2, we used the model of Grandi et al. [29]. An alternative is the model of O'Hara et al. [64] and a huge collection of models is available at the CellML project (CellML.org).
12. The dynamics of cardiac electrophysiology are introduced in numerous papers and books; a recent comprehensive review is provided by Qu et al. [71]. The book by Katz [41] is a standard reference in cardiac physiology and the book by Glass et al. [28] is a standard reference in the modeling of the heart. Numerical methods for the simulation of cardiac electrophysiology are presented by Sundnes et al. [93] (see also [25, 67]).

Chapter 2
One-Dimensional Calcium Release

The contraction of a single cardiac cell is initiated by an increase in the transmembrane potential leading to opening of the so-called L-type calcium channels (LCCs). When these channels are open, calcium flows into a rather small space called the dyadic cleft (often simply referred to as the dyad), leading to a locally increased concentration of Ca^{2+} ions. This increased concentration leads to the opening of the ryanodine receptors (RyRs), which control the flow of calcium from the internal stores referred to as the sarcoplasmic reticulum (SR). This process is referred to as the calcium-induced calcium release (CICR) and is of vital importance in the functioning of the heart. A schematic description of the process is given in Fig. 2.1.

This CICR process is one of the focal points of interest in these notes. We shall develop a model coupling the effects alluded to in Fig. 2.1. However, in this first chapter we shall simplify the process quite a bit by assuming that we just have three spaces: the SR, the dyad, and the cytosol (see Fig. 2.2). This simplification means that we assume that there is very fast diffusion between the network SR (NSR) domain and the junctional SR (JSR) domain such that the associated concentrations are identical. Furthermore, we ignore the L-type channels and assume that the concentrations in both the SR and the cytosol are constant. This leads to a one-dimensional model, in the sense that only the concentration of the dyad changes. The model is useful because it helps illustrate the tools we need in our analysis of the full CICR process and illustrates the properties of optimal drugs that will be more or less inherited in more complex models.

Our aim is therefore to understand in some detail what is going on in the process illustrated in Fig. 2.1. However, this figure is in itself a huge simplification of the complex CICR process. The cell consists of 10,000 to 20,000 dyads, each dyad having up to 100 RyRs, and human ventricles consist of billions of cells. Our aim is to focus entirely on a very small but essential element in the CICR mechanism.

We model the release of Ca^{2+} ions from the SR to the dyad by formulating a stochastic differential equation governing the concentration of Ca^{2+} ions in the

A. Tveito, G.T. Lines, *Computing Characterizations of Drugs for Ion Channels and Receptors Using Markov Models*, Lecture Notes in Computational Science and Engineering 111, DOI 10.1007/978-3-319-30030-6_2

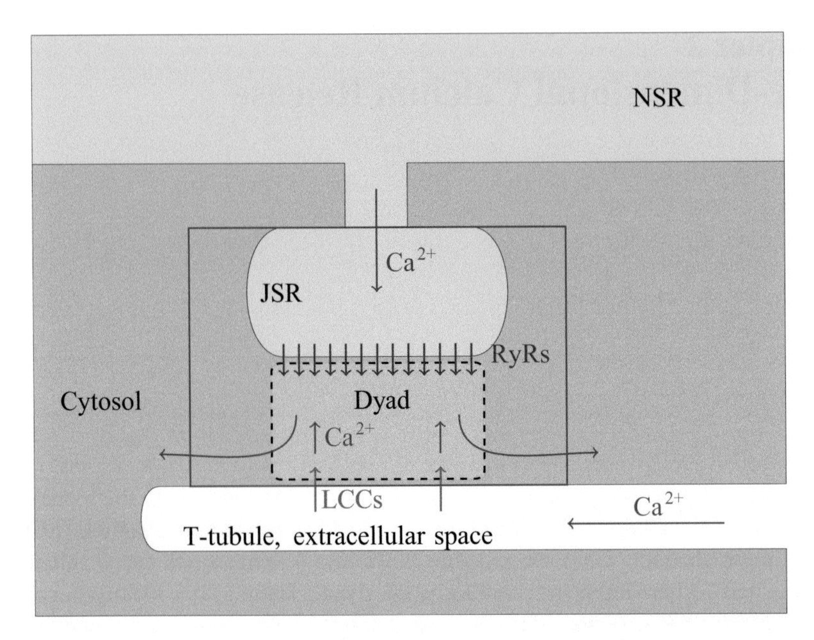

Fig. 2.1 This figure illustrates the components involved in the CICR: the T-tubule, the dyad, the SR represented by the JSR and NSR, and the cytosol. Calcium ions can enter the dyad from the T-tubule through LCCs and from the SR through the RyRs. The figure is taken from Winslow et al. [105]. In this chapter, we concentrate on the dynamics in the box surrounded by a *thin red line*. Thus we assume that the concentration of the JSR and NSR are identical and constant and we ignore the LCCs. We also assume that all the RyRs are in the same state and therefore can be treated as one channel (see also Notes at page 53)

dyad. The model will be studied both numerically and analytically and we show how the solution's properties depend on the parameters defining the model. Next, we will derive a deterministic partial differential equation (PDE) giving the probability density function of the states of the Markov model. Although the transition from a stochastic model to a deterministic model for the probability density functions is classical by now, we will spend some time deriving the equations in detail because the transition from stochastic to deterministic is such a wonderful piece of insight. Furthermore, we will provide detailed comparisons of Monte Carlo simulations based on the stochastic model and the probability density functions. In subsequent chapters, we will develop the model further by using two small spaces, the dyad and the JSR (see Fig. 2.1), allowing for different concentrations of Ca^{2+} ions. This leads to a two-dimensional (2D) problem.

Finally, we will take the LCCs into account. This leads to a 2D problem depending on one parameter: the transmembrane potential.

In these notes, we will use the concept of dimension in two different, but related, ways. In the first version of the stochastic model of CICR, we will model only the concentration of Ca^{2+} in the dyad and we will refer to the model as one dimensional (1D). When a deterministic model governing the probability density function of the states of the Markov model is derived, that model is also 1D in the sense that it depends on one spatial variable; the concentration of Ca^{2+}. Next we move to two concentrations (in the dyad and the JSR), leading to a 2D stochastic model in the sense that it is a 2×2 system of stochastic ordinary differential equations. The associated model governing the deterministic probability density functions is also 2D in the sense that the model depends on two spatial variables: the concentration of Ca^{2+} in the dyad and in the JSR. So the general rule is that the number of different concentrations allowed in the system of stochastic ordinary differential equations carries over to the spatial dimension of the deterministic system of PDEs governing the probability density functions of the states involved in the Markov model. Furthermore, the number of states in the Markov model decides the number of equations in the deterministic system of PDEs.

2.1 Stochastic Model of Calcium Release

Suppose that the cytosolic Ca^{2+} concentration is given by c_0 and the SR concentration is given by c_1; we assume both to be constant and that $c_1 \gg c_0$. We want to model the concentration $\bar{x} = \bar{x}(t)$ in the dyad located between the cytosol and the SR (see Fig. 2.2). Throughout these notes, we will use a bar to indicate stochastic variables.

We assume that there is stochastic release from the SR to the dyad, and diffusion from the dyad to the cytosol. Let v_r denote the speed of release (when the channel is open) and let v_d be the speed of diffusion; both are non-negative. Then a stochastic model of the concentration $\bar{x} = \bar{x}(t)$ in the dyad is given by

$$\bar{x}'(t) = \bar{\gamma}(t)v_r(c_1 - \bar{x}) + v_d(c_0 - \bar{x}), \tag{2.1}$$

where the function $\bar{\gamma} = \bar{\gamma}(t)$ takes on the value zero (closed) or one (open), and the dynamics of the function are governed by a Markov model of the form

$$C \underset{k_{co}}{\overset{k_{oc}}{\leftrightarrows}} O, \tag{2.2}$$

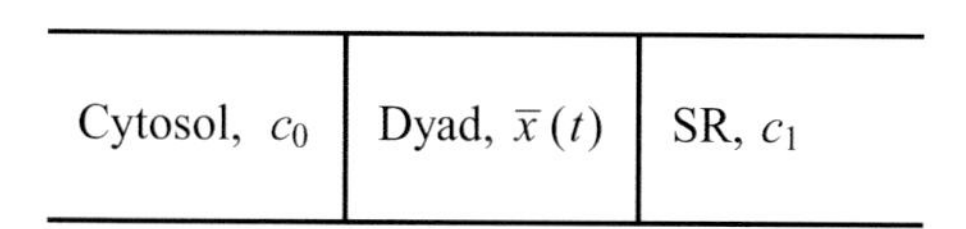

Fig. 2.2 Illustration of the model studied in the present chapter: The Ca^{2+} concentration is high in the SR and low in the cytosol. Release from the SR is governed by a Markov model and the concentration can be diffused from the dyad to the cytosol

with k_{oc} and k_{co} as reaction rates that may depend on the concentration. Markov models were introduced on page 4 but let us recall that the reaction rates k_{oc} and k_{co} basically indicate the tendency of a channel to change state. So, if the channel is open, the probability that the channel changes from open to closed in a very short time interval Δt is given by $\Delta t k_{oc}$ and, similarly, if the channel is closed, $\Delta t k_{co}$ is the probability that it becomes open in the time interval Δt. This means that the higher the rate k_{co}, the more likely it is that the channels are open. This property will be used repeatedly in what follows.

2.1.1 Bounds of the Concentration

Suppose that at time $t = t_0$, the channel is closed ($\gamma = 0$), that the concentration is given by $x(t_0) = x_0$, and that the channel remains closed for $t \leqslant t_0 + \Delta t$. Then, in the interval $t_0 \leqslant t \leqslant t_0 + \Delta t$, the dynamics are given by the deterministic equation[1]

$$x'(t) = v_d(c_0 - x)$$

and thus

$$x(t) = c_0 + e^{v_d(t_0 - t)}(x_0 - c_0)$$

in this time interval. Therefore, for a closed channel, the concentration $x(t)$ of the dyad approaches c_0 (the cytosolic concentration) at an exponential rate. The decay is faster for larger values of the diffusion velocity v_d. By consulting Fig. 2.2 we see that this is quite reasonable; if we close the release from the SR, the concentration of the dyad will gradually approach the concentration of the cytosol.

Next, we consider the case of an open channel,

$$x'(t) = v_r(c_1 - x) + v_d(c_0 - x), \tag{2.3}$$

and again we assume that $x(t_0) = x_0$. We can rewrite this in the form

$$x'(t) = (v_r + v_d)(c_+ - x),$$

where

$$c_+ = \frac{v_r c_1 + v_d c_0}{v_r + v_d},$$

[1]Note that when we consider the case of a given value γ, the model becomes deterministic and we remove the overbar that indicates a variable is stochastic.

and find that the solution is given by

$$x(t) = c_+ + e^{(v_r+v_d)(t_0-t)} (x_0 - c_+) .$$

Therefore, when the channel is open, we observe that the concentration $x(t)$ of the dyad approaches c_+ at an exponential rate. Furthermore, we note that the rate increases with $v_r + v_d$. Note also that

$$c_+ = c_1 + \frac{v_d (c_0 - c_1)}{v_r + v_d} < c_1. \tag{2.4}$$

So, to summarize, when the channel is open, the concentration approaches $c_+ < c_1$ and when it is closed, the concentration approaches c_0.

For a given state of the channel (open or closed), the concentration profile is monotone and therefore there is no way the solution can become less than c_0 or larger than c_+. We therefore have

$$c_0 \leqslant \bar{x}(t) \leqslant c_+ \tag{2.5}$$

for all time, provided that this bound holds initially.

Note that since $c_1 \gg c_0$, we have

$$c_+ \approx \frac{v_r}{v_r + v_d} c_1$$

and therefore c_+ approaches c_1 if

$$\frac{v_d}{v_r} \longrightarrow 0.$$

Suppose, for instance, that we keep v_r fixed and we let v_d approach zero. Then c_+ approaches c_1, which is reasonable since calcium will be poured into the dyad, but the connection to the cytosol is almost closed and thus the dyadic concentration will increase until it reaches an equilibrium with the SR concentration.

2.1.2 An Invariant Region for the Solution

The invariant region (2.5) deserves a comment, since it will become quite useful later. Suppose that the initial concentration of the dyad is somewhere in the interval defined by c_0 and c_+. Then, we have seen that if the channel is either closed or open, the solution remains in this interval as long as the channel does not change state. When the channel changes state, say, at time $t = \Delta t$, we have a new initial condition in the interval c_0 and c_+ and we can solve the equation deterministically once more and the solution will remain in the interval. The process can be repeated over and over and the solution will always remain in the interval c_0 and c_+. This property is useful, because it directly implies that the probability of being outside this interval is zero, which is what we need when we want to define boundary conditions for the model defining probability density functions.

2.1.3 A Numerical Scheme

To perform stochastic simulations, we discretize the equation

$$\bar{x}'(t) = \bar{\gamma}(t)v_r(c_1 - \bar{x}) + v_d(c_0 - \bar{x}) \tag{2.6}$$

to obtain the explicit scheme

$$x_{n+1} = x_n + \Delta t\,(\gamma_n v_r(c_1 - x_n) + v_d(c_0 - x_n)) \tag{2.7}$$

where γ_n takes on the value zero (closed) or one (open). The value of γ_n is computed as follows: Let σ_n be a random number in the unit interval. Assume that $\gamma_{n-1} = 0$. Then, if $k_{co}\Delta t > \sigma_n$, we set $\gamma_n = 1$, but if this condition does not hold, we set $\gamma_n = 0$. Similarly, assume that $\gamma_{n-1} = 1$. Then, if $k_{oc}\Delta t > \sigma_n$, we set $\gamma_n = 0$, but if this condition does not hold, we set $\gamma_n = 1$.

2.1.4 An Invariant Region for the Numerical Solution

We want to ensure that the numerical scheme provides solutions mimicking the properties of the analytical solutions. Therefore, we want to confirm that the invariant region for model (2.6) also holds for the numerical solutions. For this to hold, we have to assume that the time step is restricted as follows:

$$\Delta t < \frac{1}{v_r + v_d}. \tag{2.8}$$

To derive the invariant region, we define

$$F(x) = x + \Delta t\,(\gamma_n v_r(c_1 - x) + v_d(c_0 - x))$$

and note that

$$F'(x) = 1 - \Delta t\,(\gamma_n v_r + v_d) \geqslant 1 - \Delta t\,(v_r + v_d) > 0.$$

If we assume that $c_0 \leqslant x_n \leqslant c_+$, we obtain

$$x_{n+1} = F(x_n) \geqslant F(c_0) = c_0 + \Delta t\,(\gamma_n v_r(c_1 - c_0)) \geqslant c_0$$

and

$$\begin{aligned} x_{n+1} &= F(x_n) \\ &\leqslant F(c_+) \\ &= c_+ + \Delta t\,(\gamma_n v_r(c_1 - c_+) + v_d(c_0 - c_+)) \\ &\leqslant c_+ + \Delta t\,(v_r(c_1 - c_+) + v_d(c_0 - c_+)) \\ &= c_+, \end{aligned}$$

where we have used the fact that

$$c_+ = \frac{v_r c_1 + v_d c_0}{v_r + v_d}.$$

Therefore, by induction, we have $c_0 \leqslant x_n \leqslant c_+$ for all time.

2.1.5 *Stochastic Simulations*

We use the scheme (2.7) to compute the concentration governed by the model (2.6), using the parameters given in Table 2.1. The numerical results are given in Fig. 2.3 for time running from 0 to 100 ms. In Fig. 2.4, we show the same solution but focus on the time interval from 20 to 30 ms. The lower graph indicates when the channel is open (high value) and when it is closed (low value). We observe from the concentration profile that the solution increases whenever the channel is open and reduces whenever the channel is closed and we also observe that the solution remains in the interval $[c_0, c_+]$ for all time, where

$$c_+ = \frac{v_r c_1 + v_d c_0}{v_r + v_d} = 91\ \mu\text{M}.$$

Table 2.1 Parameter values for model (2.6) used in the computations presented in Figs. 2.3 and 2.4

v_d	1 ms^{-1}
v_r	0.1 ms^{-1}
c_0	0.1 μM
c_1	1,000 μM
$k_{co}(x)$	$0.1x$ $\text{ms}^{-1}\ \mu\text{M}^{-1}$
k_{oc}	1 ms^{-1}

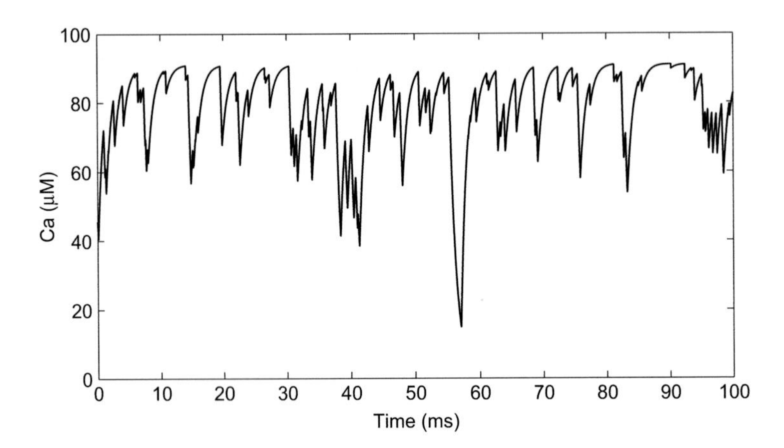

Fig. 2.3 Code: 1D/figure_mc.m. The calcium concentration of the dyad as a function of time. The numerical solution is computed using scheme (2.7) using $\Delta t = 1$ μs and $x(0) = (c_+ + c_0)/2 = 45.55$ μM. Furthermore, we assume that the channel is closed initially, so $\gamma(0) = 0$

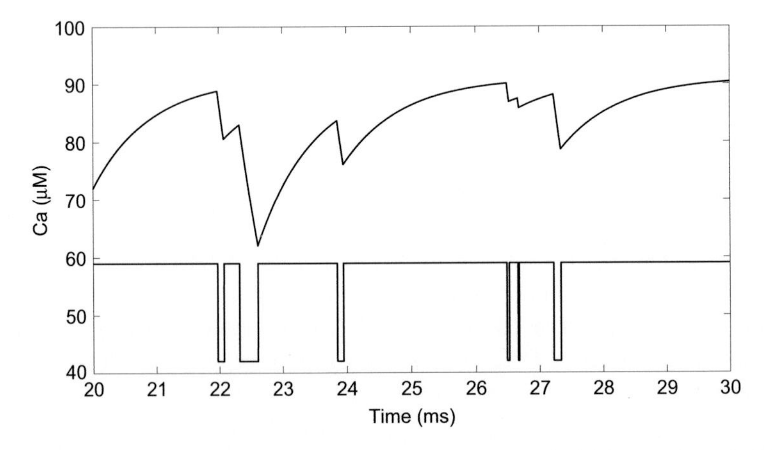

Fig. 2.4 The concentration profile is taken from Fig. 2.3 above. Here we show the solution restricted to the time interval ranging from $t = 20$ to $t = 30$ ms. In the lower part of the figure we indicate whether the channel is open (high value) or closed (low value). Seen together, the figure illustrates that the concentrations increase when the channel is open, and decrease when the channel is closed

2.2 Deterministic Systems of PDEs Governing the Probability Density Functions

We have seen that model (2.6) can be studied using Monte Carlo simulations based on the numerical scheme (2.7). Such simulations clearly give some insight into the dynamics. In addition to the simulations shown above, we can use the numerical scheme to see the effect of changing the rates of the Markov model and the other parameters of the model. However, it is tricky to compare solutions of simulations based on stochastic processes because the results vary from simulation to simulation anyway. So we are faced with the following question: Is the difference in solutions from one computation to another due to stochastic effects or are they due to changes of parameters? This matter becomes especially pertinent when we introduce theoretical drugs, because we want to compare solutions with and without application of the theoretical drug. It is tempting to derive some sort of statistics based on the simulation results and then compare the solutions computed based on two sets of parameters based on the statistics.

By running numerous simulations, we can add the results and compute probability density functions based on the stochastic simulations. Exactly how this can be done will be explained below. However, it turns out that the probability density functions can also be computed by solving a deterministic system of PDEs. In this section we show how to derive this system of PDEs. We will see below that this is quite useful, because it is much easier to compare solutions of deterministic differential equations than stochastic solutions. By analyzing the deterministic system of PDEs we can also, analytically, derive properties of the process that would be very hard to derive based on direct analysis of the stochastic model (2.6).

2.2.1 *Probability Density Functions*

Let $\rho_o = \rho_o(x,t)$ be the probability density functions of the channel being in an open state. This means that, at time t, the probability of the channel being open and the concentration $\bar{x} = \bar{x}(t)$ being in the interval $(x, x + \Delta x)$ is given by

$$P_o\{x < \bar{x}(t) < x + \Delta x\} = \int_x^{x+\Delta x} \rho_o(\xi,t)\,d\xi. \tag{2.9}$$

Similarly, the probability of the concentration $\bar{x} = \bar{x}(t)$ being in the interval $(x, x + \Delta x)$ and the channel being closed is given by

$$P_c\{x < \bar{x}(t) < x + \Delta x\} = \int_x^{x+\Delta x} \rho_c(\xi,t)\,d\xi, \tag{2.10}$$

where ρ_c is the probability density function of the channel being in the closed state. Note that

$$\int (\rho_o(\xi,t) + \rho_c(\xi,t))\,d\xi = 1, \tag{2.11}$$

where the integral is over all possible concentrations. In particular, if the initial concentration is in the invariant region given by $[c_0, c_+]$, then the integral goes over this interval.

The probability density functions ρ_o and ρ_c contain a great deal of information about the process under consideration. At every point in time, we can understand how likely it is that the concentration is in a certain interval for a given state of the channel. It is therefore of great interest to be able to compute these functions.

2.2.2 *Dynamics of the Probability Density Functions*

Now, we are interested in understanding how ρ_o and ρ_c change dynamically. Consider ρ_o and suppose that, for a given x and t, the density $\rho_o(x, t)$ is known. Over a small time interval, several things can happen that will affect the density: a) the channel can change from open to closed (reducing ρ_o), b) the channel can change from closed to open (increasing ρ_o), and, finally, c) the concentration can move from outside the interval $(x, x + \Delta x)$ to inside this interval or the concentration can move from inside the interval $(x, x + \Delta x)$ to outside this interval.

Here cases a) and b) are handled by the Markov model and we will return to that issue below, but we will start by taking care of the change in probability density due to changes in concentration. It turns out that this part will be governed by an advection[2] equation and we will start by considering two very special cases illustrating how the probability is advected in the absence of a Markov model.

2.2.3 *Advection of Probability Density*

We start by considering two very special cases in which we just assume that the channel is always open or the channel is always closed.

2.2.3.1 Advection in a Very Special Case: The Channel Is Kept Open for All Time

Let us also assume that the probability density function is known at time $t = 0$ and that it is given by a very simple function,

$$\rho_o(x, 0) = 1/h \text{ for } x \in \tilde{\Omega} = [\tilde{c} - h/2, \tilde{c} + h/2], \tag{2.12}$$

[2] Advection means the transport of a conserved quantity.

and $\rho_o = 0$ for values of x outside the interval $\tilde{\Omega}$. Here h is assumed to be a given positive number and $\tilde{c} = \frac{1}{2}(c_0 + c_+)$, where we recall that

$$c_+ = \frac{v_r c_1 + v_d c_0}{v_r + v_d}.$$

Note that, since we know that channel is open, we have $\rho_c = 0$ for all values of x and, since we have somehow forced the channel to remain open, nothing will happen to ρ_c.

If we pick any initial concentration x_0 in the interval $\tilde{\Omega}$, we know that the concentration will develop according to the ordinary differential equation

$$x_o'(t; x_0) = a_o(x) = (v_r + v_d)(c_+ - x), \tag{2.13}$$

whose solution is given by

$$x_o(t; x_0) = c_+ + e^{-t(v_r + v_d)}(x_0 - c_+);$$

see the discussion on page 26. In Fig. 2.5 we plot $x_o(t; x_0)$ as a function of t for ten values of initial data x_0 in the interval $\tilde{\Omega}$, using $h = 20\ \mu$M. The figure illustrates that the probability density function ρ_o, in this special case of a forced open channel, is simply advected in time and the advection is clearly governed by the speed of $x = x(t)$, which is given by $x'(t) = a_o(x)$.

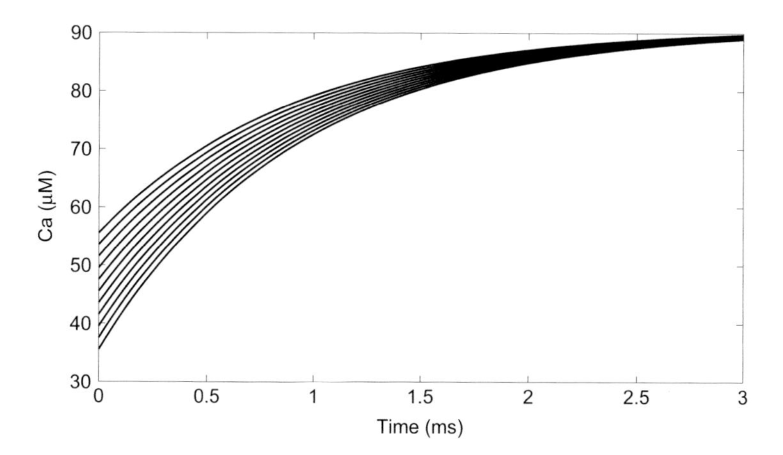

Fig. 2.5 Ten solutions of the ordinary differential equation (2.13) with data from Table 2.1. The figure illustrates that when the channel is kept open and the initial data are of the form given by (2.12) (with $h = 20\ \mu$M), the probability density is simply advected toward greater values of the concentration x

2.2.3.2 Advection in Another Very Special Case: The Channel Is Kept Closed for All Time

We can certainly repeat the considerations above for the probability density function of the closed state. In that case we assume that

$$\rho_c(x,0) = 1/h \text{ for } x \in \tilde{\Omega} = [\tilde{c} - h/2, \tilde{c} + h/2] \tag{2.14}$$

and $\rho_c = 0$ for values of x outside the interval $\tilde{\Omega}$. Again we pick any initial concentration x_0 in the interval $\tilde{\Omega}$ and recall that the concentration evolves as

$$x_c'(t; x_0) = a_c(x) = v_d (c_0 - x), \tag{2.15}$$

whose solution is given by

$$x_c(t; x_0) = c_0 + e^{-tv_d} (x_0 - c_0).$$

In Fig. 2.6 we plot $x_c(t; x_0)$ as a function of t for ten values of initial data x_0 in the interval $\tilde{\Omega}$. Again we observe that the probability density function is simply advected according to the speed of $x = x(t)$, which is given by $x' = a_c(x)$.

2.2.3.3 Advection: The General Case

We have seen how the probability density functions evolve in two very special cases. Next we consider the general case of how the probability density functions are

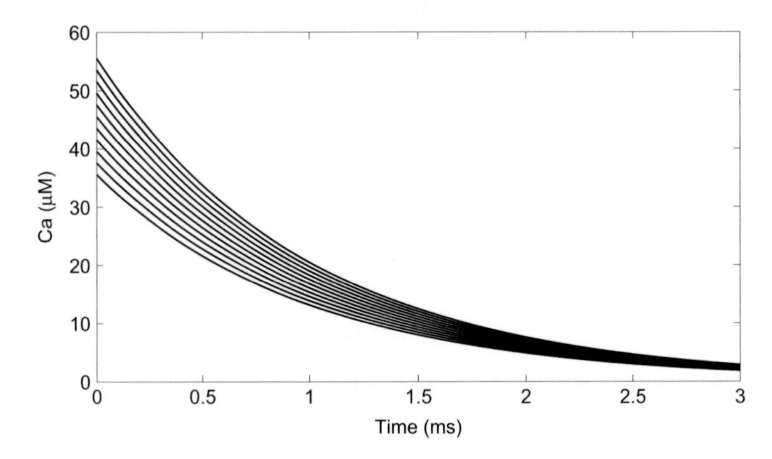

Fig. 2.6 Ten solutions of the ordinary differential equation (2.15). The figure illustrates that when the channel is kept closed and the initial data are of the form given by (2.14), the probability density is advected toward smaller values of the concentration x. As above we have used $h = 20\ \mu\text{M}$

advected when the state of the channel is kept fixed, and we focus on the probability density function of the open state.

Let $J_o(x,t)$ denote the flux per time of the probability across the point x at time t. A positive flux at x indicates a flux of probability into the domain $(x, x+\Delta x)$ and a positive flux at $x+\Delta x$ indicates a flux of probability out of the interval. This gives

$$\frac{d}{dt}P_o\left\{x < \bar{x}(t) < x+\Delta x\right\} = J_o(x,t) - J_o(x+\Delta x, t). \tag{2.16}$$

It now follows from (2.9) that

$$\begin{aligned}\frac{J_o(x,t) - J_o(x+\Delta x,t)}{\Delta x} &= \frac{d}{dt}\frac{1}{\Delta x}\int_x^{x+\Delta x} \rho_o\left(\xi,t\right)d\xi \\ &= \frac{1}{\Delta x}\int_x^{x+\Delta x}\frac{\partial \rho_o}{\partial t}\left(\xi,t\right)d\xi\end{aligned}$$

and, therefore, by going to the limit in Δx, we have

$$\frac{\partial \rho_o\left(x,t\right)}{\partial t} = -\frac{\partial J_o(x,t)}{\partial x}. \tag{2.17}$$

The flux is given by the product of velocity times density: $J_o = \rho_o v$, where in our case the velocity is given by $v = x'(t)$, so the flux will be

$$J_o = \rho_o(x,t)x'(t).$$

By recalling that, when the channel is open, we have

$$x'(t) = a_o(x) = v_r(c_1 - x) + v_d(c_0 - x),$$

we obtain

$$J_o = a_o(x)\rho_o = \left(v_r(c_1 - x) + v_d(c_0 - x)\right)\rho_o. \tag{2.18}$$

It follows from (2.17) and (2.18) that we have the conservation equation

$$\frac{\partial \rho_o\left(x,t\right)}{\partial t} + \frac{\partial}{\partial x}(a_o\rho_o) = 0, \tag{2.19}$$

where we account only for the advection of probability.

2.2.4 Changing States: The Effect of the Markov Model

We have now handled the advection of the probability listed as c) above and how changes due to the opening or closing of the channel affect the probability density function remains to be seen. Recall that the reaction scheme of the Markov model is given by

$$C \underset{k_{co}}{\overset{k_{oc}}{\leftrightarrows}} O \tag{2.20}$$

and suppose that the channel is open at time t. If we ignore the advection of concentration, handled above, we find that the probability density changes as follows from time t to time $t + \Delta t$:

$$\rho_o(x, t + \Delta t) = \rho_o(x, t) - \Delta t k_{oc} \rho_o(x, t) + \Delta t k_{co} \rho_c(x, t).$$

By going to the limit in Δt and combining this result with the conservation equation above, we obtain

$$\frac{\partial \rho_o (x, t)}{\partial t} + \frac{\partial}{\partial x}(a_o \rho_o) = k_{co} \rho_c(x, t) - k_{oc} \rho_o(x, t),$$

which governs the dynamics of the open probability density function.

2.2.5 The Closed State

We can carry out the same derivation of an equation modeling the dynamics of the probability density function of the closed state. The only change is that in the closed state we have

$$x'(t) = v_d(c_0 - x)$$

and therefore the associated flux is given by

$$J_c = v_d(c_0 - x)\rho_c. \tag{2.21}$$

2.2.6 *The System Governing the Probability Density Functions*

To summarize, we have the coupled system

$$\frac{\partial \rho_o}{\partial t} + \frac{\partial}{\partial x}(a_o \rho_o) = k_{co}\rho_c - k_{oc}\rho_o, \qquad (2.22)$$

$$\frac{\partial \rho_c}{\partial t} + \frac{\partial}{\partial x}(a_c \rho_c) = k_{oc}\rho_o - k_{co}\rho_c,$$

where

$$a_o = v_r(c_1 - x) + v_d(c_0 - x), \qquad (2.23)$$

$$a_c = v_d(c_0 - x).$$

This is a coupled system of PDEs; it is linear and first order and special care must be taken in solving it numerically, since it develops steep gradients. For ease of reference, we will sometimes call this the PDF system and its solutions are sometimes labeled the PDF solutions.

2.2.6.1 Boundary Conditions

The boundary conditions are set up to avoid the leak of probability across the boundary. Hence we need the fluxes $a_o\rho_o$ and $a_c\rho_c$ to be zero for $x = c_0$ and $x = c_+$. Note that $a_o(c_+) = a_c(c_0) = 0$, so we require that $\rho_o(c_0) = 0$ and $\rho_c(c_+) = 0$.

These conditions are fine as long as we know that the concentration is always in the interval bounded by c_0 and c_+. However, we may be interested in studying initial concentrations outside this interval.[3] Then we can extend the computational domain and use zero Dirichlet boundary conditions on the new computational domain.

2.3 Numerical Scheme for the PDF System

The dynamics of the probability density functions are governed by system (2.22), a system of linear advection-reaction equations. Numerical methods for such equations are thoroughly covered by LeVeque [48]. To describe the method, we

[3]We have seen above that the interval bounded by c_0 and c_+ is invariant in the sense that if the initial condition of the stochastic model (2.1) is in this interval, then the solution remains in the same interval for all time. We may, of course, however, pick an initial condition outside that interval, which motivates examination of the probability density functions using a larger domain. In these notes, however, we will stick to the invariant region.

consider the simple model

$$\rho_t + (a\rho)_x = h\rho, \tag{2.24}$$

where a and h are smooth functions of x. We let ρ_i^n denote an approximation of ρ at time $t = n\Delta t$ for $x \in [x_{i-1/2}, x_{i+1/2})$, where $x_i = c_0 + i\Delta x$, with

$$\Delta x = \frac{c_+ - c_0}{M}$$

for an integer $M > 1$. The numerical approximation is defined by the scheme

$$\rho_i^{n+1} = \rho_i^n - \frac{\Delta t}{\Delta x}\left((a\rho)_{i+1/2}^n - (a\rho)_{i-1/2}^n\right) + \Delta t h_i \rho_i^n, \tag{2.25}$$

where

$$(a\rho)_{i+1/2}^n = \max(a_{i+1/2}, 0)\rho_i^n + \min(a_{i+1/2}, 0)\rho_{i+1}^n \tag{2.26}$$

and $a_{i+1/2} = a(x_{i+1/2})$. In an appendix to this chapter (see page 50), we will go a bit deeper into the problem of computing solutions to the problem (2.22).

2.4 Rapid Convergence to Steady State Solutions

The PDF solutions rapidly reach a steady state solution. This is illustrated in Fig. 2.7. As initial conditions, we have $\rho_o(x,0) = \rho_c(x,0) = 0$, except $\rho_c(x,0) = 1/h$ for $x \in \tilde{\Omega} = [\tilde{c} - h/2, \tilde{c} + h/2]$, with $h = (c_+ - c_0)/20$, and where we recall that $\tilde{c} = \frac{1}{2}(c_0 + c_+)$. We have used $\Delta x = 0.1136$ mV and $\Delta t = 11.36$ ns. Furthermore, discrete initial conditions are normalized in order to ensure that

$$\Delta x \sum_{i,j} \rho_{i,j} = 1, \tag{2.27}$$

where $\rho = \rho_o + \rho_c$. In the upper panel, we show the solution for the first 10 ms and we observe rapid convergence toward a steady state solution. In the lower panel, we show the same results but for a small (and interesting) part of the concentration ranging from 80 to 91 μM. The solution seems to be almost in steady state after 6–8 ms. Because of this property of the solution of PDF system (2.22), we will often concentrate on steady state solutions.

In Fig. 2.8 we show the solution for $\rho_c(x,t)$. Here we have plotted the logarithm of the distribution to highlight the small but significant probability densities for the channel being closed at high concentrations and again we note rapid convergence toward equilibrium.

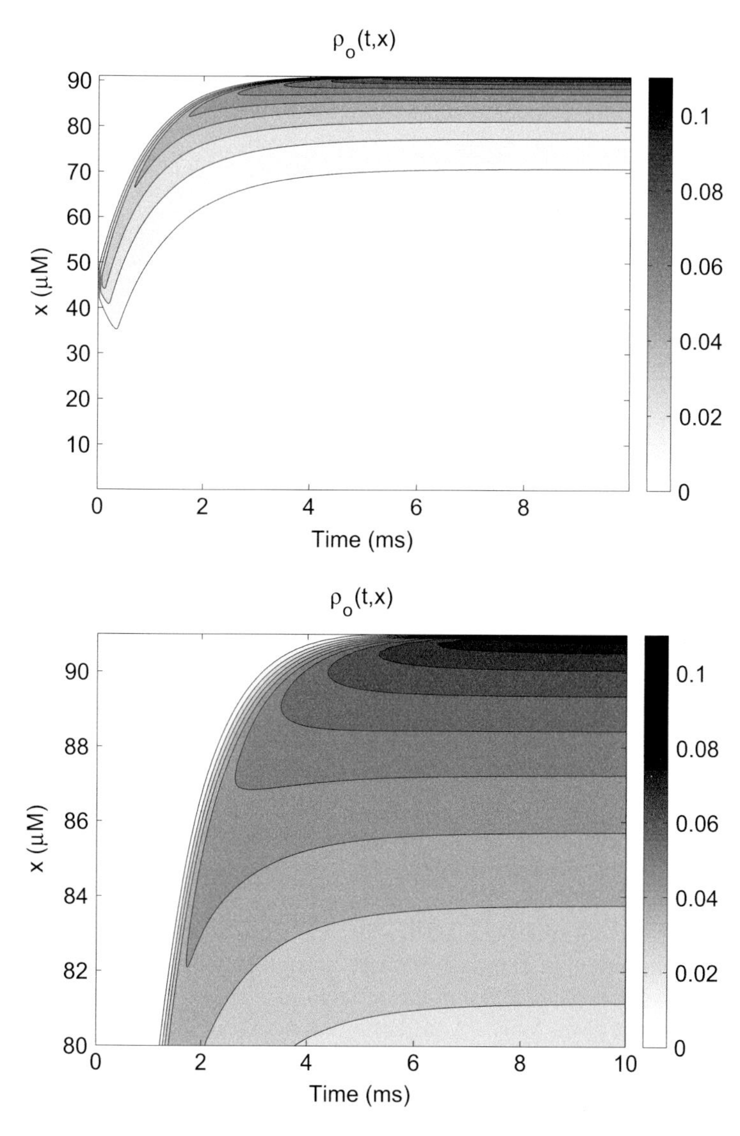

Fig. 2.7 Convergence to the steady state solution of ρ_o for PDF system (2.22). *Upper panel*: Dynamics of the open probability for all relevant values of the calcium concentration. *Lower panel*: Solution for concentrations in the interval 80–91 μM. Convergence to steady state is quite rapid

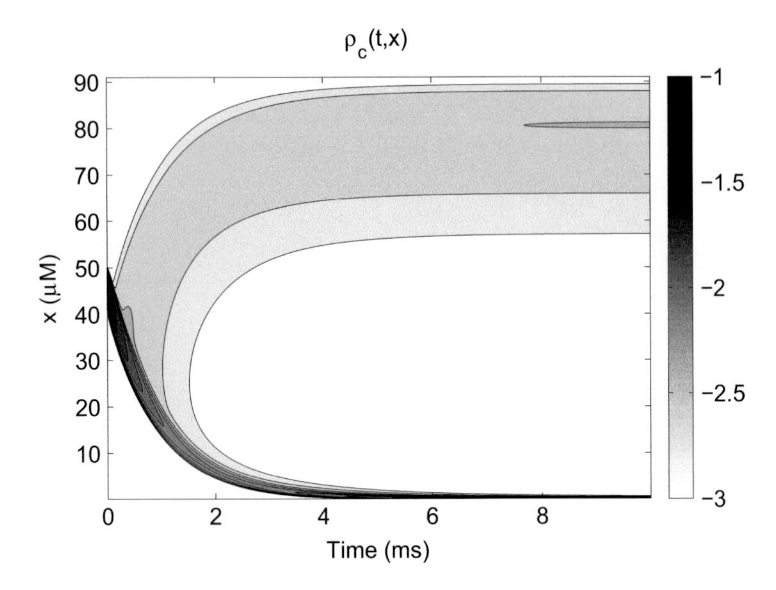

Fig. 2.8 The figure shows the probability density function of the closed state. In order to highlight small values of the probability densities, we show $\log(\rho_c(x,t))$

2.5 Comparison of Monte Carlo Simulations and Probability Density Functions

We are now in a position to study the release process illustrated in Fig. 2.2 using two different approaches: We can use Monte Carlo simulations and solve the stochastic differential equation (2.1) or we can compute the probability density functions of the process by solving system (2.22). In Fig. 2.9, we compare the numerical results obtained using these two approaches. Here, the probability density functions are computed using scheme (2.25) and the Monte Carlo simulations are based on the numerical scheme given by (2.7). In the figure, we show the solution of the PDF system at time $t^* = 1$ s. The Monte Carlo-based solution is computed by dividing the interval $[c_0, c_+]$ into 100 intervals and then counting the number of open states in each interval. The counting is performed over a period of time where we assume that the histogram has reached a stationary shape. In Fig. 2.9 the counting is based on the time interval running from $t = t^*/2$ to $t = t^*$, with $t^* = 1$ s. By considering the simulations shown in Fig. 2.7, we know that in this interval the probability density functions have reached their steady state solutions. In the figure, the histogram is computed running 500 Monte Carlo simulations. The figure clearly shows that the probability density approach gives the average of a large number of Monte Carlo simulations. We will see this repeated over and over in this text.

At steady state, we observe that it is quite unlikely that we have a low concentration combined with an open channel and it is quite likely that we have a large concentration (close to $c_+ = 91$ μM) combined with an open channel. There

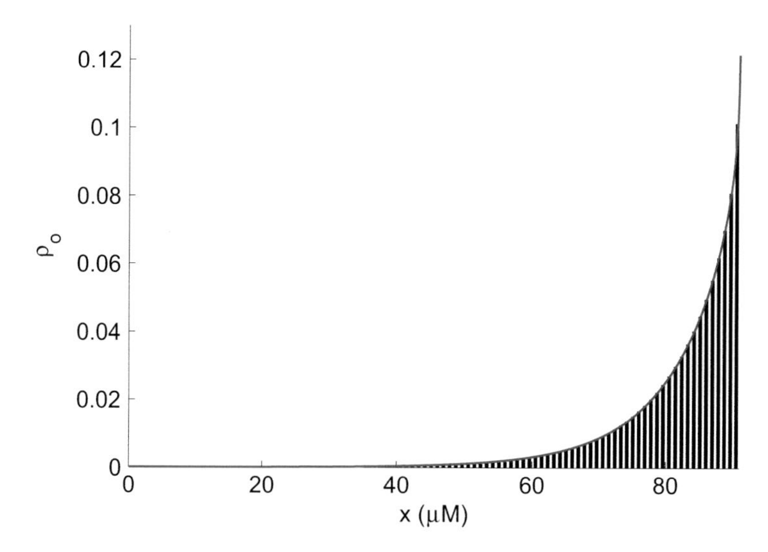

Fig. 2.9 Numerical solution of PDF system (2.22) (*red*) at time $t = t^* = 1$ s compared with the result of Monte Carlo simulations based on scheme (2.7) (*histogram*)

is a boundary layer close to the upper possible concentration, which means that the channel tends to be open and the concentration tends to be close to its maximum value.

In order to further illustrate the connection between the Monte Carlo simulations and the solution of the PDF system, we show four arbitrary solutions in the time interval from 900 to 1000 ms computed by the stochastic scheme (2.7). The solutions are given in Fig. 2.10 and we note that all the solutions are quite close to the upper level c_+ of the calcium concentration and the channel tends to be open.

2.6 Analytical Solutions in the Stationary Case

In the stationary case, we can derive analytical solutions of the PDF system. We start the derivation by recalling that the open and closed probability densities are governed by the following system of PDEs:

$$\frac{\partial \rho_o}{\partial t} + \frac{\partial}{\partial x}(a_o \rho_o) = k_{co}\rho_c - k_{oc}\rho_o, \tag{2.28}$$

$$\frac{\partial \rho_c}{\partial t} + \frac{\partial}{\partial x}(a_c \rho_c) = k_{oc}\rho_o - k_{co}\rho_c, \tag{2.29}$$

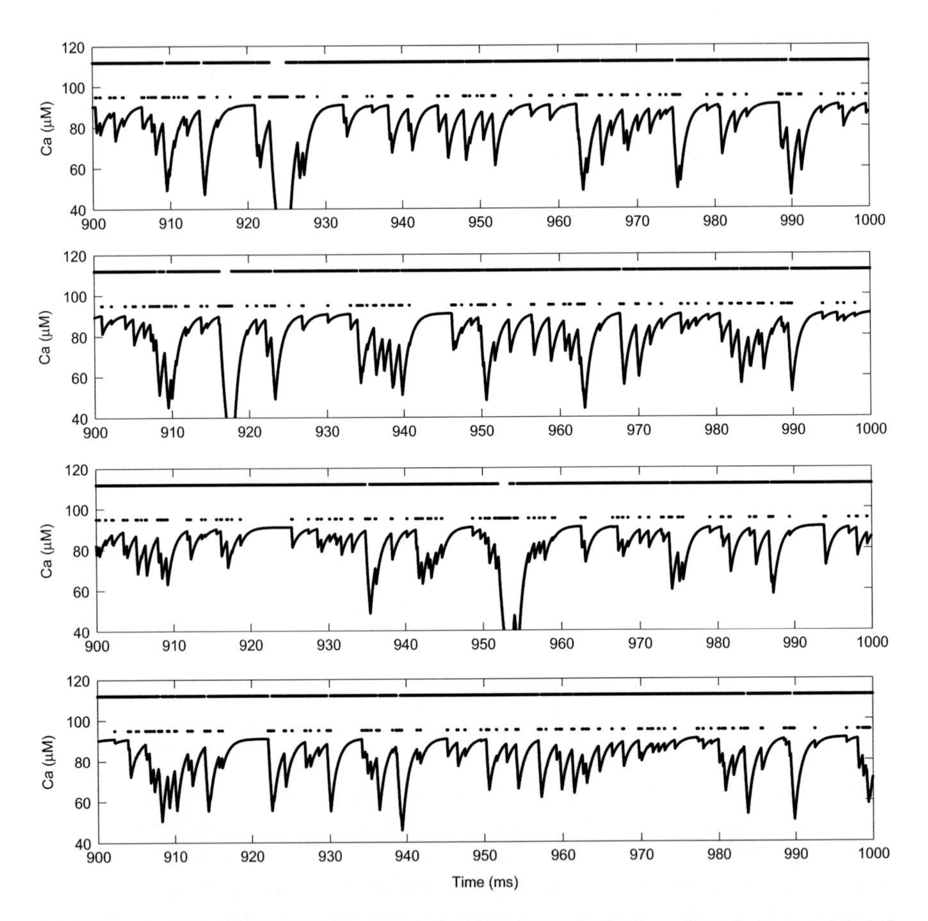

Fig. 2.10 Four simulations based on the stochastic scheme (2.7) where the solutions are plotted from 900 to 1,000 ms. The *lower curves* give the concentrations and we note that the concentrations are quite large but limited above by the upper limit given by $c_+ = 91$ μM. The *upper two lines* indicate whether the channel is open (*upper*) or closed (*lower*); we see that the channel is open most of the time. These results fit well with the results presented in Fig. 2.9, where the probability density functions are plotted

where

$$a_o = v_r(c_1 - x) + v_d(c_0 - x), \tag{2.30}$$
$$a_c = v_d(c_0 - x).$$

We consider the system for $x \in [c_0, c_+]$, where

$$c_+ = c_1 + \frac{v_d\,(c_0 - c_1)}{v_r + v_d}.$$

In the computations reported above, we saw that the solutions converge rapidly toward steady state solutions. The steady state solutions are given by the system

$$\frac{\partial}{\partial x}(a_o \rho_o) = k_{co}\rho_c - k_{oc}\rho_o, \tag{2.31}$$

$$\frac{\partial}{\partial x}(a_c \rho_c) = k_{oc}\rho_o - k_{co}\rho_c. \tag{2.32}$$

By adding these equations, we find that

$$\frac{\partial}{\partial x}(a_o \rho_o + a_c \rho_c) = 0. \tag{2.33}$$

Therefore, by invoking the boundary conditions, we have

$$a_o \rho_o + a_c \rho_c = 0. \tag{2.34}$$

Here it is useful to recall that $a_c < 0$ and $a_o > 0$ for $x \in (c_0, c_+)$ and thus we have

$$\rho_c = -\frac{a_o}{a_c}\rho_o. \tag{2.35}$$

The system can therefore be reduced to a scalar equation of the form

$$\frac{\partial}{\partial x}(a_o \rho_o) = -\left(k_{co}\frac{a_o}{a_c} + k_{oc}\right)\rho_o. \tag{2.36}$$

By differentiation, we can write this equation in the standard form

$$\rho_o' = -a(x)\rho_o, \tag{2.37}$$

with

$$a(x) = \frac{k_{co}}{a_c} + \frac{k_{oc}}{a_o} + \frac{a_o'}{a_o}.$$

We define the function $A = A(x)$ as

$$A'(x) = -a(x),$$

and find that

$$\left(e^{-A(x)}\rho_o\right)' = 0$$

and therefore

$$\rho_o = c e^{A(x)},$$

where c is a constant. We can find c by observing that

$$\begin{aligned} 1 &= \int_{c_0}^{c+} (\rho_o + \rho_c)\, dx \\ &= \int_{c_0}^{c+} \left(1 - \frac{a_o}{a_c}\right) \rho_o dx \\ &= c \int_{c_0}^{c+} \left(1 - \frac{a_o}{a_c}\right) e^{A(x)} dx \end{aligned}$$

and therefore

$$c = \left(\int_{c_0}^{c+} \left(1 - \frac{a_o}{a_c}\right) e^{A(x)} dx \right)^{-1}. \tag{2.38}$$

Recall that $v_d = 1\ \text{ms}^{-1}$, $c_0 = 0.1\ \mu\text{M}$, $v_r = 0.1\ \text{ms}^{-1}$, $c_1 = 1{,}000\ \mu\text{M}$, $k_{oc} = 1\ \text{ms}^{-1}$, and $k_{co} = (x/10)\ \text{ms}^{-1}(\mu\text{M})^{-1}$ and that the fluxes are defined by (2.30). For these data, we have the analytical solution

$$\rho_o(x) = K e^{x/10} (91 - x)^{-\frac{0.1}{1.1}} (x - 0.1)^{0.01},$$

$$\rho_c(x) = 1.1 K e^{x/10} (91 - x)^{\frac{1}{1.1}} (x - 0.1)^{-0.99},$$

where $K \approx 1.0073 \cdot 10^{-5}$.

2.7 Numerical Solution Accuracy

Since we have a steady state analytical solution, we can evaluate the accuracy of the numerical method under consideration. However, to do so, we will first clarify how we compute stationary solutions using the numerical scheme.

2.7.1 Stationary Solutions Computed by the Numerical Scheme

The numerical scheme (2.25) can be written in matrix form:

$$\rho^{n+1} = (I + \Delta t A)\, \rho^n.$$

The scheme is constructed such that if a discrete version of the integral condition (2.11) holds at time $t = 0$, it will hold for all subsequent time steps. More precisely, if we define

$$r^n = \Delta x \sum_{i=1}^{M} (\rho_{o,i}^n + \rho_{c,i}^n), \tag{2.39}$$

and $r^0 = 1$, then, by the construction of the scheme, we have $r^n = 1$ for all $n \geq 1$. Since the solution we are considering converges rapidly to a stationary solution, it is useful to be able to compute the stationary solution directly. The stationary version of the scheme reads

$$\rho = (I + \Delta t A)\,\rho$$

but here we have to make sure that the condition $r^n = 1$ is added to obtain a unique solution. When this condition is added, the stationary version of the system can be written in the form

$$B\phi = b.$$

An alternative to this method is to observe that the stationary solution is characterized by $A\rho = 0$. Therefore, using Matlab terminology, we can find the stationary solution by first computing

$$z = \text{null}(A)$$

and then set

$$\rho = \frac{z}{\Delta x \sum_i z_i}.$$

2.7.2 *Comparison with the Analytical Solution: The Stationary Solution*

The numerical and analytical solutions are compared in Fig. 2.11. In the numerical scheme, we use $\Delta x = 0.909\ \mu\text{M}$ and we observe that the analytical and numerical solutions are almost indistinguishable. In Table 2.2, we show the error as the mesh is refined. In the table, we measure only the errors of inner nodes to avoid evaluating the analytical solution at singular points. We define $[c_0 + \delta x, c_+ - \delta x]$ as the inner interval, where δx is the mesh parameter Δx used in the coarsest simulation in the convergence study. The difference between the analytical solution ρ and numerical

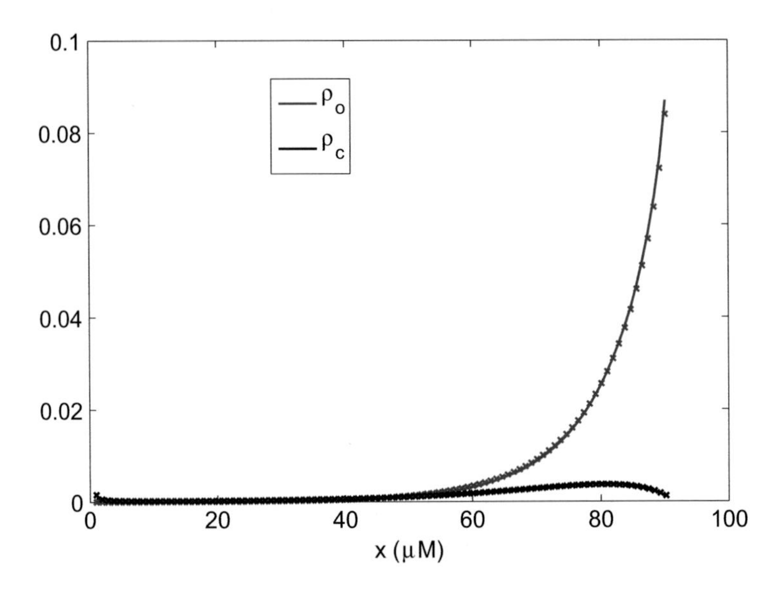

Fig. 2.11 Comparison of the numerical and analytical solutions of the steady state problem (2.31) and (2.32). Numerical solutions are marked with ×

Table 2.2 Error of the numerical computations as the mesh is refined. The convergence is first order

Δ x	Error	Error/Δx
0.909	0.086	0.095
0.455	0.036	0.078
0.227	0.016	0.072
0.114	0.008	0.069
0.057	0.004	0.066
0.028	0.002	0.064
0.014	0.001	0.063

solution $\hat{\rho}$ is measured by

$$\|\hat{\rho} - \rho\| = |\hat{\rho}_o - \rho_o|/|\rho_o| + |\hat{\rho}_c - \rho_c|/|\rho_c| \tag{2.40}$$

where $|x| = \sqrt{\sum_i x_i^2}$ and i runs over the nodes in the inner interval.

2.8 Increasing the Reaction Rate from Open to Closed

In Fig. 2.12 (upper panel), we increase the reaction rate k_{oc} from one to three. This means that the channel is much more prone to be closed and we see that this changes the probability density function ρ_o considerably. For completeness, we also plot the closed probability density functions (lower panel) and observe that, when

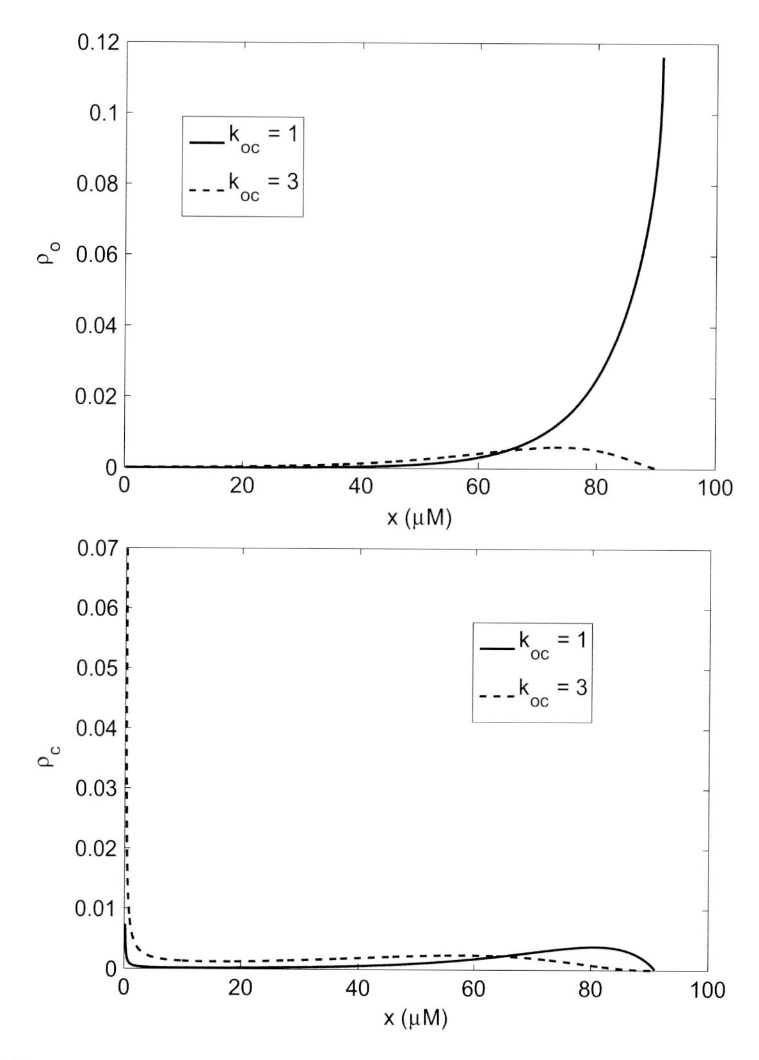

Fig. 2.12 *Upper panel*: Comparison of the open probability density function for the cases $k_{oc} = 1$ ms^{-1} and $k_{oc} = 3$ ms^{-1}. When k_{oc} is increased, the open probability is significantly reduced for high concentrations. *Lower panel*: Comparison of the closed probability density function for the cases $k_{oc} = 1$ ms^{-1} and $k_{oc} = 3$ ms^{-1}. When k_{oc} is increased, the closed probability is significantly increased for low concentrations

k_{oc} is increased, there is a high probability of the channel being closed and the concentration being quite low. All the other parameters used in the model are as specified on page 29.

2.9 Advection Revisited

In the derivation of system (2.22) above governing the probability density functions of the states of the Markov model, we found it useful to consider a case representing the pure advection of probability density. Let us now see that we can find the same solution using system (2.22), that is,

$$\frac{\partial \rho_o}{\partial t} + \frac{\partial}{\partial x}(a_o \rho_o) = k_{co}\rho_c - k_{oc}\rho_o, \qquad (2.41)$$
$$\frac{\partial \rho_c}{\partial t} + \frac{\partial}{\partial x}(a_c \rho_c) = k_{oc}\rho_o - k_{co}\rho_c,$$

where, as usual,

$$a_o = v_r(c_1 - x) + v_d(c_0 - x), \qquad (2.42)$$
$$a_c = v_d(c_0 - x);$$

see page 37. Let us assume that $\rho_c(x, 0) = 0$ and that

$$\rho_o(x, 0) = 1/h \text{ for } x \in \tilde{\Omega} = [\tilde{c} - h/2, \tilde{c} + h/2] \qquad (2.43)$$

and $\rho_o = 0$ for values of x outside the interval $\tilde{\Omega}$; for other notation see page 32. Furthermore, we assume that $k_{oc} = 0\ \text{ms}^{-1}$ (if the channel is open, it remains open) and $k_{co} = 1\ \text{ms}^{-1}$. Then, the solution of system (2.41) with the given initial conditions is given by[4]

$$(\rho_o, \rho_c) = (r, 0) \qquad (2.44)$$

where r solves the pure advection equation

$$r_t + (ar)_x = 0 \qquad (2.45)$$

with $a(x) = a_o(x)$ and the initial condition $r(x, 0) = \rho_o(x, 0)$.

In Fig. 2.13 we show the solution ρ_o of this problem in the left panel and in the right panel we repeat the solution given in Fig. 2.5, where the pure advection case was studied by solving a series of ordinary differential equations; see page 33.

For completeness, we also consider pure advection in the case where the channel is always closed. In this case we put $k_{co} = 0\ \text{ms}^{-1}$ and $k_{oc} = 1\ \text{ms}^{-1}$ and we use the initial conditions given by (2.14). In Fig. 2.14 we show (left panel) the solution

[4] To see that (ρ_o, ρ_c) given by (2.44) solves system (2.41), it is sufficient to insert (ρ_o, ρ_c) into the system to verify that it is a solution.

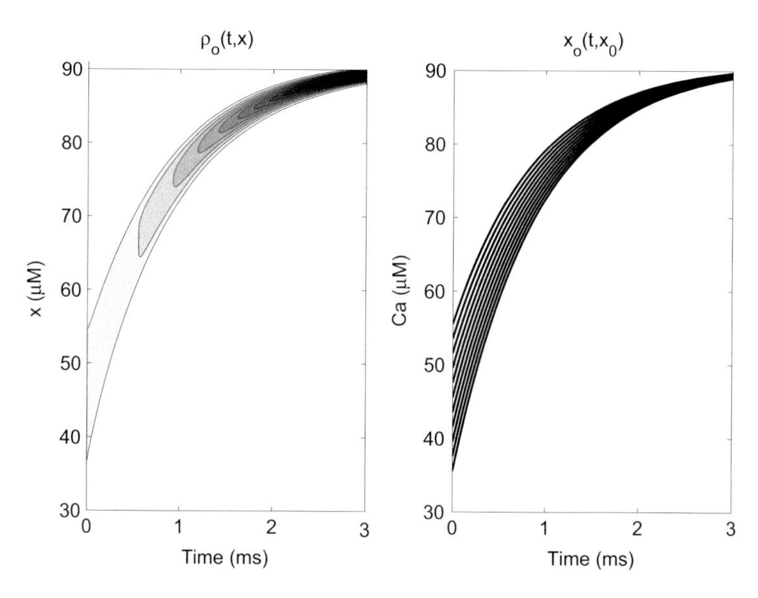

Fig. 2.13 *Left panel*: Solution of system (2.41) using $k_{oc} = 0\ \text{ms}^{-1}$ and $k_{co} = 1\ \text{ms}^{-1}$ and the initial condition (2.43) computed by solving (2.45) using the mesh parameters $\Delta x = 0.114\ \mu\text{M}$ and $\Delta t = 0.0114\ \mu\text{s}$. *Right panel*: Ten solutions of (2.13) given in Fig. 2.5 above

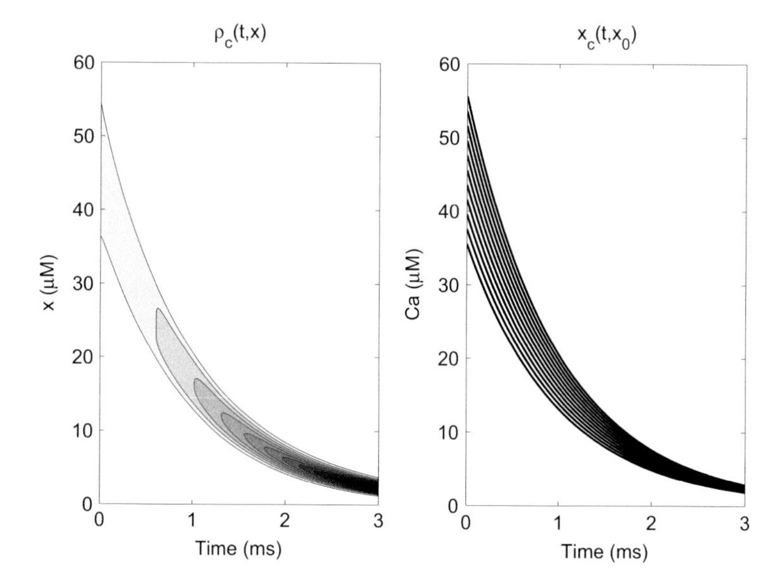

Fig. 2.14 *Left panel*: Solution of system (2.41) using $k_{co} = 0\ \text{ms}^{-1}$ and $k_{oc} = 1\ \text{ms}^{-1}$ and the initial condition (2.14) computed by solving (2.45) using the mesh parameters $\Delta x = 0.114\ \mu\text{M}$ and $\Delta t = 0.0114\ \mu\text{s}$. *Right panel*: Ten solutions of (2.15) given in Fig. 2.6 above

ρ_c of this problem computed by solving the pure advection problem

$$r_t + (ar)_x = 0 \tag{2.46}$$

with $a(x) = a_c(x)$ and $r(x,0) = \rho_c(x,0)$. We also show (right panel) the solution of the pure advection problem computed by solving a series of ordinary differential equations, as explained on page 34.

2.10 Appendix: Solving the System of Partial Differential Equations

In this chapter, we derived the system

$$\begin{aligned} \frac{\partial \rho_o}{\partial t} + \frac{\partial}{\partial x}(a_o \rho_o) &= k_{co}\rho_c - k_{oc}\rho_o, \\ \frac{\partial \rho_c}{\partial t} + \frac{\partial}{\partial x}(a_c \rho_c) &= k_{oc}\rho_o - k_{co}\rho_c, \end{aligned} \tag{2.47}$$

where

$$\begin{aligned} a_o &= v_r(c_1 - x) + v_d(c_0 - x), \\ a_c &= v_d(c_0 - x); \end{aligned} \tag{2.48}$$

see page 37. We also briefly sketched a numerical method for solving it; see (2.25). The numerical solution of systems of this form is used repeatedly in these notes, so solution methods deserve a little more attention. In this appendix we will present one way of solving the system; by consulting literature in numerical methods for solving PDEs, the reader will find a huge number of alternatives. The numerical solution of systems of this form is an active field of research and we will by no means argue that the method we present here is any better than other methods. Our focus is simplicity.

2.10.1 Operator Splitting

By breaking this system down into smaller parts, we will see that it is actually quite straightforward to solve numerically. Let us start by writing the system in the form

$$\rho_t + (A\rho)_x = K\rho \tag{2.49}$$

where

$$\rho = \begin{pmatrix} \rho_o \\ \rho_c \end{pmatrix}, \ A = \begin{pmatrix} a_o & 0 \\ 0 & a_c \end{pmatrix}, \text{ and } K = \begin{pmatrix} -k_{oc} & k_{co} \\ k_{oc} & -k_{co} \end{pmatrix}. \tag{2.50}$$

Then one way of solving this system is to introduce operator splitting. Using first-order operator splitting, we can solve the system (2.49) in two steps. Assume that the solution is given by ρ^n at time $t_n = n\Delta t$. Then the first step is to solve the system

$$\rho_t + (A\rho)_x = 0 \tag{2.51}$$

from $t = t_n$ to $t = t_n + \Delta t$ using $\rho(t_n) = \rho^n$ as the initial condition. Next we define the initial condition $u(t_n) = \rho(t_{n+1})$ (which we just computed) and then solve the system of ordinary differential equations given by

$$u_t = Ku \tag{2.52}$$

from $t = t_n$ to $t = t_n + \Delta t$. Finally, we define

$$\rho_{n+1} = u(t_{n+1}) \tag{2.53}$$

and thereby we have an approximate solution at time $t = t_{n+1}$ and the procedure can be repeated.

Now the problem of solving system (2.47) is reduced to solving a linear hyperbolic problem of the form (2.51) and a linear system of ordinary differential equations of the form (2.52). Methods for solving the latter can be found in any introductory text in numerical methods for PDEs. The explicit and implicit Euler methods are particularly popular because of their simplicity (see, e.g., [96]). In our computations, we use either the explicit or the implicit Euler method or we use the ODE15s method provided by Matlab (www.mathworks.com).

2.10.2 *The Hyperbolic Part*

Systems of hyperbolic equations can in general be hard to solve, but the present system takes on a particularly simple form. We observe that the two equations in (2.51) simply decouple and take the form

$$\begin{aligned} \frac{\partial \rho_o}{\partial t} + \frac{\partial}{\partial x}(a_o \rho_o) &= 0, \\ \frac{\partial \rho_c}{\partial t} + \frac{\partial}{\partial x}(a_c \rho_c) &= 0; \end{aligned} \tag{2.54}$$

thus it is sufficient to discuss how to solve a scalar equation of the form

$$u_t + (au)_x = 0. \tag{2.55}$$

This problem is further simplified by the fact that the function a has a uniform sign. This is obviously true for $a = a_c = v_d(c_0 - x)$ since $x \in (c_0, c_+)$, where we recall that

$$c_+ = \frac{v_r c_1 + v_d c_0}{v_r + v_d} \tag{2.56}$$

and therefore $a_c \leq 0$ for all relevant values of x. Similarly,

$$a = a_o = v_r(c_1 - x) + v_d(c_0 - x) = (v_r + v_d)(c_+ - x) \tag{2.57}$$

and therefore $a_o \geq 0$ for all relevant values of x.

We mentioned above that a scalar equation of the form

$$u_t + (au)_x = 0 \tag{2.58}$$

can be solved using the scheme

$$u_i^{n+1} = u_i^n - \frac{\Delta t}{\Delta x}\left((au)_{i+1/2}^n - (au)_{i-1/2}^n\right), \tag{2.59}$$

where

$$(au)_{i+1/2}^n = \max(a_{i+1/2}, 0)u_i^n + \min(a_{i+1/2}, 0)u_{i+1}^n \tag{2.60}$$

and $a_{i+1/2} = a(x_{i+1/2})$; see (2.25) on page 37. For the probability density function of the open state ρ_o with $a = a_o \geq 0$, we obtain

$$(a_o\rho_o)_{i+1/2}^n = a_{o,i+1/2}\rho_{o,i}^n \tag{2.61}$$

and for the probability density function of the closed state ρ_c with $a = a_c \leq 0$, we obtain

$$(a_c\rho_c)_{i+1/2}^n = a_{c,i+1/2}\rho_{c,i+1}^n. \tag{2.62}$$

The numerical schemes of the hyperbolic part given by (2.51) therefore read

$$\rho_{o,i}^{n+1} = \rho_{o,i}^n - \frac{\Delta t}{\Delta x}\left(a_{o,i+1/2}\rho_{o,i}^n - a_{o,i-1/2}\rho_{o,i-1}^n\right) \tag{2.63}$$

and

$$\rho_{c,i}^{n+1} = \rho_{c,i}^{n} - \frac{\Delta t}{\Delta x}\left(a_{c,i+1/2}\rho_{c,i+1}^{n} - a_{c,i-1/2}\rho_{c,i}^{n}\right). \tag{2.64}$$

2.10.3 The Courant–Friedrichs–Lewy Condition

For hyperbolic problems of the form

$$u_t + (au)_x = 0 \tag{2.65}$$

it is well known that a certain condition must be imposed on the time step in order to avoid spurious oscillations. The condition states that

$$\frac{\Delta t}{\Delta x} \max_x |a(x)| \leq 1; \tag{2.66}$$

see LeVeque [48] for a derivation of the Courant–Friedrichs–Lewy condition. Note that in our case the condition

$$\Delta t \leq \frac{\Delta x}{(v_r + v_d)(c_+ - c_0)} \tag{2.67}$$

covers both the equations of the decoupled system (2.54). This is a stability condition for the hyperbolic part of the problem. If we solve the ordinary differential equation part (2.52) using an implicit scheme, that part is unconditionally stable. Nevertheless, the ordinary differential equation part usually requires smaller time steps than the hyperbolic part in order to obtain sufficient accuracy.

2.11 Notes

1. Figure 2.1 is taken from Winslow et al. [105]. The figure will be used many times in this text as we gradually consider more complex models of CICR. A detailed description of the CICR mechanism and associated models is given by Winslow, Greenstein, Tankskanen, and Chen in [105] and [104].
2. A review of possible pathological changes arising in the vicinity of the dyad is given by Louch et al. [55] and calcium signaling in the developing cardiomyocyte is reviewed by Louch et al. [54]. Cardiac calcium signaling is reviewed by Bers [5].
3. The goal of the calcium dynamics of a cardiac cell is to enable the well coordinated contraction of cardiac muscle. Cardiac excitation contraction is reviewed by Bers [3, 4].

4. A detailed model of a calcium release unit is presented by Hake et al. [30] and Chai et al. [9] used the largest computer in the world (in 2013) to simulate the calcium dynamics of a single sarcomere at the nanometer scale. Simulations of the calcium dynamics of a whole cardiac cell are presented by Nivala et al. [60] and Li et al. [49, 51]. The dynamics was analyzed in [98] using a model developed by Swietach et al. [95].
5. The derivation in Sect. 2.2 of the system of deterministic differential equations based on the stochastic release equations is motivated by the derivation of Nykamp and Tranchina [63].
6. The probability density function approach used to model calcium concentrations is taken from Huertas and Smith [35].
7. As mentioned in the beginning of this chapter, the model illustrated in Fig. 2.2 relies on a series of simplifying assumptions. One additional simplification underlying the model given in (2.1) is that we assume that there is just one channel. In reality, the RyRs come in clusters of 10–20 channels, but here we assume that the effect of these channels can be added together in one big channel taking on the states of the Markov model in question. This is a major simplification that makes it possible to deal with the problem. The case of many interacting channels is dealt with by Bressloff [6] (page 112) for the case of a Markov model consisting of only two states (closed and open).
8. For readers who need to refresh basic notions of differential equations, we recommend a look at the books by Logan [53], Strauss [91] or [96, 100]. As mentioned several times above, we recommend LeVeque [48] for an introduction to the numerical solution of hyperbolic problems.
9. Systems of PDEs written in the form (2.22) appear in many different applications; see Bressloff [6], where other methods of analysis are also presented.
10. An introduction to operator splitting and an explanation of why it works are given by, for example, LeVeque [48]. Operator splitting for the monodomain equation of electrophysiology was used by Qu and Garfinkel [70] and the accuracy was analyzed by Schroll et al. [80]. Application to the bidomain model was presented by Keener and Bogar [45] and by Sundnes et al. [94].

Chapter 3
Models of Open and Closed State Blockers

So far we have studied a one-dimensional model of calcium-induced calcium release. The analysis started with a stochastic differential equation modeling release from internal storage to the dyad. We found that this model could be analyzed using Monte Carlo simulations or a system of deterministic partial differential equations giving the probability density functions of the open and the closed states. Furthermore, we found analytical solutions of the stationary solutions of the probability density system.

The aim of the present chapter is to introduce mathematical models of a drug and then show how the parameters defining the drug can be computed so that it works as well as possible. For simplicity, we will focus on closed to open mutations (CO-mutations; see page 16), but it will become clear how to handle open to closed mutations (OC-mutations) in later chapters.

Let us start by recalling that the Markov model governing the states of the channel is given by

$$C \underset{k_{co}}{\overset{k_{oc}}{\leftrightarrows}} O. \tag{3.1}$$

When a CO-mutation is present, we introduce the mutation severity index μ and replace the reaction rate k_{co} by μk_{co},

$$C \underset{\mu k_{co}}{\overset{k_{oc}}{\leftrightarrows}} O. \tag{3.2}$$

Obviously, $\mu = 1$ represents the wild type case and the size of $\mu > 1$ gives the strength of the mutation. By recalling what the Markov model means, we see that the mutation increases the probability of going from the closed to the open state and thus the open state probability will increase.

A. Tveito, G.T. Lines, *Computing Characterizations of Drugs for Ion Channels and Receptors Using Markov Models*, Lecture Notes in Computational Science and Engineering 111, DOI 10.1007/978-3-319-30030-6_3

In this chapter, we will study theoretical open and closed state blockers. We recall from Chap. 1 that open and closed state blockers can be presented in the forms

$$C \underset{\mu k_{co}}{\overset{k_{oc}}{\leftrightarrows}} O \underset{k_{ob}}{\overset{k_{bo}}{\leftrightarrows}} B \tag{3.3}$$

and

$$B \underset{k_{bc}}{\overset{k_{cb}}{\leftrightarrows}} C \underset{\mu k_{co}}{\overset{k_{oc}}{\leftrightarrows}} O, \tag{3.4}$$

respectively. The reasoning behind this way of modeling the effect of a drug was discussed on page 18 above; see in particular Fig. 1.9. Basically, we assume that the drug introduces a new conformational state of the channel protein that can be attained via the open state (for open state blockers) or via the closed state (for closed state blockers). The blocked states are always assumed to be non-conducting.

The mathematical problem of finding a suitable theoretical drug is now to find the parameters k_{bc} and k_{cb} for the closed state blockers and k_{bo} and k_{ob} for the open state blockers such that the effect of the mutation is reduced as much as possible. We will see that this problem is much easier using the probability density approach than using Monte Carlo simulations.

To compute optimal drugs for the CO-mutation, we will first consider the equilibrium states of the reactions. For closed state blockers, we can use the equilibrium considerations to reduce the number of free parameters from two to one. In principle, this can also be done for open state blockers, but some averaging is needed in the process and optimality is not obtained. For the closed state blocker, we can use the steady state system derived above to completely characterize both parameters of the drug to obtain optimality and computations will show that the resulting drug is theoretically extremely good and asymptotically perfect in the sense that it completely reverses the effect of the mutation. We are also able to derive a good open state blocker, but the method is less satisfactory and the results are not as good as for the closed state blocker.

3.1 Markov Models of Closed State Blockers for CO-Mutations

We start the derivation of theoretical drugs by considering closed state blockers. The reaction scheme of a closed state blocker takes the form

$$B \underset{k_{bc}}{\overset{k_{cb}}{\leftrightarrows}} C \underset{\mu k_{co}}{\overset{k_{oc}}{\leftrightarrows}} O, \tag{3.5}$$

where the reaction rates of the drug given by k_{cb} and k_{bc} must be determined so that the mutated cell behaves as similarly to the wild type cell as possible. We regard these parameters as free and we seek to compute them to obtain optimal efficiency of the theoretical drug. Allow us also to briefly repeat that this is basically our definition of a theoretical drug as discussed on page 18.

3.1.1 Equilibrium Probabilities for Wild Type

Consider the Markov model given by

$$C \underset{k_{co}}{\overset{k_{oc}}{\leftrightarrows}} O$$

and let o denote the probability of being in the open state and c the probability of being in the closed state. Suppose the channel just flickers between open and closed and nothing else happens. Then the equilibrium probabilities are characterized by

$$k_{co}c = k_{oc}o. \tag{3.6}$$

This means that the channel keeps on flickering in equilibrium and the probabilities of the open and closed states satisfy the relation (3.6). From this relation it follows that

$$c = \frac{k_{oc}}{k_{co}}o$$

and then, since $o + c = 1$, we obtain

$$o = \left(1 + \frac{k_{oc}}{k_{co}}\right)^{-1}.$$

3.1.2 Equilibrium Probabilities for the Mutant Case

In the CO-mutation case, we assume that the rate from C to O is increased and we define

$$k_{co,\mu} = \mu k_{co}, \tag{3.7}$$

where $\mu \geqslant 1$ and $\mu = 1$ denotes wild type. The equilibrium open probability of the mutant is given by

$$o_{\mu} = \left(1 + \frac{k_{oc}}{\mu k_{co}}\right)^{-1},$$

which clearly increases with increasing values of μ.

3.1.3 Equilibrium Probabilities for Mutants with a Closed State Drug

The equilibrium probabilities of reaction (3.5) are characterized by

$$\mu k_{co} c = k_{oc} o,$$
$$k_{bc} b = k_{cb} c;$$

so

$$c = \frac{k_{oc}}{\mu k_{co}} o,$$
$$b = \frac{k_{cb}}{k_{bc}} c = \frac{k_{cb}}{k_{bc}} \frac{k_{oc}}{\mu k_{co}} o,$$

and, since $o + c + b = 1$, we obtain

$$\left(1 + \frac{k_{oc}}{\mu k_{co}} + \frac{k_{cb}}{k_{bc}} \frac{k_{oc}}{\mu k_{co}}\right) o = 1.$$

So

$$o = \left(1 + \frac{k_{oc}}{\mu k_{co}} \left(1 + \frac{k_{cb}}{k_{bc}}\right)\right)^{-1}.$$

Define

$$\delta_c = \frac{k_{cb}}{k_{bc}} \tag{3.8}$$

and note that, in equilibrium, the wild type open probability is given by

$$o = \left(1 + \frac{k_{oc}}{k_{co}}\right)^{-1}$$

and the drugged mutant open probability is given by

$$o_{\mu,\delta_c} = \left(1 + \frac{k_{oc}}{k_{co}} \frac{1+\delta_c}{\mu}\right)^{-1}.$$

Now, we want to choose the drug characterization δ_c such that $o_{\mu,\delta_c} \approx o$ and this can clearly be achieved by requiring that

$$\frac{1+\delta_c}{\mu} \approx 1$$

or

$$\delta_c \approx \mu - 1.$$

So we obtain the characterization

$$k_{cb} = (\mu - 1)k_{bc}. \tag{3.9}$$

This means that, for the closed state blocker, we reduced the number of parameters characterizing the blocker from two to one. We will use the probability density approach to determine the remaining degree of freedom.

3.2 Probability Density Functions in the Presence of a Closed State Blocker

The probability density approach to the stochastic model in the presence of a closed state drug is

$$\begin{aligned}
\frac{\partial \rho_o}{\partial t} + \frac{\partial}{\partial x}(a_o \rho_o) &= \mu k_{co} \rho_c - k_{oc} \rho_o, \\
\frac{\partial \rho_c}{\partial t} + \frac{\partial}{\partial x}(a_c \rho_c) &= k_{oc} \rho_o - (\mu k_{co} + k_{cb})\, \rho_c + k_{bc} \rho_b, \\
\frac{\partial \rho_b}{\partial t} + \frac{\partial}{\partial x}(a_c \rho_b) &= k_{cb} \rho_c - k_{bc} \rho_b,
\end{aligned}$$

where

$$\begin{aligned}
a_o &= v_r(c_1 - x) + v_d(c_0 - x), \\
a_c &= v_d(c_0 - x).
\end{aligned}$$

From (3.9), the parameters of the drug are related by

$$k_{cb} = (\mu - 1)\, k_{bc}; \tag{3.10}$$

so the system is

$$\begin{aligned}
\frac{\partial \rho_o}{\partial t} + \frac{\partial}{\partial x}(a_o \rho_o) &= \mu k_{co} \rho_c - k_{oc} \rho_o, \\
\frac{\partial \rho_c}{\partial t} + \frac{\partial}{\partial x}(a_c \rho_c) &= k_{oc} \rho_o - (\mu k_{co} + (\mu - 1)\, k_{bc})\, \rho_c + k_{bc} \rho_b, \\
\frac{\partial \rho_b}{\partial t} + \frac{\partial}{\partial x}(a_c \rho_b) &= (\mu - 1)\, k_{bc} \rho_c - k_{bc} \rho_b.
\end{aligned}$$

In the stationary case, we obtain the system

$$\frac{\partial}{\partial x}(a_o \rho_o) = \mu k_{co} \rho_c - k_{oc} \rho_o, \tag{3.11}$$

$$\frac{\partial}{\partial x}(a_c \rho_c) = k_{oc} \rho_o - (\mu k_{co} + (\mu - 1)\, k_{bc})\, \rho_c + k_{bc} \rho_b, \tag{3.12}$$

$$\frac{\partial}{\partial x}(a_c \rho_b) = (\mu - 1)\, k_{bc} \rho_c - k_{bc} \rho_b. \tag{3.13}$$

In this system, the mutation severity is given by μ and the drug is characterized by a single parameter given by k_{bc}. For a given value of μ our aim is now to compute the value of k_{bc} such that the probability density function of the open state given by this system is as similar as possible to the probability density function of the open state in the case of $\mu = 1$, that is, the wild type solution when no drug is applied.

3.2.1 Numerical Simulations with the Theoretical Closed State Blocker

We consider a mutation characterized by $\mu = 3$ and we apply closed state blockers (see reaction scheme (3.5)) with parameters satisfying the relation (3.10). In Fig. 3.1, we show the results of these simulations using the Monte Carlo approach: The lower panel of the figure is the same as the upper panel, except that we focus on concentrations ranging from 80 to 91 µM . We observe significant differences between the wild type solution and the solution representing the mutation. Furthermore, we observe that the drug works quite well. Similar results are given in Fig. 3.2, where the computations are based on the probability density approach: Here the lower panel focuses on very high concentrations ranging from 89 to 91 µM. We also see

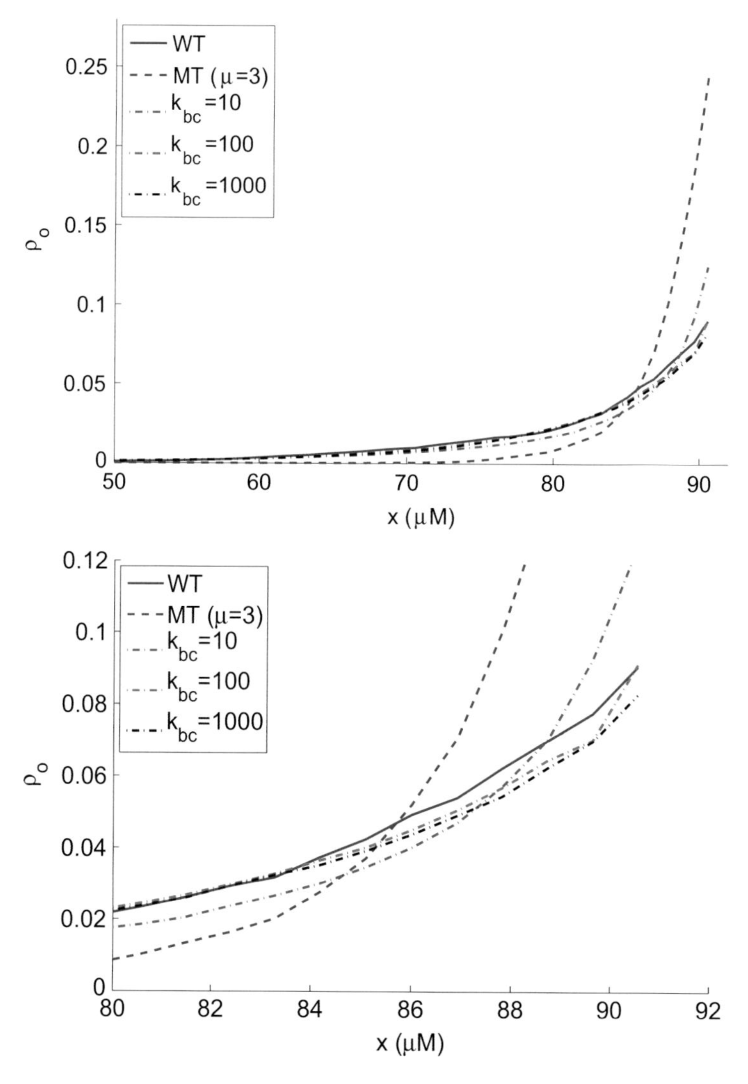

Fig. 3.1 Monte Carlo simulations using the theoretical closed state blocker given by the reaction scheme (3.5), where the reaction rates are related by (3.10) and the mutation severity index is given by $\mu = 3$. The lower panel focuses on higher levels of concentrations

that the closed state drug improves as the value of k_{bc} increases. In fact, the result seems to indicate that the drug is asymptotically perfect in the sense that the solution converges toward the wild type solution when $k_{bc} \to \infty$. Model parameters for these simulations are given in Table 3.1.

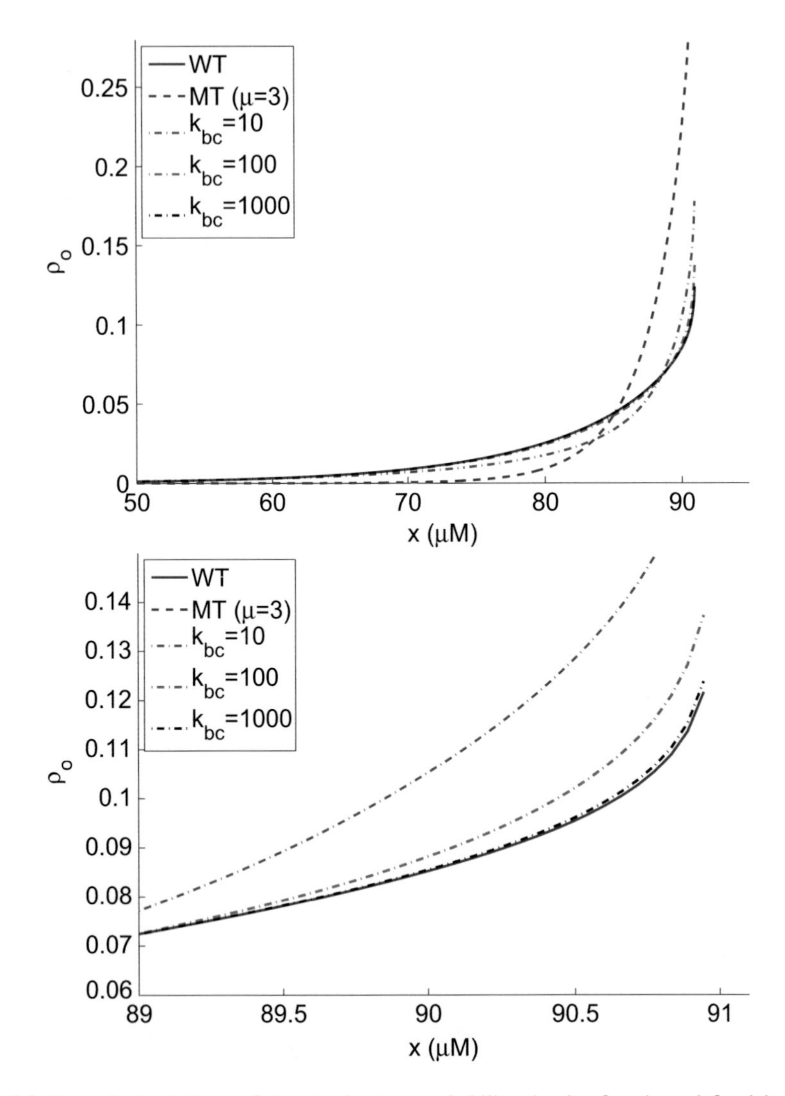

Fig. 3.2 Numerical solutions of the steady state probability density functions defined by the system (3.11)–(3.13), where the reaction rates are related by (3.10) and the mutation severity index is given by $\mu = 3$. The *lower panel* focuses on higher levels of concentrations. Note that the concentration axis of this figure is different from that of the *lower panel* of Fig. 3.1

Table 3.1 Parameter values for the undrugged case

v_d	1 ms^{-1}
v_r	0.1 ms^{-1}
c_0	0.1 μM
c_1	1,000 μM
$k_{co}(x)$	$0.1x$ ms^{-1} μM^{-1}
k_{oc}	1 ms^{-1}

3.3 Asymptotic Optimality for Closed State Blockers in the Stationary Case

In the simulations above, we observed that the closed state blocker worked well and that the drug became more effective as the value of k_{bc} increased. Our aim is now to indicate that, when $k_{bc} \rightarrow \infty$, the drug will completely repair the mutation. It is worth mentioning that the possibility of making a drug with $k_{bc} = \infty$ is quite unlikely, but the asymptotic result is still of theoretical interest.

Consider the steady state system

$$\frac{\partial}{\partial x}(a_o \rho_o) = \mu k_{co} \rho_c - k_{oc} \rho_o, \tag{3.14}$$

$$\frac{\partial}{\partial x}(a_c \rho_c) = k_{oc} \rho_o - (\mu k_{co} + (\mu - 1) k_{bc}) \rho_c + k_{bc} \rho_b, \tag{3.15}$$

$$\frac{\partial}{\partial x}(a_c \rho_b) = (\mu - 1) k_{bc} \rho_c - k_{bc} \rho_b. \tag{3.16}$$

By adding all the equations, we obtain

$$\frac{\partial}{\partial x}(a_o \rho_o + a_c (\rho_c + \rho_b)) = 0. \tag{3.17}$$

From the boundary conditions, we obtain

$$a_o \rho_o + a_c (\rho_c + \rho_b) = 0 \tag{3.18}$$

and therefore

$$\rho_c = \frac{-1}{a_c}(a_o \rho_o + a_c \rho_b), \tag{3.19}$$

where we recall that $a_c < 0$ for $x \in (c_0, c_+)$. Now, the system (3.14)–(3.16) can be rewritten in the form

$$\frac{\partial}{\partial x}(a_o \rho_o) = -\mu k_{co} \rho_b - \left(\frac{\mu k_{co} a_o}{a_c} + k_{oc}\right) \rho_o, \tag{3.20}$$

$$\frac{1}{k_{bc}} \frac{\partial}{\partial x}(a_c \rho_b) = -(\mu - 1) \frac{a_o}{a_c} \rho_o - \mu \rho_b. \tag{3.21}$$

We are interested in solutions of this system as k_{bc} becomes very large and we therefore note that, in the limit as $k_{bc} \rightarrow \infty$, the second equation yields

$$\rho_b = -\frac{(\mu - 1)}{\mu} \frac{a_o}{a_c} \rho_o \tag{3.22}$$

and therefore the first equation becomes

$$\frac{\partial}{\partial x}(a_o\rho_o) = -\mu k_{co}\rho_b - \left(\frac{\mu k_{co}a_o}{a_c} + k_{oc}\right)\rho_o \tag{3.23}$$

$$= k_{co}(\mu - 1)\frac{a_o}{a_c}\rho_o - \left(\frac{\mu k_{co}a_o}{a_c} + k_{oc}\right)\rho_o \tag{3.24}$$

$$= -\left(k_{co}\frac{a_o}{a_c} + k_{oc}\right)\rho_o. \tag{3.25}$$

So

$$\frac{\partial}{\partial x}(a_o\rho_o) = -\left(k_{co}\frac{a_o}{a_c} + k_{oc}\right)\rho_o. \tag{3.26}$$

Recall that the wild type model is

$$\frac{\partial}{\partial x}(a_o\rho_o) = -\left(k_{co}\frac{a_o}{a_c} + k_{oc}\right)\rho_o \tag{3.27}$$

(see (2.36)). By comparing (3.26) and (3.27), we see that when the drug is chosen to be of the form

$$k_{cb} = (\mu - 1)\,k_{bc}$$

and when we let $k_{bc} \to \infty$, the drug *completely* repairs the probability density functions of the mutated cell.

3.4 Markov Models for Open State Blockers

Next, we want to consider models of open state blockers. The reaction scheme of an open state blocker for the mutant reads

$$C \underset{\mu k_{co}}{\overset{k_{oc}}{\leftrightarrows}} O \underset{k_{ob}}{\overset{k_{bo}}{\leftrightarrows}} B.$$

The equilibrium probabilities are now characterized by

$$\mu k_{co}c = k_{oc}o,$$

$$k_{bo}b = k_{ob}o;$$

so

$$c = \frac{k_{oc}}{\mu k_{co}} o,$$

$$b = \frac{k_{ob}}{k_{bo}} o,$$

and since $o + c + b = 1$, we have

$$\left(1 + \frac{k_{oc}}{\mu k_{co}} + \frac{k_{ob}}{k_{bo}}\right) o = 1.$$

We now define the open state blocker characterization

$$\delta_o = \frac{k_{ob}}{k_{bo}}$$

and note that the open probability is given by

$$o_{\mu,\delta_o} = \left(1 + \frac{k_{oc}}{\mu k_{co}} + \delta_o\right)^{-1}.$$

Since the wild type open probability is given by

$$o = \left(1 + \frac{k_{oc}}{k_{co}}\right)^{-1},$$

we want to choose the drug such that $o_{\mu,\delta_o} \approx o$ and we therefore require

$$\frac{k_{oc}}{\mu k_{co}} + \delta_o \approx \frac{k_{oc}}{k_{co}}$$

or

$$\delta_{o,\mu} \approx \frac{k_{oc}}{k_{co}} \frac{\mu - 1}{\mu}, \tag{3.28}$$

where we recall that the mutation severity index $\mu \geqslant 1$. Since $\mu = 1$ is the wild type case, we note that in that case $\delta_o = 0$ is the optimal drug, which makes sense; there is no need to drug the wild type. However, for mutant cells, we have $\mu > 1$ and the characterization (3.28) of δ_o depends on the dyad calcium concentration, x. We will therefore use direct optimization to find suitable open state blockers.

3.4.1 *Probability Density Functions in the Presence of an Open State Blocker*

The probability density model in the presence of an open state drug is

$$\frac{\partial \rho_o}{\partial t} + \frac{\partial}{\partial x}(a_o \rho_o) = \mu k_{co} \rho_c - (k_{oc} + k_{ob}) \rho_o + k_{bo} \rho_b, \quad (3.29)$$

$$\frac{\partial \rho_c}{\partial t} + \frac{\partial}{\partial x}(a_c \rho_c) = k_{oc} \rho_o - \mu k_{co} \rho_c, \quad (3.30)$$

$$\frac{\partial \rho_b}{\partial t} + \frac{\partial}{\partial x}(a_c \rho_b) = k_{ob} \rho_o - k_{bo} \rho_b, \quad (3.31)$$

where we recall that

$$a_o = v_r(c_1 - x) + v_d(c_0 - x),$$
$$a_c = v_d(c_0 - x).$$

In the stationary case, we obtain the system

$$\frac{\partial}{\partial x}(a_o \rho_o) = \mu k_{co} \rho_c - (k_{oc} + k_{ob}) \rho_o + k_{bo} \rho_b, \quad (3.32)$$

$$\frac{\partial}{\partial x}(a_c \rho_c) = k_{oc} \rho_o - \mu k_{co} \rho_c, \quad (3.33)$$

$$\frac{\partial}{\partial x}(a_c \rho_b) = k_{ob} \rho_o - k_{bo} \rho_b. \quad (3.34)$$

We let both k_{ob} and k_{bo} be free parameters and use the *Fminsearch* function in Matlab to optimize these parameters by minimizing the discrete l_2 difference[1] between the wild type and mutant ρ_o. The resulting parameters are $k_{ob} = 0.28\ \mathrm{ms}^{-1}$, and $k_{bo} = 1.63\ \mathrm{ms}^{-1}$ and the associated numerical results are given in Fig. 3.3, marked as *opt*.

3.5 Open Blocker Versus Closed Blocker

In Fig. 3.4, we compare the results of the best open state blocker (referred to as *opt* in Fig. 3.3) and closed state blocker, using $k_{bc} = 1{,}000\ \mathrm{ms}^{-1}$ (see Fig. 3.2). We clearly see that the closed state blocker is better; in fact, at this resolution of

[1]The discrete l_2 difference between two vectors is given by $\|u - v\|_2 = (\sum_i (u_i - v_i)^2)^{1/2}$.

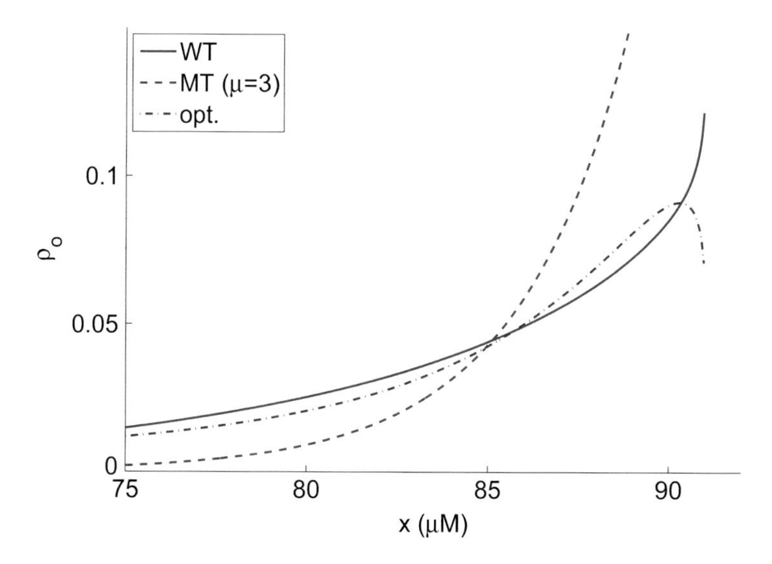

Fig. 3.3 Graphs of the numerical solutions using open state blockers. The open state blockers are based on optimization using the *Fminsearch* function in Matlab. In the simulation marked with *opt*, both parameters k_{ob} and k_{bo} are used in the minimization

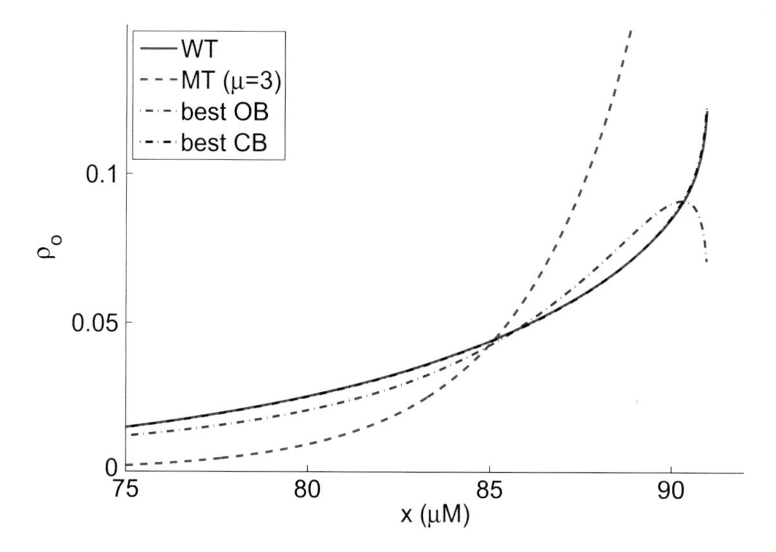

Fig. 3.4 Comparison of the best open state blocker and closed state blocker using $k_{bc} = 1{,}000$ ms^{-1} (see Table 3.2 for all the parameters of the two drugs). It is hard to distinguish between the wild type solution and the solution of the mutant case where the closed state blocker is applied

Table 3.2 Parameter values for the drugs used in Fig. 3.4

k_{ob}	0.28 ms^{-1}
k_{bo}	1.63 ms^{-1}
k_{cb}	2,000 ms^{-1}
k_{bc}	1,000 ms^{-1}

the graphs, it is hard to distinguish the wild type solution from the solution of the mutant case where the closed state blocker is applied.

3.6 CO-Mutations Does Not Change the Mean Open Time

To understand why the closed state blocker is much better than the open state blocker for CO-mutations, it is useful to recall that the mean open time of the Markov model

$$C \underset{\mu k_{co}}{\overset{k_{oc}}{\leftrightarrows}} O \tag{3.35}$$

is given by

$$\tau_o = \frac{1}{k_{oc}}.$$

Thus the mean open time is independent of the mutation. If a closed state blocker is introduced as

$$B \underset{k_{bc}}{\overset{k_{cb}}{\leftrightarrows}} C \underset{\mu k_{co}}{\overset{k_{oc}}{\leftrightarrows}} O, \tag{3.36}$$

we clearly see that the mean open time is still given by

$$\tau_o = \frac{1}{k_{oc}}.$$

On the other hand, for an open state blocker of the form

$$C \underset{\mu k_{co}}{\overset{k_{oc}}{\leftrightarrows}} O \underset{k_{ob}}{\overset{k_{bo}}{\leftrightarrows}} B, \tag{3.37}$$

the mean open time is changed and reads

$$\tau_o = \frac{1}{k_{oc} + k_{ob}}.$$

With a closed state blocker used to repair a CO-mutation, the mean open time is kept constant, as it should, but it is changed using an open state blocker. Consequently, it is hard to see how to derive an efficient open state blocker for a CO-mutation.

3.7 Notes

1. In this chapter we focused on CO-mutations (see page 16) and, for such mutations, closed state blockers are best suited from a theoretical perspective. We will see later that OC-mutations are more easily repaired using open state blockers.
2. The argument of asymptotic optimality given on page 63 is not a rigorous proof. To prove it mathematically, we have to take the boundary layer into consideration. Our derivation assumes smooth solutions but that assumption does not hold at the boundary.
3. In this section, we used probability density formulations for systems with more than two states. The general case of many states is presented in Appendix C of Huertas and Smith [35].
4. The mean open time will be introduced and analyzed in Chap. 13. In the present chapter we just used very basic properties.
5. We mentioned above that we used the function *Fminsearch* in Matlab to solve a minimization problem; see page 66. The *Fminsearch* function uses the Melder-Nead [58] algorithm studied by Lagarias et al. [46]. The method is very powerful and will be used routinely in these notes.
6. It is an underlying assumption for Markov models that the states of the model correspond to the conformational states of the channel protein. This should not be interpreted literally; rather, it has proved to be a useful modeling technique. A thorough discussion on the modeling of ion channels using Markov models and the models relation to the states of the protein is provided by Rudy and Silva [75].

Chapter 4
Properties of Probability Density Functions

The physical processes we study in this text are modeled using models including stochastic terms. Direct numerical simulations based on such stochastic models give results that are hard to interpret and it is therefore common to run many simulations and compute the average, and we have also seen that we can derive models governing the probability density functions. These are powerful tools that provide insight in the processes. In this chapter we will see that it is useful to have specific numbers that characterize stochastic variables and associated probability density functions. We encountered the equilibrium probability of being in the open or closed state (see, e.g., page 57) and we introduced probability density functions (see, e.g., page 30). Here we shall derive some specific (and common) characteristics of the probability density functions and discuss how these characteristics can be used to gain an understanding of calcium release. We will also show how the characteristics relate to the concepts already introduced and we will discuss how the characteristics vary as functions of the mutation severity index. Finally, we will show how the statistical characterizations can be used to evaluate the properties of theoretical drugs.

4.1 Probability Density Functions

Let us briefly recall the models under consideration. We consider the model

$$\bar{x}'(t) = \bar{\gamma}(t)v_r(c_1 - \bar{x}) + v_d(c_0 - \bar{x}) \tag{4.1}$$

of the calcium concentration of the dyad (see Fig. 2.1). Recall that v_r denotes the speed of release from the sarcoplasmic reticulum (SR) to the dyad, v_d denotes the speed of diffusion from the dyad to the cytosol, c_0 is the concentration of calcium

A. Tveito, G.T. Lines, *Computing Characterizations of Drugs for Ion Channels and Receptors Using Markov Models*, Lecture Notes in Computational Science and Engineering 111, DOI 10.1007/978-3-319-30030-6_4

ions in the cytosol, and c_1 is the calcium concentration in the SR; both c_0 and c_1 are assumed to be constant. The stochastic function $\bar{\gamma} = \bar{\gamma}(t)$ can be either zero (closed state) or one (open state) and the state is governed by the Markov model

$$C \underset{k_{co}}{\overset{k_{oc}}{\leftrightarrows}} O, \tag{4.2}$$

where k_{oc} and k_{co} are the rates associated with the Markov model. As discussed above, the probability density functions of the states of the Markov model are governed by the following system of partial differential equations:

$$\frac{\partial \rho_o}{\partial t} + \frac{\partial}{\partial x}(a_o \rho_o) = k_{co}\rho_c - k_{oc}\rho_o, \tag{4.3}$$

$$\frac{\partial \rho_c}{\partial t} + \frac{\partial}{\partial x}(a_c \rho_c) = k_{oc}\rho_o - k_{co}\rho_c, \tag{4.4}$$

where, as above, ρ_o and ρ_c are the probability density functions of the open and closed states, respectively. Furthermore, we recall that

$$a_o = v_r(c_1 - x) + v_d(c_0 - x), \tag{4.5}$$

$$a_c = v_d(c_0 - x). \tag{4.6}$$

The system of partial differential equations given by (4.3) and (4.4) is solved on the computational domain given by $\Omega = [c_0, c_+]$, where

$$c_+ = \frac{v_r c_1 + v_d c_0}{v_r + v_d},$$

and the boundary conditions are set up to ensure that there is no leak of probability across the boundaries (see page 37).

4.2 Statistical Characteristics

For the probability density functions given by the system (4.3) and (4.4), we can introduce the common statistical concepts of probability, expectation, and standard deviation. The probabilities of being in the open and closed states are given by

$$\pi_o = \int_\Omega \rho_o dx \text{ and } \pi_c = \int_\Omega \rho_c dx, \tag{4.7}$$

respectively. It is worth noting that these values are time dependent but independent of space (concentration). Furthermore, the sum of these probabilities adds up to one,

$$\pi_o(t) + \pi_c(t) = 1,$$

for all time. The expected values of the concentration are given by

$$E_o = \frac{1}{\pi_o}\int_\Omega x\rho_o dx \text{ and } E_c = \frac{1}{\pi_c}\int_\Omega x\rho_c dx \tag{4.8}$$

under the condition that the channels are open and closed, respectively. Finally, the standard deviations σ_o and σ_c are given by

$$\sigma_o^2 = \frac{1}{\pi_o}\int_\Omega x^2\rho_o dx - E_o^2, \tag{4.9}$$

$$\sigma_c^2 = \frac{1}{\pi_c}\int_\Omega x^2\rho_c dx - E_c^2. \tag{4.10}$$

We will show below how changes in the Markov model affect these characteristics and how the characteristics are influenced by the theoretical drugs. Generally, we have to solve the system (4.3) and (4.4) and then compute the statistical properties. However, we will see that in the special case in which the rate functions defining the Markov model, k_{oc} and k_{co}, are constant; we can compute some of the characteristics analytically. We will therefore start by considering such a case.

4.3 Constant Rate Functions

We consider the system (4.3) and (4.4) in the special case that both k_{oc} and k_{co} are constants (independent of the concentration x). If we integrate (4.3) and (4.4) over the interval Ω, we obtain the system

$$\pi_o' = k_{co}\pi_c - k_{oc}\pi_o, \tag{4.11}$$

$$\pi_c' = k_{oc}\pi_o - k_{co}\pi_c, \tag{4.12}$$

where we use the boundary conditions that state that there is no flux of probability across the boundaries.

4.3.1 Equilibrium Probabilities

When this system reaches equilibrium, the probabilities satisfy

$$k_{co}\pi_c = k_{oc}\pi_o \tag{4.13}$$

and since $\pi_o + \pi_c = 1$, we find that

$$\pi_o = \frac{k_{co}}{k_{oc} + k_{co}}, \tag{4.14}$$

$$\pi_c = \frac{k_{oc}}{k_{oc} + k_{co}}, \tag{4.15}$$

which we recognize as the probabilities o and c, respectively, derived directly from the equilibrium of the Markov model on page 57. This relation explains the connection between these two ways of considering the probability of being in a given state of the Markov model, but it is important to note that this relation only holds when the rate functions are constant.

4.3.2 Dynamics of the Probabilities

In the special case with only two states of the Markov model and constant rate functions, we can analytically compute how the probabilities evolve in time. If we use the fact that $\pi_o(t) + \pi_c(t) = 1$ for all time, we find that the system (4.11) and (4.12) can be reduced to one equation written in the form

$$\pi_o' = (k_{co} + k_{oc}) \left(\frac{k_{co}}{k_{co} + k_{oc}} - \pi_o \right). \tag{4.16}$$

Suppose we know that the channel is closed at $t = 0$; then $\pi_o(0) = 0$ and we find the solution

$$\pi_o(t) = \frac{k_{co}}{k_{co} + k_{oc}} \left(1 - e^{-(k_{co}+k_{oc})t} \right). \tag{4.17}$$

We note that if the channel is closed at $t = 0$, the open probability reaches the equilibrium given by

$$\frac{k_{co}}{k_{co} + k_{oc}}$$

at an exponential rate in time and the exponent is given by $k_{co} + k_{oc}$ so that equilibrium is reached faster for higher rates.

4.3.3 Expected Concentrations

We still consider constant rate functions. In that case, we will show that the expected concentration in the case of open or closed channels can be obtained by solving a 2×2 linear system of ordinary differential equations. We start by considering the system defining the probability density functions,

$$\frac{\partial \rho_o}{\partial t} + \frac{\partial}{\partial x}(a_o\rho_o) = k_{co}\rho_c - k_{oc}\rho_o, \tag{4.18}$$

$$\frac{\partial \rho_c}{\partial t} + \frac{\partial}{\partial x}(a_c\rho_c) = k_{oc}\rho_o - k_{co}\rho_c. \tag{4.19}$$

Since

$$E_o\pi_o = \int_\Omega x\rho_o dx \text{ and } E_c\pi_c = \int_\Omega x\rho_c dx, \tag{4.20}$$

we find, using (4.18), that

$$(E_o\pi_o)_t = \int_\Omega x\frac{\partial \rho_o}{\partial t}dx \tag{4.21}$$

$$= -\int_\Omega x\frac{\partial}{\partial x}(a_o\rho_o)\,dx + k_{co}\int_\Omega x\rho_c dx - k_{oc}\int_\Omega x\rho_o dx \tag{4.22}$$

$$= -\int_\Omega x\frac{\partial}{\partial x}(a_o\rho_o)\,dx + k_{co}\pi_c E_c - k_{oc}\pi_o E_o. \tag{4.23}$$

Here the integral can be handled using integration by parts. The domain Ω is defined by the interval $[x_-, x_+] = [c_0, c_+]$ and we recall that $a_o\rho_o = a_c\rho_c = 0$ at $x = x_-$ and at $x = x_+$. Therefore, by using the definition of a_o given in (4.5), we obtain

$$-\int_{x_-}^{x_+} x\frac{\partial}{\partial x}(a_o\rho_o)\,dx = -\left[x\,(a_o\rho_o)\right]_{x_-}^{x_+} + \int_{x_-}^{x_+} a_o\rho_o dx \tag{4.24}$$

$$= (v_r c_1 + v_d c_0)\,\pi_o - (v_r + v_d)\,\pi_o E_o. \tag{4.25}$$

Consequently, we obtain

$$(E_o\pi_o)_t = (v_r c_1 + v_d c_0)\,\pi_o + k_{co}\pi_c E_c - (v_r + v_d + k_{oc})\,\pi_o E_o. \tag{4.26}$$

Similarly, we have

$$(E_c\pi_c)_t = \int_\Omega x\frac{\partial \rho_c}{\partial t}dx \tag{4.27}$$

$$= -\int_\Omega x\frac{\partial}{\partial x}(a_c\rho_c)\,dx + k_{oc}\int_\Omega x\rho_o dx - k_{co}\int_\Omega x\rho_c dx \tag{4.28}$$

$$= -\int_\Omega x\frac{\partial}{\partial x}(a_o\rho_o)\,dx + k_{oc}\pi_o E_o - k_{co}\pi_c E_c \tag{4.29}$$

and, by the definition (4.6) of a_c, we find that

$$-\int_{x_-}^{x_+}\frac{\partial}{\partial x}(a_c\rho_c)\,xdx = -\left[(a_c\rho_c)\,x\right]_{x_-}^{x_+} + \int_{x_-}^{x_+} a_c\rho_c dx \tag{4.30}$$

$$= v_d c_0 \pi_c - v_d \pi_c E_c. \tag{4.31}$$

We therefore obtain

$$(E_c\pi_c)_t = v_d c_0 \pi_c + k_{oc}\pi_o E_o - (v_d + k_{co})\,\pi_c E_c. \tag{4.32}$$

Since we have already found explicit formulas for π_o and π_c, we can define

$$e_o = E_o\pi_o \text{ and } e_c = E_c\pi_c \tag{4.33}$$

and solve the system

$$e_o' = (v_r c_1 + v_d c_0)\,\pi_o + k_{co}e_c - (v_r + v_d + k_{oc})\,e_o, \tag{4.34}$$

$$e_c' = v_d c_0 \pi_c + k_{oc}e_o - (v_d + k_{co})\,e_c. \tag{4.35}$$

When π_o, π_c, and e_o, e_c are computed, of course computing the expectations E_o and E_c is straightforward.

4.3.4 Numerical Experiments

In Figs. 4.1 and 4.2, we illustrate the properties derived above by presenting the results of numerical computations. The parameters used in the computations are given in Table 4.1. In Fig. 4.1, we show how the probability defined by (4.7) evolves as a function of time. The solid line is the exact solution given by the formula (4.17) and the crosses are based on the numerical solution of the system (4.3) and (4.4), where the probability defined by (4.7) is replaced by a Riemann sum based on the numerical solution. In Fig. 4.2, we show the evolution of the expected concentration for the open (solid) or closed (dashed) state, based on solving the system of

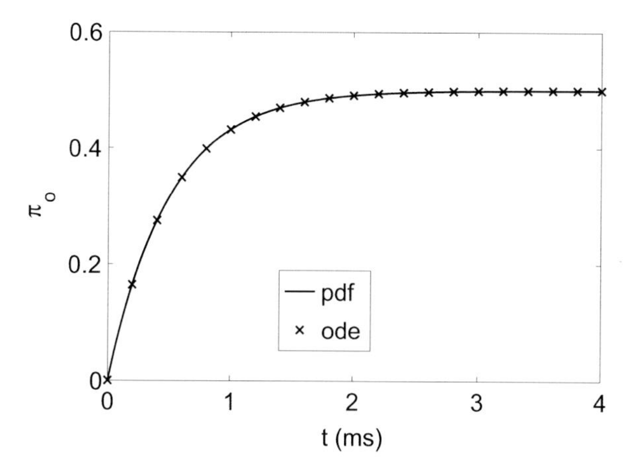

Fig. 4.1 Comparison of the theoretically derived open probability given by (4.17) with the numerical solution of the probability density functions defined by the system (4.3) and (4.4). In the latter case, the integrals (4.7) are replaced by Riemann sums

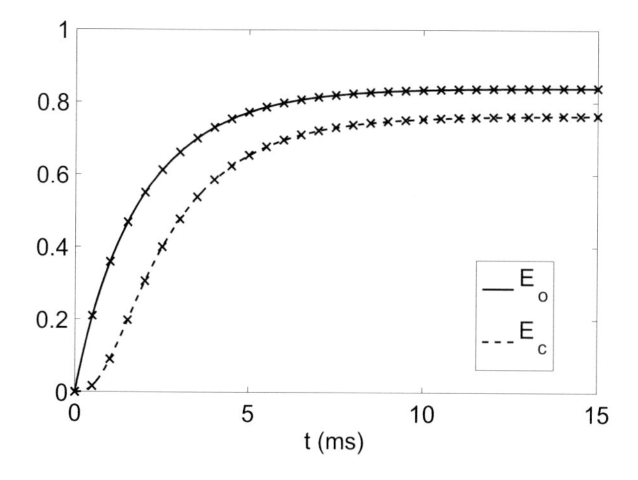

Fig. 4.2 Comparison of the theoretically derived expectations given by (4.33), where e_o and e_c are solutions of the system (4.34) and (4.35), with the numerical solution of the probability density functions defined by the system (4.3) and (4.4). In the latter case, the integrals (4.8) are replaced by Riemann sums

ordinary differential equations given by (4.34) and (4.35) and then computing the expectations from (4.33) and the solution of (4.16). The crosses are based on the numerical solution of the system (4.3) and (4.4) and the expected values of the concentration defined by (4.8) are again replaced by a Riemann sum based on the numerical solution.

Table 4.1 Parameter values for the model of (4.1) and (4.2)

v_d	$0.1\ \text{ms}^{-1}$
v_r	$1.0\ \text{ms}^{-1}$
c_0	0 mM
c_1	1 mM
k_{co}	$1\ \text{ms}^{-1}$
k_{oc}	$1\ \text{ms}^{-1}$

4.3.5 Expected Concentrations in Equilibrium

In the case of constant rates, we derived the following system describing the evolution of the expected concentrations for open or closed channels, respectively,

$$e_o' = (v_r c_1 + v_d c_0)\,\pi_o + k_{co} e_c - (v_r + v_d + k_{oc})\,e_o, \tag{4.36}$$

$$e_c' = v_d c_0 \pi_c + k_{oc} e_o - (v_d + k_{co})\,e_c, \tag{4.37}$$

where we recall that

$$e_o = E_o \pi_o \text{ and } e_c = E_c \pi_c. \tag{4.38}$$

The stationary solution of this system is given as the solution of the following linear 2×2 system of equations:

$$\begin{pmatrix} k_{oc} + v_r + v_d & -k_{co} \\ -k_{oc} & k_{co} + v_d \end{pmatrix} \begin{pmatrix} e_o \\ e_c \end{pmatrix} = \begin{pmatrix} (v_r c_1 + v_d c_0)\,\pi_o \\ v_d c_0 \pi_c \end{pmatrix}, \tag{4.39}$$

where π_o and π_c are equilibrium probabilities given by (4.14) and (4.15). The solution of this system in terms of a formula becomes messy, but if we consider the specific parameters used in the computations (see Table 4.1), we find that the equilibrium expectations are given by

$$E_o = 0.8397\ \text{mM}, \tag{4.40}$$

$$E_c = 0.7634\ \text{mM}, \tag{4.41}$$

which compares well with our observations in Fig. 4.2.

4.4 Markov Model of a Mutation

Mutations may change the release mechanism and thus seriously alter the function of the calcium-induced calcium release. Mutations in the RyR2 gene can lead to changes in the receptor function, increasing the open probability.

Table 4.2 Parameter values for the model (4.43) and (4.44)

v_d	$1\ \text{ms}^{-1}$
v_r	$0.1\ \text{ms}^{-1}$
c_0	$0.1\ \mu\text{M}$
c_1	$1{,}000\ \mu\text{M}$
k_{co}	$0.1\ \text{ms}^{-1}\mu\text{M}^{-1}$
k_{oc}	$1\ \text{ms}^{-1}$

As mentioned above, one way to model the increased open probability is to define

$$k_{co,\mu} = \mu k_{co}, \tag{4.42}$$

where μ is referred to as the mutation severity index. This is a CO-mutation (see page 16) and it does not affect the mean open time. The parameter $\mu = 1$ denotes the wild type case and larger values of μ indicate more severe mutations. Basically, since $k_{co,\mu} > k_{co}$ for $\mu > 1$, the mutation will lead to an increased probability of being in the open state.

The system governing the open and closed probability densities now takes the form

$$\frac{\partial \rho_o}{\partial t} + \frac{\partial}{\partial x}(a_o \rho_o) = \mu k_{co}\, x \rho_c - k_{oc} \rho_o, \tag{4.43}$$

$$\frac{\partial \rho_c}{\partial t} + \frac{\partial}{\partial x}(a_c \rho_c) = k_{oc} \rho_o - \mu k_{co}\, x \rho_c, \tag{4.44}$$

where, as above, we have

$$a_o = v_r(c_1 - x) + v_d(c_0 - x), \tag{4.45}$$

$$a_c = v_d(c_0 - x).$$

Note that in this model the opening rate depends on the concentration x. Model parameters are given in Table 4.2.

In Fig. 4.3, we show the results of Monte Carlo simulations (histograms) and solutions of the probability density system (4.43) and (4.44) (red solid line) for the wild type case ($\mu = 1$) and mutant case ($\mu = 3$). As above, we see that these two computational approaches give more or less the same answer. It is more interesting to observe the effect of the mutation. We see that the mutation tends to shift the open probability density function toward the upper boundary, where the function becomes very large. This shows that, in the case of mutation, it is very likely to have a high concentration *and* an open channel—much more likely than in the wild type case.

The statistical characteristics introduced above are given in Table 4.3. We note that the total open probability π_o increases from 0.811 for the wild type to 0.962 for the mutant. Also, we note that the expected concentration, E_o, for open channels is

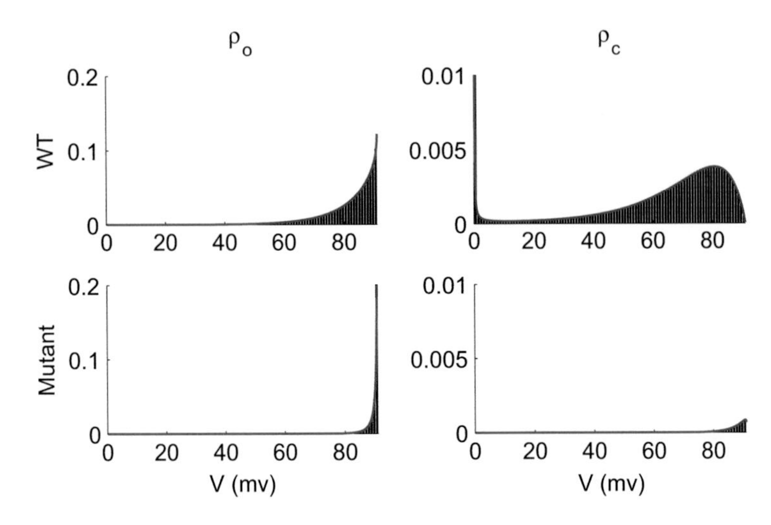

Fig. 4.3 *Upper panel*: Wild type open (*left*) and closed (*right*) probability density functions computed using Monte Carlo simulations (histogram) and by solving the probability density system (*red line*). The integral of the open probability density function is 0.811 (0.189 for the closed state probability density function). *Lower panel*: Similar figure as for the mutant case ($\mu = 3$). The integral of the open probability density function is 0.962 (0.038 for the closed state probability density function)

Table 4.3 Statistical properties of the wild type and mutant cases

Case	π_o	E_o	σ_o	π_c	E_c	σ_c
Wild type	0.811	81.91	9.50	0.189	43.04	35.26
Mutant	0.962	87.95	3.20	0.038	84.34	4.85

given by 81.91 μM for the wild type and 87.95 μM for the mutant. The standard deviation, on the other hand, is significantly reduced (by a factor of three) in the mutant case compared to the wild type. The probability of being in the closed state decreases by a factor of five in the mutant case compared to the wild type, whereas the expected concentration is doubled and the standard deviation is reduced by a factor of seven.

4.4.1 How Does the Mutation Severity Index Influence the Probability Density Function of the Open State?

We have seen a few examples indicating how changes in the reaction rates k_{co} and k_{oc} change the probability density functions. Since we are able to solve the stationary case analytically, this issue can be studied in great detail. Let us start by recalling that we model the effect of the mutation by introducing a severity index μ. The stationary model is then

$$\frac{\partial}{\partial x}(a_o \rho_o) = \mu k_{co} x \rho_c - k_{oc} \rho_o, \tag{4.46}$$

$$\frac{\partial}{\partial x}(a_c \rho_c) = k_{oc} \rho_o - \mu k_{co} x \rho_c, \tag{4.47}$$

where we recall that $\mu = 1$ is the wild type case. We discussed above how to solve the steady state model analytically (see Sect. 2.6, page 41) and we can use the analytical solution to investigate how the mutation affects the probability density functions. Since the steady state open probability density function is given by the solution of

$$\rho_o' = -\alpha(x) \rho_o$$

with

$$\alpha(x) = \frac{\mu k_{co} x}{v_d (c_0 - x)} - \frac{v_p - k_{oc}}{v_p (c_+ - x)},$$

where

$$v_p = v_r \frac{c_1 - c_0}{c_+ - c_0},$$

we have solutions of the form

$$\rho_{o,\mu}(x) = K_\mu e^{\frac{\mu k_{co} x}{v_d}} (c_+ - x)^{\frac{k_{oc}}{v_p} - 1} (x - c_0)^{\frac{c_0 \mu k_{co}}{v_d}}, \tag{4.48}$$

where K_μ is a constant given by the somewhat complicated expression

$$1/K_\mu = (c_+ - c_0)^{a+b} e^a \Gamma(a) \Gamma(b) ({}_1F_1(a, a+b, c) + k_{oc} \frac{v_p - v_d}{v_d v_p} {}_1F_1(a, a+b+1, c)).$$

Here ${}_1F_1$ is Kummer's regularized hypergeometric function and

$$a = c_0 \mu k_{co}/v_d, b = k_{oc}/v_p, c = (c_+ - c_0) \mu k_{co}/v_d.$$

It is useful to consider the ratio of the mutant solution to the wild type solution and we find that

$$\frac{\rho_{o,\mu}(x)}{\rho_{o,1}(x)} = \frac{K_\mu}{K_1} e^{\frac{(\mu-1) x k_{co}}{v_d}} (x - c_0)^{\frac{(\mu-1) c_0 k_{co}}{v_d}}.$$

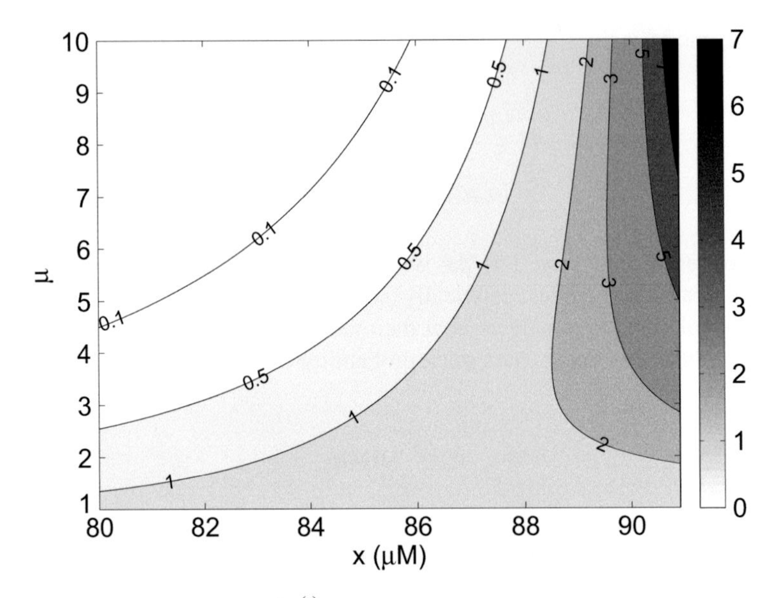

Fig. 4.4 Contours of the function $\frac{\rho_{o,\mu}(x)}{\rho_{o,1}(x)}$. Note that the open probability density function of the mutant is much greater than the open probability density function of the wild type for large values of the concentration and for large values of the mutation severity index μ

In Fig. 4.4, we graph this relation as a function of the severity index μ and the concentration x. We observe that, close to the maximum concentration, the open probability density function of the mutant is much larger than for the wild type.

4.4.2 Boundary Layers

As seen in both the numerical and analytical solutions above, the probability density functions may have singularities at the endpoints. It is easily seen from (4.48) that $\rho_{o,\mu}$ has a singularity at the endpoint $x = c_+$ whenever

$$\frac{k_{oc}}{v_p} < 1.$$

Similarly, we find that the closed probability density function is given by

$$\rho_{c,\mu}(x) = K_\mu \frac{v_p}{v_d} e^{\frac{\mu x k_{co}}{v_d}} (c_+ - x)^{\frac{k_{oc}}{v_p}} (x - c_0)^{\frac{\mu c_0 k_{co}}{v_d} - 1},$$

which has a singularity at $x = c_0$ whenever

$$\frac{\mu c_0 k_{co}}{v_d} < 1.$$

4.5 Statistical Properties as Functions of the Mutation Severity Index

We have seen, using numerical computations and analytical considerations, how the mutation severity index changes the probability density functions. In this section, we shall look with more detail into how the index changes the statistical properties of the probability density functions. Again, we consider a case where the rates k_{oc} and k_{co} are constants.

4.5.1 *Probabilities*

We recall that the open probability, defined as

$$\pi_o = \int_{\Omega} \rho_o dx, \tag{4.49}$$

evolves as

$$\pi_o(t) = \frac{k_{co}}{k_{co} + k_{oc}} \left(1 - e^{-(k_{co}+k_{oc})t}\right) \tag{4.50}$$

for wild type parameters in the case of $\pi_o(0) = 0$. If we introduce the mutation severity index in the Markov model (see (4.42)), we find that the open probability evolves as

$$\pi_{o,\mu}(t) = \frac{\mu k_{co}}{\mu k_{co} + k_{oc}} \left(1 - e^{-(\mu k_{co}+k_{oc})t}\right) \tag{4.51}$$

and thus the mutant case shows faster convergence toward a higher probability than the wild type case. In Fig. 4.5, we show the graphs of π_o and $\pi_{o,\mu}$ in the case of $\mu = 3$ and $\mu = 10$; the other parameters are given in Table 4.4.

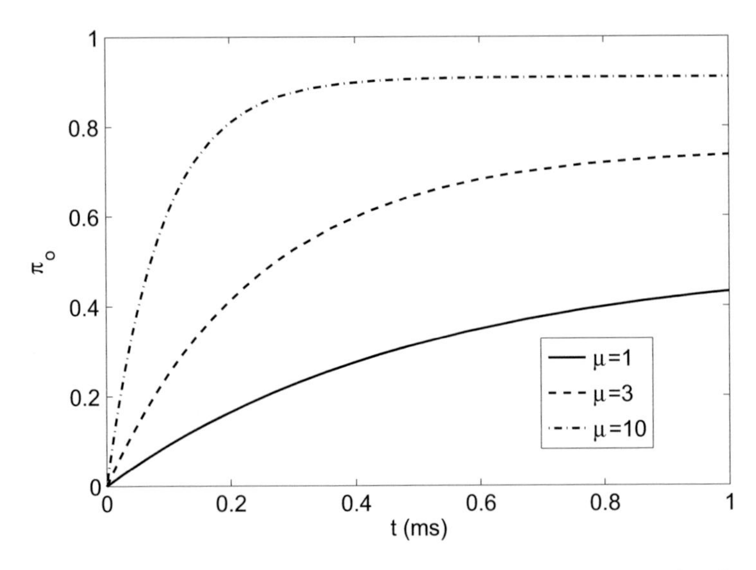

Fig. 4.5 The open probability π_o defined by (4.49) with $\mu = 1$ (wild type), $\mu = 3$, and $\mu = 10$. The mutation increases the equilibrium open probability and reduces the time to reach equilibrium

Table 4.4 Parameter values for the model (4.1) and (4.2) (copied from Table 4.1)

v_d	0.1 ms^{-1}
v_r	1.0 ms^{-1}
c_0	0 mM
c_1	1 mM
k_{co}	1 ms^{-1}
k_{oc}	1 ms^{-1}

4.5.2 Expected Calcium Concentrations

We defined the expected calcium concentrations in the case of open and closed channels as

$$E_o = \frac{1}{\pi_o} \int_\Omega x \rho_o dx \text{ and } E_c = \frac{1}{\pi_c} \int_\Omega x \rho_c dx. \tag{4.52}$$

Recall that π_o and π_c, are given by explicit formulas and that we introduced

$$e_o = E_o \pi_o \text{ and } e_c = E_c \pi_c. \tag{4.53}$$

For constant rates k_{oc} and k_{co}, the expectations can be found by solving the system of ordinary differential equations

$$e_o' = (v_r c_1 + v_d c_0)\,\pi_o + k_{co} e_c - (v_r + v_d + k_{oc})\, e_o, \tag{4.54}$$

$$e_c' = v_d c_0 \pi_c + k_{oc} e_o - (v_d + k_{co})\, e_c, \tag{4.55}$$

and then computing

$$E_o(t) = \frac{e_o(t)}{\pi_o(t)} \text{ and } E_c(t) = \frac{e_c(t)}{\pi_c(t)}.$$

In Fig. 4.6, we show the expected values of the calcium concentration for wild type data when the channel is open (solid, red) and closed (solid, blue), as well as mutant-type data ($\mu = 3$) when the channel is open (dotted, red) and closed (dotted, blue). In the computation using mutant data, we simply replace k_{co} with μk_{co}. However, keep in mind that this affects the formulas defining the probabilities π_o and π_c as well.

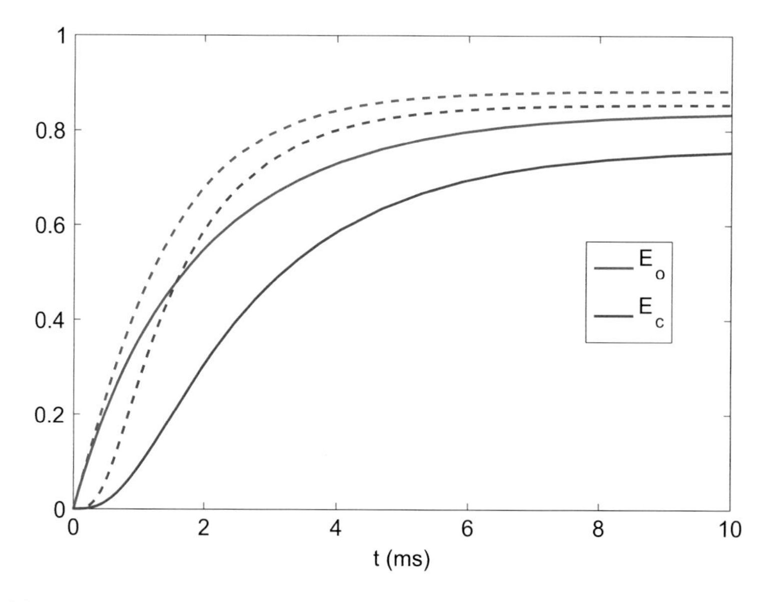

Fig. 4.6 Expected values of the concentration for wild type (*dotted lines*) and mutant (*solid lines*) cases as a function of time. In the mutant case, we used $\mu = 3$

4.5.3 Expected Calcium Concentrations in Equilibrium

As explained above, the equilibrium version of the expected concentrations E_o and E_c can be found by solving the following 2×2 linear system of equations:

$$\begin{pmatrix} k_{oc} + v_r + v_d & -\mu k_{co} \\ -k_{oc} & \mu k_{co} + v_d \end{pmatrix} \begin{pmatrix} e_o \\ e_c \end{pmatrix} = \begin{pmatrix} (v_r c_1 + v_d c_0)\,\pi_o \\ v_d c_0 \pi_c \end{pmatrix} \tag{4.56}$$

and then computing

$$E_o = \frac{e_o}{\pi_o} \text{ and } E_c = \frac{e_c}{\pi_c},$$

where π_o and π_c are equilibrium probabilities given by (4.14) and (4.15),

$$\pi_o = \frac{\mu k_{co}}{k_{oc} + \mu k_{co}}, \tag{4.57}$$

$$\pi_c = \frac{k_{oc}}{k_{oc} + \mu k_{co}}. \tag{4.58}$$

In Fig. 4.7, we plot the expectations as a function of the mutation severity index. The red line represents the expected value of the calcium concentration when the channel is open and the blue line represents the expected value of the calcium concentration

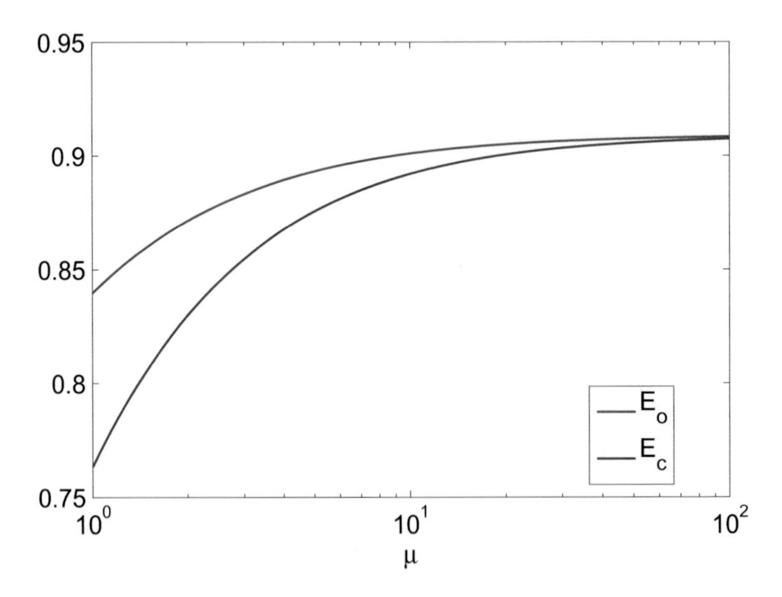

Fig. 4.7 Steady state of E_o and E_c as a function of the mutation severity index

when the channel is closed. Here, we use the parameters given in Table 4.4. The graphs start at $\mu = 1$, which represents the wild type case.

4.5.4 What Happens as $\mu \longrightarrow \infty$?

When the mutation severity index goes to infinity, we force the channel to be open more or less all the time. If we consider the stochastic model

$$\bar{x}'(t) = \bar{\gamma}(t)v_r(c_1 - \bar{x}) + v_d(c_0 - \bar{x})$$

as $\mu \longrightarrow \infty$, we know that the channel is generally open, so we have $\bar{\gamma}(t) \approx 1$. Therefore, we obtain the model

$$\bar{x}'(t) \approx v_r(c_1 - \bar{x}) + v_d(c_0 - \bar{x}).$$

As we have seen earlier, the equilibrium version of this equation is given by

$$x = c_+ = \frac{v_r c_1 + v_d c_0}{v_r + v_d} \approx 0.91 \text{ mM}$$

and this is what we see from the graphs of Fig. 4.7.

We can also see this from system (4.56). For the parameters given in Table 4.4, we have

$$\pi_o = \frac{\mu}{1+\mu} \text{ and } \pi_c = \frac{1}{1+\mu}$$

and therefore the system (4.56) takes the form

$$\begin{pmatrix} 2.1 & -\mu \\ -1 & \mu + 0.1 \end{pmatrix} \begin{pmatrix} e_o \\ e_c \end{pmatrix} = \begin{pmatrix} \frac{\mu}{1+\mu} \\ 0 \end{pmatrix}, \tag{4.59}$$

which, in terms of E_o and E_c, reads

$$\begin{pmatrix} 2.1 & -\mu \frac{\pi_c}{\pi_o} \\ -\pi_o & (\mu + 0.1)\pi_c \end{pmatrix} \begin{pmatrix} E_o \\ E_c \end{pmatrix} = \begin{pmatrix} 1 \\ 0 \end{pmatrix}. \tag{4.60}$$

If we let $\mu \longrightarrow \infty$, we obtain the system

$$\begin{pmatrix} 2.1 & -1 \\ -1 & 1 \end{pmatrix} \begin{pmatrix} E_o \\ E_c \end{pmatrix} = \begin{pmatrix} 1 \\ 0 \end{pmatrix} \tag{4.61}$$

and the solution

$$E_o = E_c \approx 0.91 \text{ mM}.$$

4.6 Statistical Properties of Open and Closed State Blockers

We have seen above that open and closed state theoretical blockers can significantly reduce the effect of the mutation. Computations have shown that closed state blockers repair the effect of the mutation as the parameter k_{bc} goes to infinity. This effect is also shown by a direct mathematical argument. For the open state blocker, we have seen that fairly good results can be obtained when the parameters of the drug are optimized, but perfect results can probably not be obtained for a CO-mutation because of the change of the mean open time described above. In this section, we present the statistical properties of the two types of drugs. The properties are presented in Table 4.5. In the table we observe that the total open probability (see Sect. 4.2, page 72) of the open state in the wild type case is 0.811. This increases to 0.962 for the mutant case ($\mu = 3$). When the closed state blocker is applied and the factor k_{bc} is increased, we see that the open probability is repaired by the drug. The same effect holds for the expected concentration E_o of the open state; it is completely repaired by the closed state blocker for large values of k_{bc}. This also holds for the standard deviation. For the open state blocker, we do not obtain a sufficient effect by increasing k_{bo}, but when both parameters of the drug are optimized, the open probability and the expected concentration of the open state are almost completely repaired. The open state blocker is, however, unable to repair the standard deviation.

Table 4.5 Statistical properties of the closed and open state blockers

Case	π_o	E_o	σ_o
Closed blocker, k_{bc}=10	0.739	82.47	10.59
Closed blocker, k_{bc}=100	0.805	81.97	9.66
Closed blocker, k_{bc}=1,000	0.811	81.91	9.52
Open blocker, k_{bo}=1	0.935	86.85	6.45
Open blocker, k_{bo}=10	0.936	85.97	4.89
Open blocker, k_{bo}=100	0.936	85.80	3.44
Optimized open blocker	0.817	80.09	13.10
Wild type, no drug	0.811	81.91	9.50
Mutant, no drug	0.962	87.95	3.20

4.7 Stochastic Simulations Using Optimal Drugs

We derived closed state and open state blockers with the parameters summarized in Table 3.2. In Fig. 4.8, we show the solutions of the stochastic model

$$\bar{x}'(t) = \bar{\gamma}(t)v_r(c_1 - \bar{x}) + v_d(c_0 - \bar{x}) \tag{4.62}$$

computed using the scheme

$$x_{n+1} = x_n + \Delta t\left(\gamma_n v_r(c_1 - x_n) + v_d(c_0 - x_n)\right), \tag{4.63}$$

where the dynamics of the stochastic function γ are given by the Markov model. The wild type solution is given in the upper-left part of the solution and we observe significantly larger variations than for the solution in the mutant case (upper right). The effect of the mutation is well repaired by both drugs. Note that since a random number is used in every time step, the solutions will never coincide, no matter how good the drug is. This illustrates the difficulty of comparing stochastic solutions and shows that comparison using probability density functions and derived statistics is much easier.

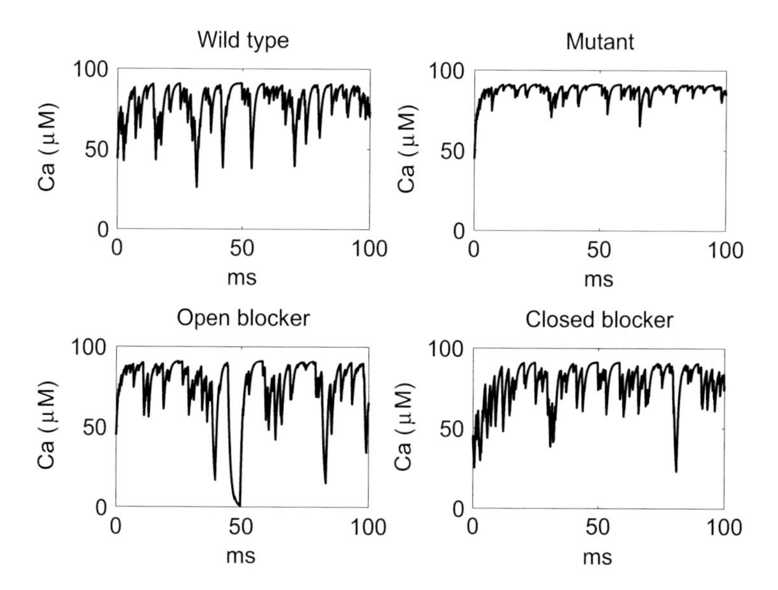

Fig. 4.8 Simulations based on the stochastic model (4.62) computed using scheme (4.63). In the mutant case, we use $\mu = 3$. The parameters specifying the drugs are given in Table 3.2

4.8 Notes

1. The mean open time will be introduced and analyzed in Chap. 13. In the present chapter, we have just used the very basic properties.
2. The statistical properties discussed in this chapter are taken from Williams et al. [103].

Chapter 5
Two-Dimensional Calcium Release

The essence of calcium-induced calcium release is once more illustrated in Fig. 5.1. This figure is very similar to Fig. 2.1 on page 24 except that the box surrounded by a thin red line is now slightly extended. This is meant to illustrate that the model is now extended to account for changes in the calcium concentration of the junctional sarcoplasmic reticulum (JSR) space (see Fig. 5.1); so we now consider a two-dimensional (2D) model where the concentration of the dyad ($\bar{x} = \bar{x}(t)$) and the JSR ($\bar{y} = \bar{y}(t)$) vary, recalling that the bar notation indicates stochastic variables. The concentration of the cytosol and the network sarcoplasmic reticulum (NSR) are still kept constant and we still ignore L-type calcium currents. An illustration of the mathematical model under consideration is given in Fig. 5.2.

The basic steps of the analysis of the 2D problem follow the steps of the analysis of the one-dimensional (1D) problem. We will start our analysis of the 2D problem by formulating a 2×2 system of stochastic differential equations giving the dynamics of the calcium concentration of the dyad and of the JSR. This model will be used as a basis for Monte Carlo simulations. By following the steps above, we also derive a 2D deterministic equation describing the probability density functions of the open and closed states. A numerical method for this system will be presented and, again, we will find that it is reasonable to focus on steady state computations. The probability density model will be extended to account for open or closed state blockers and, as above, we will see that we can find very good closed state blockers for CO-mutations (see page 16).

A. Tveito, G.T. Lines, *Computing Characterizations of Drugs for Ion Channels and Receptors Using Markov Models*, Lecture Notes in Computational Science and Engineering 111, DOI 10.1007/978-3-319-30030-6_5

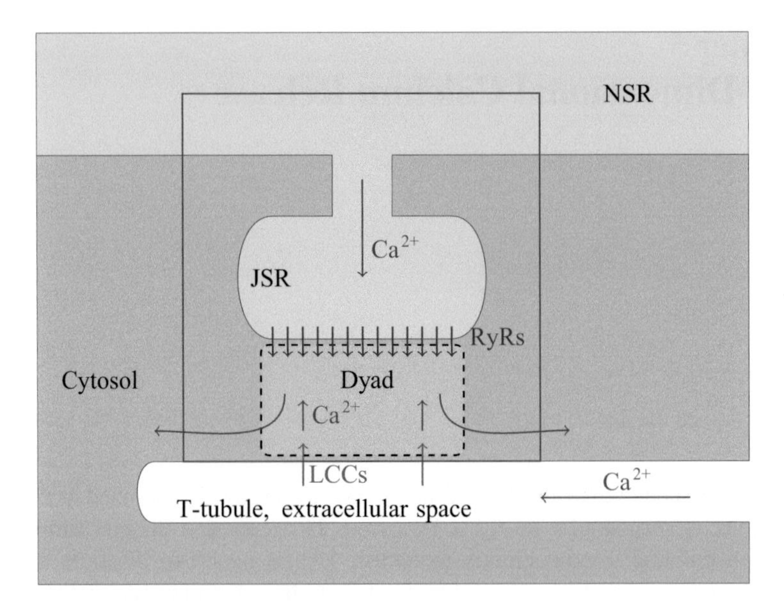

Fig. 5.1 As above, this figure illustrates the components involved in calcium-induced calcium release: the T-tubule, the dyad, the sarcoplasmic reticulum (SR) represented by the JSR and NSR and the cytosol. In this chapter, we concentrate on the dynamics in the box surrounded by a *thin red line*. We assume that the concentrations of the cytosol (c_0) and of the NSR (c_1) are constants and we ignore the LCCs. The variables of interest are the calcium concentrations of the dyad ($\bar{x} = \bar{x}(t)$) and the JSR ($\bar{y} = \bar{y}(t)$)

Cytosol, c_0	Dyad, $\bar{x}(t)$	JSR, $\bar{y}(t)$	NSR, c_1

Fig. 5.2 Sketch of a release unit. The cytosolic calcium concentration (c_0) and NSR calcium concentration (c_1) are assumed to be constant, while the concentrations of the dyad and JSR are given by $\bar{x} = \bar{x}(t)$ and $\bar{y} = \bar{y}(t)$, respectively. Note that $c_0 \ll c_1$

5.1 2D Calcium Release

The process of calcium release illustrated in Fig. 5.2 can be modeled as follows:

$$\bar{x}'(t) = \bar{\gamma}(t)v_r(\bar{y} - \bar{x}) + v_d(c_0 - \bar{x}), \tag{5.1}$$

$$\bar{y}'(t) = \bar{\gamma}(t)v_r(\bar{x} - \bar{y}) + v_s(c_1 - \bar{y}), \tag{5.2}$$

where v_r denotes the rate of release from the JSR to the dyad, v_d denotes the speed of calcium diffusion from the dyad to the cytosol, and v_s denotes the speed of calcium diffusion from the NSR to the JSR. Furthermore, $\bar{\gamma}(t)$ is a stochastic variable taking on two possible values, zero and one, with (as above) zero denoting a closed channel and one denoting an open channel. The dynamics of $\bar{\gamma}$ are governed by the Markov model under consideration. Furthermore, we always assume that

$$c_1 \gg c_0 \text{ and } v_r, v_d, v_s > 0. \tag{5.3}$$

For the 2D case, we also assume[1] that

$$v_d v_s \geq v_r^2. \tag{5.4}$$

5.1.1 *The 1D Case Revisited: Invariant Regions of Concentration*

Suppose the speed of diffusion, v_s, from the JSR to the NSR becomes very large. From (5.2), we observe that the limiting case when $v_s \to \infty$ yields $y = c_1$ and thus the problem is in 1D and can be written

$$\bar{x}'(t) = \bar{\gamma}(t)v_r\left(c_1 - \bar{x}\right) + v_d\left(c_0 - \bar{x}\right),$$

which is exactly the problem we discussed in Chap. 2 (page 25). We analyzed this equation and saw that, when the channel is closed ($\gamma = 0$), the solution tends toward the equilibrium point represented by

$$x = c_0$$

and, when the channel is open, the equilibrium solution is given by

$$x = c_+ = (1 - \alpha)\,c_1 + \alpha c_0,$$

where

$$\alpha = \frac{v_d}{v_r + v_d}.$$

Based on this, we concluded that if the initial concentration is in the interval $[c_0, c_+]$, the solution will always remain in this interval. The reason for this is that if the channel is closed, the solution will decrease toward c_0 and, if the channel is open, the solution will increase toward c_+. For closed channels, c_0 is a stable equilibrium and, similarly, if the channel is open, c_+ is a stable equilibrium.

[1]This is a technical assumption needed in an argument below.

5.1.2 *Stability of Linear Systems*

Before we consider the 2D case, we need to recall some basic properties of linear systems of ordinary differential equations. For a system of the form

$$x'(t) = Ax,$$

where A is a matrix and the unknown x is a vector, we know that the equilibrium solution $x = 0$ is stable, provided that the real part of all the eigenvalues of A is negative. However, the systems under consideration here are of the form

$$x'(t) = Ax + b, \tag{5.5}$$

where b is a known vector. In the case of a non-singular matrix A, the equilibrium solution is given by

$$x^* = -A^{-1}b \tag{5.6}$$

and we are interested in the stability of this solution. To assess the stability, we define

$$e = x - x^*$$

and observe that

$$e'(t) = x'(t) = Ax + b = Ax - Ax^* = Ae$$

and, of course, $e = 0$ is a stable equilibrium of the system

$$e' = Ae,$$

provided that the real part of all the eigenvalues of A are negative. Therefore, the equilibrium solution (5.6) of the system (5.5) is stable under the same condition. With these observations at hand, we are ready to try to understand the dynamics of the system (5.1) and (5.2).

5.1.3 *Convergence Toward Two Equilibrium Solutions*

Our aim is now to understand the dynamics of the 2D case and we start by considering the system when the channel is closed.

5.1.3.1 Equilibrium Solution for Closed Channels

In this case, the system (5.1) and (5.2) is quite simple, since there is no communication between the dyad and the JSR. The system is

$$x'(t) = v_d (c_0 - x), \tag{5.7}$$

$$y'(t) = v_s (c_1 - y), \tag{5.8}$$

and the stable equilibrium solution of this system is given by

$$x_c = c_0,$$

$$y_c = c_1.$$

5.1.3.2 Equilibrium Solution for Open Channels

The more interesting case is when the channel is open. Then the system reads

$$x'(t) = v_r (y - x) + v_d (c_0 - x), \tag{5.9}$$

$$y'(t) = v_r (x - y) + v_s (c_1 - y), \tag{5.10}$$

and the equilibrium solution is given by

$$x_o = \alpha c_1 + (1 - \alpha) c_0,$$

$$y_o = \beta c_1 + (1 - \beta) c_0,$$

where

$$\alpha = \frac{v_r v_s}{v_d (v_r + v_s) + v_r v_s},$$

$$\beta = \frac{v_s (v_d + v_r)}{v_d (v_r + v_s) + v_r v_s}.$$

It is useful, but not surprising, to note that

$$y_o - x_o = (\beta - \alpha)(c_1 - c_0) = \frac{v_s v_d}{v_d (v_r + v_s) + v_r v_s} (c_1 - c_0) > 0,$$

since c_1 is assumed to be larger than c_0 (see (5.3)).

5.1.3.3 Stability of the Equilibrium Solution

Whether the equilibrium solution for open channels is stable remains to be seen. As noted above, this can be determined by invoking the eigenvalues of the system matrix, which, in this case, are given by

$$A = \begin{pmatrix} -(v_r + v_d) & v_r \\ v_r & -(v_r + v_s) \end{pmatrix}.$$

Since the matrix is symmetric, the eigenvalues are real, so it is sufficient to see if they are always non-positive. The eigenvalues are given by

$$\lambda_- = \frac{1}{2}\left(-\sqrt{(v_d - v_s)^2 + 4v_r^2} - v_d - 2v_r - v_s\right),$$
$$\lambda_+ = \frac{1}{2}\left(\sqrt{(v_d - v_s)^2 + 4v_r^2} - v_d - 2v_r - v_s\right),$$

where obviously $\lambda_- < 0$ for any $v_r, v_d, v_s > 0$. Hence, $\lambda_+ < 0$ also remains to be shown. To this end, we start by assuming that $\lambda_+ > 0$; so we assume that

$$0 < \sqrt{u} - v,$$

with

$$u = (v_d - v_s)^2 + 4v_r^2$$

and

$$v = v_d + 2v_r + v_s.$$

We can safely multiply both sides of this inequality with something positive such as $\sqrt{u} + v$ and we therefore find that

$$\begin{aligned} 0 &< \left(\sqrt{u} - v\right)\left(\sqrt{u} + v\right) \\ &= u - v^2 \\ &= -4\left(v_d v_r + v_d v_s + v_r v_s\right) \end{aligned}$$

and, since $v_r, v_d, v_s > 0$, this is a contradiction and we conclude that $\lambda_+ < 0$ for all $v_r, v_d, v_s > 0$.

5.1.4 Properties of the Solution of the Stochastic Release Model

We have found that when the channel is closed, the equilibrium solution is given by

$$x_c = c_0,$$
$$y_c = c_1,$$

which is stable. Similarly, when the channel is open, the equilibrium solution is given by

$$x_o = \alpha c_1 + (1-\alpha)\, c_0, \text{ with } \alpha = \frac{v_r v_s}{v_d\,(v_r + v_s) + v_r v_s},$$
$$y_o = \beta c_1 + (1-\beta)\, c_0, \text{ with } \beta = \frac{v_s\,(v_d + v_r)}{v_d\,(v_r + v_s) + v_r v_s},$$

and this solution is also stable. The solution of the model given by the system (5.1) and (5.2) will therefore tend toward (x_c, y_c) whenever the channel is closed and toward (x_o, y_o) whenever the channel is open. This will be illustrated in numerical simulations below.

5.1.5 Numerical Scheme for the 2D Release Model

To perform 2D stochastic simulations, we use the numerical scheme

$$x_{n+1} = x_n + \Delta t\,(\gamma_n v_r\,(y_n - x_n) + v_d\,(c_0 - x_n)), \tag{5.11}$$
$$y_{n+1} = y_n + \Delta t\,(\gamma_n v_r\,(x_n - y_n) + v_s\,(c_1 - y_n)), \tag{5.12}$$

where γ is computed according to the Markov model given by the reaction scheme

$$C \underset{k_{co}}{\overset{k_{oc}}{\leftrightarrows}} O \tag{5.13}$$

(see page 28), where k_{oc} and k_{co} are reaction rates that may depend on both the concentrations represented by $x = x(t)$ and $y = y(t)$.

Table 5.1 Values of parameters used in 2D simulations based on the scheme (5.11) and (5.12)

v_d	1 ms^{-1}
v_r	0.1 ms^{-1}
v_s	0.01 ms^{-1}
c_0	0.1 μM
c_1	1,000 μM
k_{co}	1 ms^{-1}
k_{oc}	1 ms^{-1}

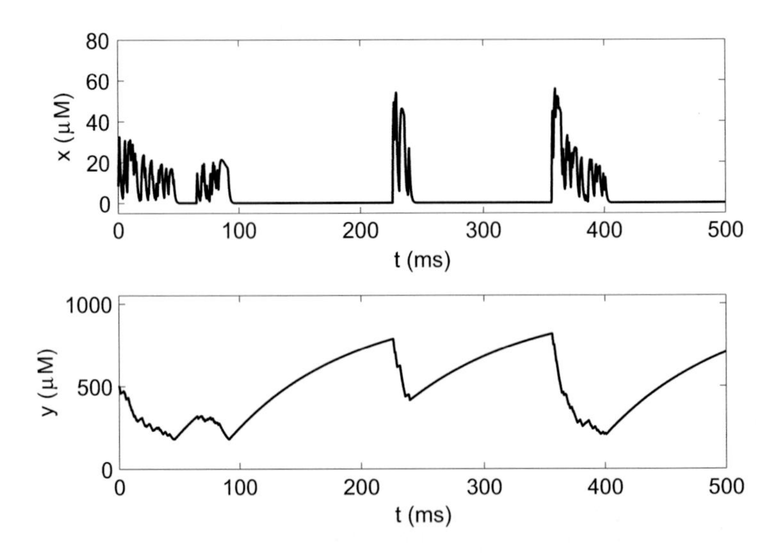

Fig. 5.3 Results of simulation using the scheme (5.11) and (5.12) with the data given in Table 5.1

5.1.5.1 Simulations Using the 2D Stochastic Model

We use the numerical scheme given by (5.11) and (5.12), where the parameters and functions involved are described in Table 5.1. The numerical solutions are given in Figs. 5.3 and 5.4. In the latter figure, we also indicate when the channel is open and closed (upper panel).

5.1.6 Invariant Region for the 2D Case

We observed in the 1D case that an invariant region for the numerical scheme used to compute approximate solutions of the stochastic model was useful for the probability density system, since it defined the interval in which to solve the system. Similarly, we will derive an invariant region for numerical solutions generated by the scheme (5.11) and (5.12) and this invariant region will define the geometry we will use to solve the probability density system.

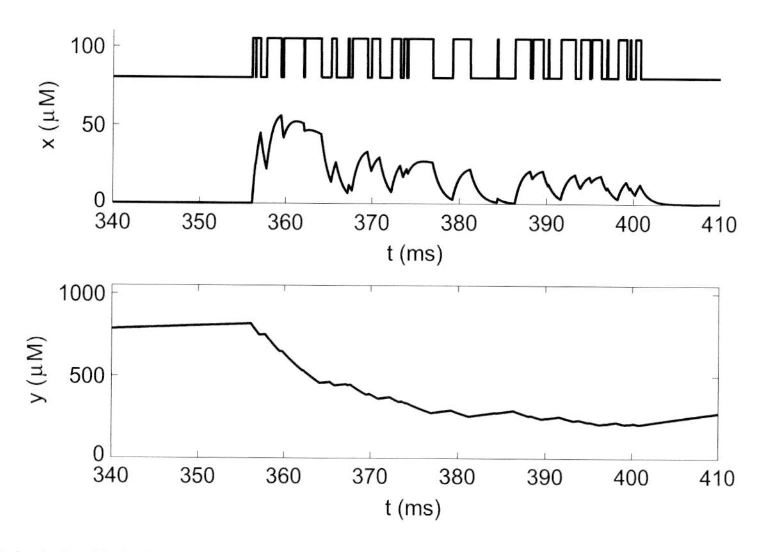

Fig. 5.4 A detailed view of the results given in Fig. 5.3. The open/closed state of the channel is indicated in the *upper panel*

Let us start by recalling the assumptions (5.3) and (5.4) and let us also assume that the time step $\Delta t > 0$ is chosen such that

$$\Delta t < \min\left(\frac{1}{v_r + v_d}, \frac{1}{v_r + v_s}\right). \tag{5.14}$$

Define

$$x_- = c_0, \tag{5.15}$$

$$x_+ = \frac{v_r c_1 + v_d c_0}{v_r + v_d}, \tag{5.16}$$

$$y_- = \frac{c_0 v_r + c_1 v_s}{v_r + v_s}, \tag{5.17}$$

$$y_+ = c_1, \tag{5.18}$$

and observe that

$$y_- - x_+ = \frac{c_0 v_r + c_1 v_s}{v_r + v_s} - \frac{v_r c_1 + v_d c_0}{v_r + v_d} = (c_1 - c_0)\frac{v_d v_s - v_r^2}{(v_r + v_s)(v_r + v_d)}.$$

It now follows from the assumptions (5.3) and (5.4) that we have

$$y_- \geqslant x_+. \tag{5.19}$$

Our aim is now to show that $\Omega = (x_-, x_+) \times (y_-, y_+)$ is an invariant region for solutions of the scheme (5.11) and (5.12). Because of (5.19), this means, in particular, that under the assumptions (5.3) and (5.4) the lowest possible calcium concentration of the JSR will always be larger than (or equal to) the highest calcium concentration of the dyad.

The numerical scheme (5.11, 5.12) can be written in the form

$$x_{n+1} = F(x_n, y_n, \gamma_n),$$
$$y_{n+1} = G(x_n, y_n, \gamma_n),$$

where

$$F(x, y, \gamma) = x + \Delta t \left(\gamma v_r \left(y - x\right) + v_d \left(c_0 - x\right)\right),$$
$$G(x, y, \gamma) = y + \Delta t \left(\gamma v_r \left(x - y\right) + v_s \left(c_1 - y\right)\right).$$

We will consider the properties of the functions F and G for x and y in the domain

$$\Omega = \{(x, y) : x_- \leq x \leq x_+,\ y_- \leq y \leq y_+\} \tag{5.20}$$

and for $0 \leq \gamma \leq 1$. Note that

$$\frac{\partial F(x, y, \gamma)}{\partial x} = 1 - \Delta t \left(\gamma v_r + v_d\right) \geq 1 - \Delta t \left(v_r + v_d\right) > 0$$

by condition (5.14). In addition, we have

$$\frac{\partial F(x, y, \gamma)}{\partial y} = \Delta t \gamma v_r \geq 0$$

and

$$\frac{\partial F(x, y, \gamma)}{\partial \gamma} = \Delta t v_r \left(y - x\right) \geq 0,$$

where we use (5.19) and (5.20). Similarly, we have

$$\frac{\partial G(x, y, \gamma)}{\partial y} = 1 - \Delta t \left(\gamma v_r + v_s\right) \geq 1 - \Delta t \left(v_r + v_s\right) > 0,$$

which is also positive by condition (5.14). Finally, we have

$$\frac{\partial G(x, y, \gamma)}{\partial x} = \Delta t \gamma v_r \geq 0$$

and

$$\frac{\partial G(x, y, \gamma)}{\partial \gamma} = \Delta t v_r (x - y) \leq 0$$

by (5.19) and (5.20). We now assume that

$$(x_n, y_n) \in \Omega.$$

Then,

$$x_{n+1} = F(x_n, y_n, \gamma_n) \geq F(x_-, y_-, 0) = x_-$$

and

$$x_{n+1} = F(x_n, y_n, \gamma_n) \leq F(x_+, y_+, 1) = x_+.$$

So we conclude that

$$x_- \leq x_{n+1} \leq x_+.$$

Similarly,

$$y_{n+1} = G(x_n, y_n, \gamma_n) \geq G(x_-, y_-, 1) = y_-$$

and

$$y_{n+1} = G(x_n, y_n, \gamma_n) \leq G(x_+, y_+, 0) = y_+;$$

so we conclude that

$$y_- \leq y_{n+1} \leq y_+.$$

We have seen that under the assumptions (5.3), (5.4), and (5.14), it follows that, if

$$(x_n, y_n) \in \Omega,$$

then also

$$(x_{n+1}, y_{n+1}) \in \Omega$$

and we therefore conclude that Ω is an invariant region for the scheme of (5.11) and (5.12). This means that the probability density system will be solved in the domain defined by Ω.

5.2 Probability Density Functions in 2D

In the 1D case considered above, we derived a model for the probability density functions. In the 2D case, we can follow exactly the same steps and arrive at a system of partial differential equations of the form

$$\frac{\partial \rho_o}{\partial t} + \frac{\partial}{\partial x}\left(a_o^x \rho_o\right) + \frac{\partial}{\partial y}\left(a_o^y \rho_o\right) = k_{co}\rho_c - k_{oc}\rho_o, \tag{5.21}$$

$$\frac{\partial \rho_c}{\partial t} + \frac{\partial}{\partial x}\left(a_c^x \rho_c\right) + \frac{\partial}{\partial y}\left(a_c^y \rho_c\right) = k_{oc}\rho_o - k_{co}\rho_c, \tag{5.22}$$

where

$$\begin{aligned} a_o^x &= v_r\,(y-x) + v_d\,(c_0 - x)\,, \\ a_o^y &= v_r\,(x-y) + v_s\,(c_1 - y)\,, \\ a_c^x &= v_d\,(c_0 - x)\,, \\ a_c^y &= v_s\,(c_1 - y)\,. \end{aligned} \tag{5.23}$$

As in 1D, ρ_o and ρ_c denote the open and closed probability density functions, respectively, satisfying the integral condition

$$\int_\Omega (\rho_o + \rho_c)\,dx\,dy = 1. \tag{5.24}$$

Here the domain can be taken to be

$$\Omega = \{(x,y) : x_- \leqslant x \leqslant x_+,\ y_- \leqslant y \leqslant y_+\} \tag{5.25}$$

and the boundary conditions are again defined to ensure that there is no flux of probability out of the domain (see page 37).

5.2.1 *Numerical Method for Computing the Probability Density Functions in 2D*

To solve the system (5.21) and (5.22), we need to define a numerical method. For the 1D model (see page 37), we used an upwind scheme as presented by LeVeque [48]. Here, we use the 2D version of the same numerical method. Consider the partial differential equation

$$\rho_t + (a\rho)_x + (b\rho)_y = g\rho$$

Table 5.2 Discretization parameters

Δt	0.001 ms
Δx	0.92 μM
Δy	9.3 μM

where a, b, and g are smooth functions of x and y. We let $\rho_{i,j}^n$ denote an approximation of ρ at time $t = n\Delta t$ for $(x, y) \in [x_{i-1/2}, x_{i+1/2}) \times [y_{j-1/2}, y_{j+1/2})$, where $x_i = x_- + i\Delta x$, $y_j = y_+ + j\Delta y$, and

$$\Delta x = \frac{x_+ - x_-}{M_x}, \quad \Delta y = \frac{y_+ - y_-}{M_y}.$$

Here M_x and M_y denote the number of grid points along the x and y axes, respectively. The numerical approximation is defined by the scheme

$$\rho_{i,j}^{n+1} = \rho_{i,j}^n - \frac{\Delta t}{\Delta x}\left((a\rho)_{i+1/2,j}^n - (a\rho)_{i-1/2,j}^n\right) \\ - \frac{\Delta t}{\Delta y}\left((b\rho)_{i,j+1/2}^n - (b\rho)_{i,j-1/2}^n\right) + \Delta t g_{i,j}\rho_{i,j}^n, \tag{5.26}$$

where

$$(a\rho)_{i+1/2,j}^n = \max(a_{i+1/2,j}, 0)\rho_{i,j}^n + \min(a_{i+1/2,j}, 0)\rho_{i+1,j}^n, \tag{5.27}$$

$$(b\rho)_{i,j+1/2}^n = \max(b_{i,j+1/2}, 0)\rho_{i,j}^n + \min(b_{i,j+1/2}, 0)\rho_{i,j+1}^n. \tag{5.28}$$

In our simulations, this scheme is used for both equations (5.21) and (5.22) above, where the right-hand sides are given by $k_{co}\rho_c - k_{oc}\rho_o$ and $k_{oc}\rho_o - k_{co}\rho_c$, respectively.

As pointed out above, the probability densities integrates to one (see (5.24)), and the discrete version of this condition reads,

$$\Delta x \Delta y \sum_{i,j} \rho_{i,j} = 1, \tag{5.29}$$

where $\rho = \rho_o + \rho_c$. Note that the initial conditions must be chosen such that this condition holds. The discretization parameters used throughout this chapter are given in Table 5.2.

5.2.2 *Rapid Decay to Steady State Solutions in 2D*

We observed in 1D that the time-dependent probability density functions converge rapidly toward steady state solutions. This is illustrated in Fig. 2.7 on page 39. In Fig. 5.5, we show snapshots of the open probability density function at times 1, 2,

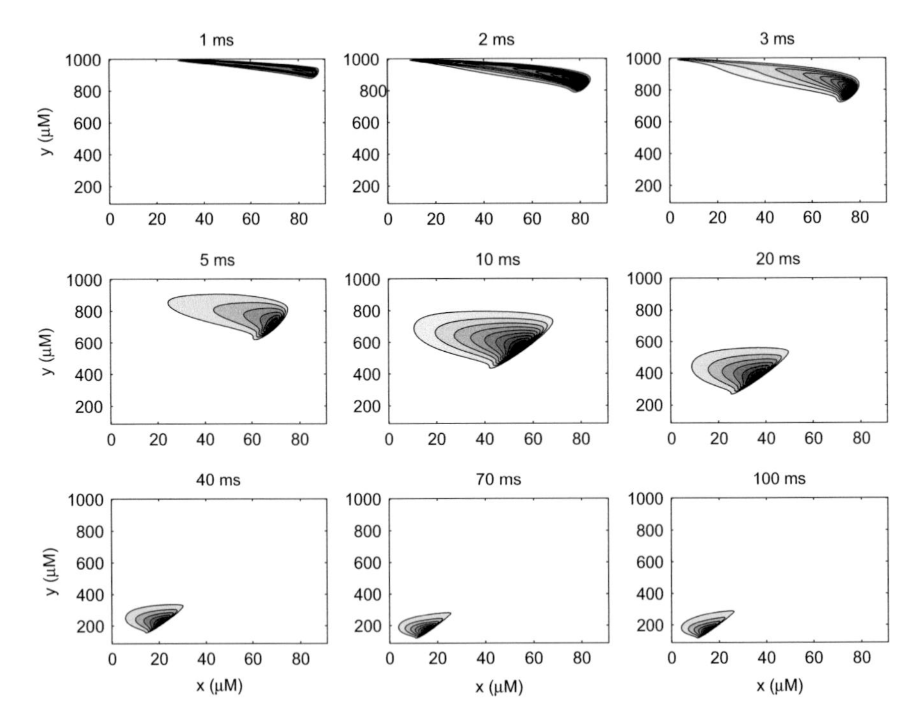

Fig. 5.5 Open probability density function ρ_o as a function of the dyad (x) and the JSR concentrations (y) for times $t = 1, 2, 3, 5, 10, 20, 40, 70$, and 100 ms. Note the convergence toward an equilibrium solution. In the computations, we use $\Delta t = 0.001$ ms, $\Delta x = 0.92$ μM, and $\Delta y = 9.3$ μM

3, 5, 10, 20, 40, 70, and 100 ms and we observe that the solution converges toward an equilibrium solution with time. This is verified in Fig. 5.6, where we plot the (weighted) norm between the dynamic and stationary solutions for time t ranging from 0 to 150 ms and we see that the solution is quite close to equilibrium at $t = 100$ ms. This observation is useful because it implies that when we assess the effect of various theoretical drugs, it is sufficient to consider steady state solutions.

5.2.3 Comparison of Monte Carlo Simulations and Probability Density Functions in 2D

As in 1D, we want to compare the probability densities ρ_o and ρ_c computed by solving the probability density system (5.21) and (5.22) using the scheme (5.26) with Monte Carlo simulations based on the stochastic differential equations (5.1) and (5.2) solved by the numerical scheme (5.11) and (5.12). The comparison is undertaken in the same manner as in 1D. We simply run a number of Monte Carlo

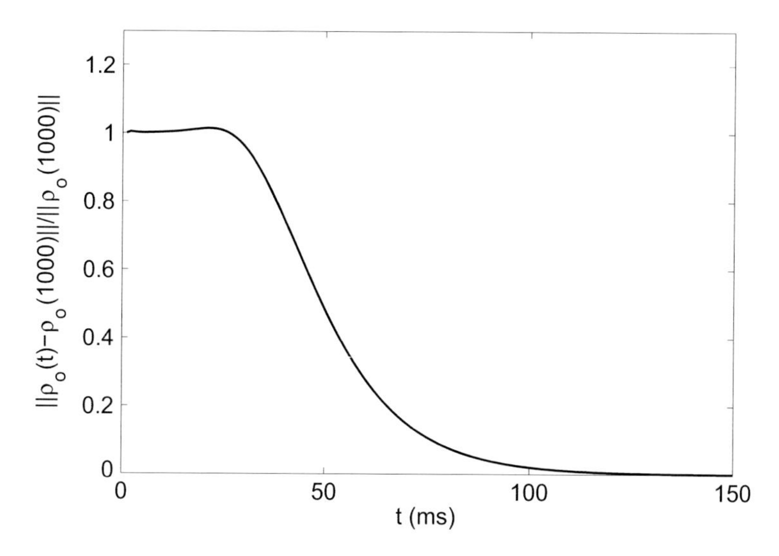

Fig. 5.6 The weighted norm of the difference between the open probability density function ρ_o at time t and at time 1,000 ms. This figure shows convergence toward an equilibrium solution

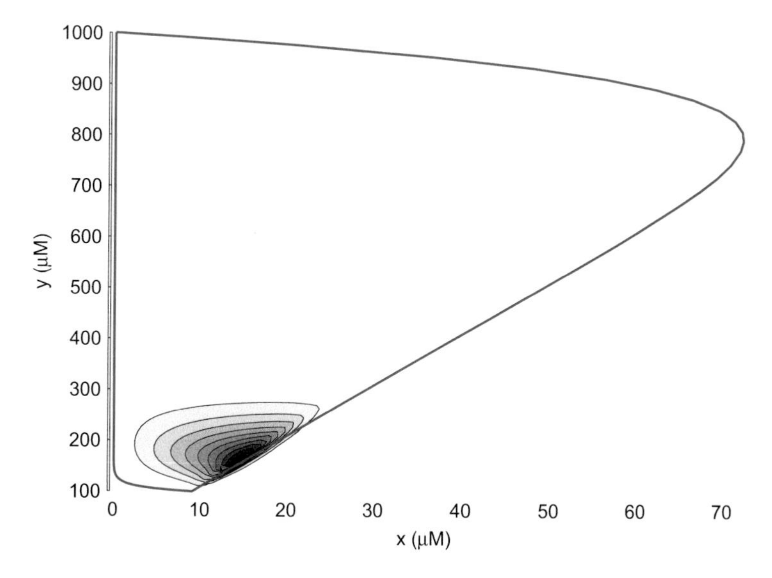

Fig. 5.7 Steady state open probability density function ρ_o computed by solving the probability density system (5.21) and (5.22). The solution is bounded (*red curve*) by solutions of the system (5.7) and (5.8) and the system (5.9) and (5.10)

simulations for a long time and count the number of open states in small rectangles. The procedure is a direct generalization of the method used in 1D (see page 40).

The numerical solution of the probability density system is given in Fig. 5.7 and the associated solution based on Monte Carlo simulations is given in Fig. 5.8. As in

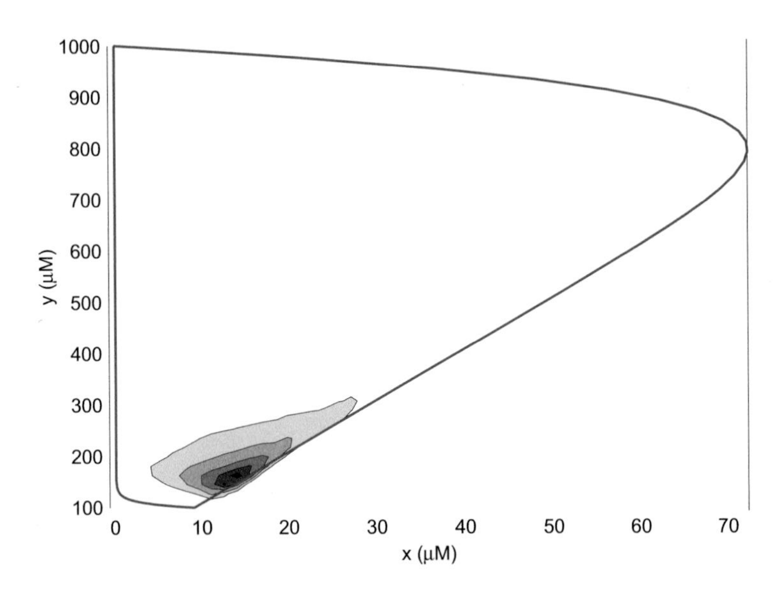

Fig. 5.8 Open probability density function ρ_o computed by Monte Carlo simulations using the scheme (5.11) and (5.12). The solution is bounded (*red curve*) by solutions of the system (5.7) and (5.8) and the system (5.9) and (5.10)

1D, we observe that the solutions are quite similar. In both these figures, we observe that the solutions stay inside a region bounded by a red curve. The red curve is computed by solving (5.7) and (5.8) for the closed state and (5.9) and (5.10) for the open state.

5.2.4 *Increasing the Open to Closed Reaction Rate in 2D*

In 1D, we observed that if we increased the reaction rate k_{oc} from open to closed, the steady state probability density functions changed considerably (see page 46). We observed that the open probability decreased and the closed probability increased significantly. In Fig. 5.9, we study the same effect in 2D and again we observe that the open probability density function is considerably decreased when k_{oc} is increased from one to three. The statistics of the solutions are given in Table 5.3 and we note that the total open probability is reduced considerably when k_{oc} is increased from one to three. The expected dyad concentration (x) does not change very much, but the expected JSR concentration (y) increases significantly and this observation holds for both open and closed channels.

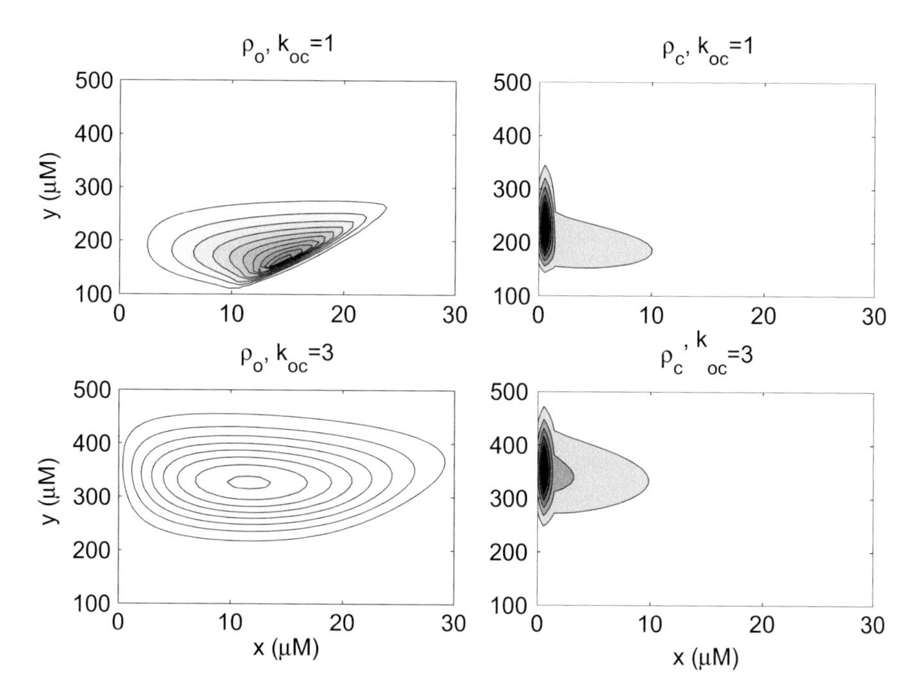

Fig. 5.9 The effect of increasing k_{oc} from one to three. The open probability density function is reduced considerably

Table 5.3 Statistical properties of the probability density functions for $k_{oc} = 1\ \text{ms}^{-1}$ and $k_{oc} = 3\ \text{ms}^{-1}$

k_{oc}	π_o	E_{x_o}	E_{y_o}	σ_{x_o}	σ_{y_o}
1	0.430	12.63	202.4	4.948	46.27
3	0.221	13.23	339.2	6.723	56.88
k_{oc}	π_c	E_{x_c}	E_{y_c}	σ_{x_c}	σ_{y_c}
1	0.570	5.12	218.2	4.842	49.90
3	0.779	5.95	348.0	5.563	57.22

5.3 Notes

1. The 2D stochastic model and the associated probability density functions are taken from Huertas and Smith [35], but some of the parameters are changed.

Chapter 6
Computing Theoretical Drugs in the Two-Dimensional Case

Let us briefly recall the difficulty we want to overcome with the theoretical drug. The difficulty is that in the prototypical reaction defined by the Markov model

$$C \underset{k_{co}}{\overset{k_{oc}}{\leftrightarrows}} O$$

the rates may change under various mutations. One case that we have focused on in these notes is CO-mutations where the reaction rate from C to O is increased. The reaction of a CO-mutation takes the form

$$C \underset{\mu k_{co}}{\overset{k_{oc}}{\leftrightarrows}} O,$$

where we assume that $\mu \geqslant 1$ is a constant. We refer to this constant as the mutation severity index and the mutation is typically worse the larger the value of μ; furthermore, $\mu = 1$ refers to the wild type case. Our aim is to devise a theoretical drug of the form

$$B_c \underset{k_{bc}}{\overset{k_{cb}}{\leftrightarrows}} C \underset{\mu k_{co}}{\overset{k_{oc}}{\leftrightarrows}} O \underset{k_{ob}}{\overset{k_{bo}}{\leftrightarrows}} B_o,$$

where the constants k_{bc}, k_{cb}, k_{bo}, and k_{ob} are used to tune the drug such that the effect of the mutation is reduced as much as possible. As above, we will consider blockers associated with the closed state, which means that $k_{ob} = 0$, or blockers associated with the open state, which means that $k_{cb} = 0$. The model and discretization parameters used throughout this chapter are given in Table 6.1.

A. Tveito, G.T. Lines, *Computing Characterizations of Drugs for Ion Channels and Receptors Using Markov Models*, Lecture Notes in Computational Science and Engineering 111, DOI 10.1007/978-3-319-30030-6_6

Table 6.1 Parameters reused from the previous chapter (i.e., Table 5.1)

v_d	1 ms^{-1}
v_r	0.1 ms^{-1}
v_s	0.01 ms^{-1}
c_0	0.1 μM
c_1	1,000 μM
k_{co}	1 ms^{-1}
k_{oc}	1 ms^{-1}
Δt	0.001 ms
Δx	0.92 μM
Δy	9.3 μM

6.1 Effect of the Mutation in the Two-Dimensional Case

When the effect of the mutation is taken into account, the probability density functions are governed by the system

$$\frac{\partial \rho_o}{\partial t} + \frac{\partial}{\partial x}\left(a_o^x \rho_o\right) + \frac{\partial}{\partial y}\left(a_o^y \rho_o\right) = \mu k_{co}\rho_c - k_{oc}\rho_o, \tag{6.1}$$

$$\frac{\partial \rho_c}{\partial t} + \frac{\partial}{\partial x}\left(a_c^x \rho_c\right) + \frac{\partial}{\partial y}\left(a_c^y \rho_c\right) = k_{oc}\rho_o - \mu k_{co}\rho_c, \tag{6.2}$$

where we recall that the fluxes are given by

$$\begin{aligned} a_o^x &= v_r\,(y-x) + v_d\,(c_0 - x)\,, \\ a_o^y &= v_r\,(x-y) + v_s\,(c_1 - y)\,, \\ a_c^x &= v_d\,(c_0 - x)\,, \\ a_c^y &= v_s\,(c_1 - y) \end{aligned} \tag{6.3}$$

(see page 102). In Fig. 6.1, we compare the solution of this system when $\mu = 1$ (wild type) and $\mu = 3$ (mutant) and in Table 6.2 we give the statistics of the solutions. The total open probability increases from 0.430 for the wild type to 0.743 for the mutant. In addition, the expected concentrations of both the dyad and the junctional sarcoplasmic reticulum (JSR) decrease considerably. In the one-dimensional (1D) case we observed that the variability of the solution decreased when the mutation was introduced. This observation seems to carry over to the two-dimensional (2D) case.

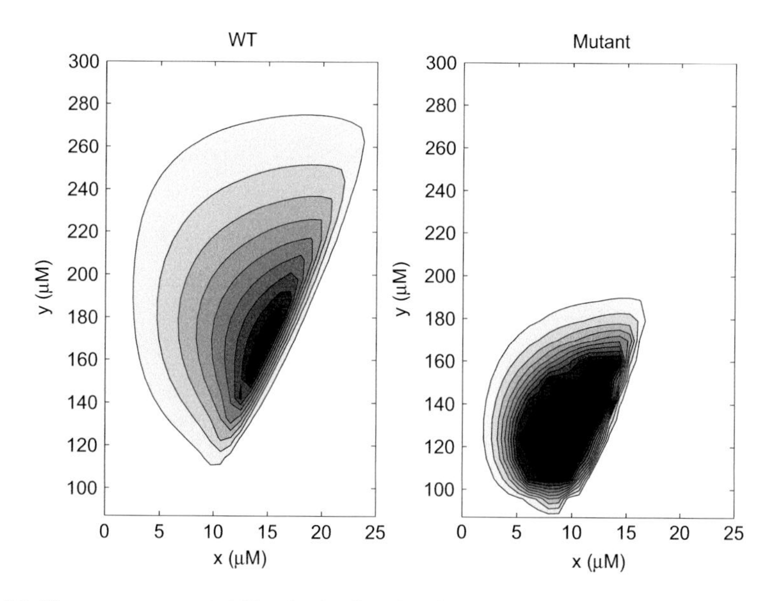

Fig. 6.1 The open state probability density function for the wild type case (*left*) and the mutant case (*right*, $\mu = 3$)

Table 6.2 Properties of the open probability density function in the wild type and mutant cases

Case	π_o	E_{x_o}	E_{y_o}	σ_{x_o}	σ_{y_o}
Wild type	0.430	12.63	202.4	4.948	46.27
Mutant	0.743	9.64	131.7	2.419	18.90

6.2 A Closed State Drug

In the 1D case, we were able to compute a characterization of the closed state drug based on considering the equilibrium solution of the reaction scheme. Since the reaction scheme is the same in the 1D and 2D problems, we can use exactly the same characterization as above. Let us first recall that the reaction scheme of the closed state drug takes the form

$$B \underset{k_{bc}}{\overset{k_{cb}}{\leftrightarrows}} C \underset{\mu k_{co}}{\overset{k_{oc}}{\leftrightarrows}} O.$$

We found above (see (3.9) on page 59) that the parameters of the closed state blocker should be related as

$$k_{cb} = (\mu - 1)k_{bc}, \tag{6.4}$$

so the optimal value of k_{bc} remains to be determined. To find the optimal value of this parameter, we need to extend the system (6.1) and (6.2) to account for the theoretical drug. When the closed state blocker is added, the steady state version of the probability density system reads

$$\frac{\partial}{\partial x}\left(a_o^x \rho_o\right) + \frac{\partial}{\partial y}\left(a_o^y \rho_o\right) = \mu k_{co}\rho_c - k_{oc}\rho_o, \tag{6.5}$$

$$\frac{\partial}{\partial x}\left(a_c^x \rho_c\right) + \frac{\partial}{\partial y}\left(a_c^y \rho_c\right) = k_{oc}\rho_o - \left(\mu k_{co} + (\mu - 1)\, k_{bc}\right)\rho_c + k_{bc}\rho_b, \tag{6.6}$$

$$\frac{\partial}{\partial x}\left(a_c^x \rho_b\right) + \frac{\partial}{\partial y}\left(a_c^y \rho_b\right) = (\mu - 1)\, k_{bc}\rho_c - k_{bc}\rho_b. \tag{6.7}$$

Our aim is now to compute the value of the single parameter k_{bc} such that the open probability density function defined by the system (6.5)–(6.7) is as close as possible to the solution of the system (6.1) and (6.2) in the case of $\mu = 1$ (i.e., the wild type case). In other words, we want to use the drug to repair the effect of the mutations in the sense that we want the open probability densities to be as close as possible to the wild type open probability densities.

In Fig. 6.2 we show the solution of the system (6.5)–(6.7) using $\mu = 3$ and $k_{bc} = 0.01, 0.1, 1,$ and $10\ \mathrm{ms}^{-1}$. As expected, we note that the solution becomes increasingly similar to the wild type solution (see Fig. 6.1) as k_{bc} increases.

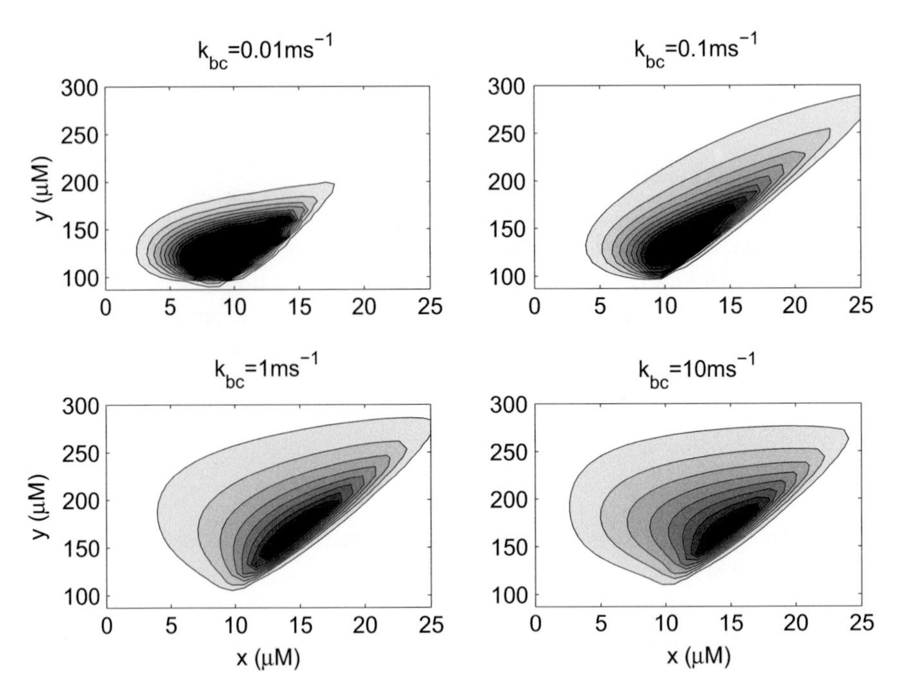

Fig. 6.2 Closed state blocker applied to the mutant case ($\mu = 3$). As the value k_{bc} increases, the probability density function approaches the wild type solution

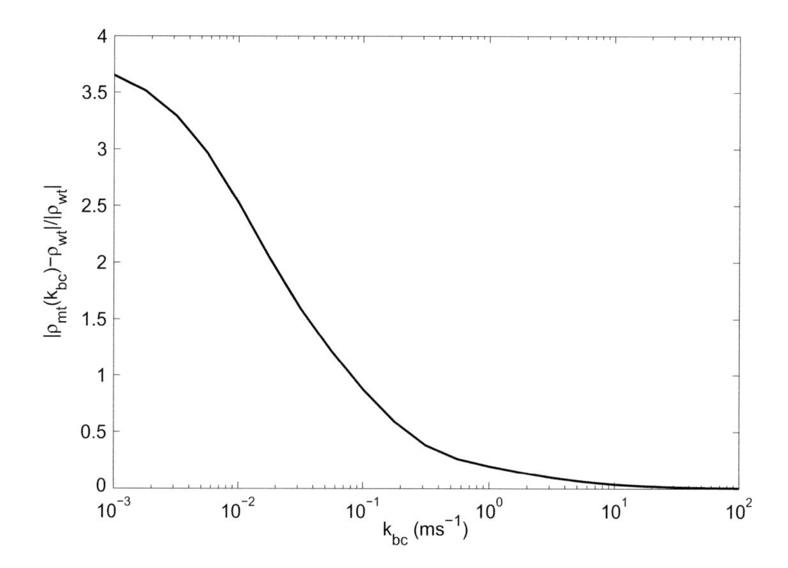

Fig. 6.3 The solution with the closed state blocker approaches the wild type case as k_{bc} increases

6.2.1 Convergence as k_{bc} Increases

Again we observe that the theoretical closed state blocker becomes more efficient for larger values of k_{bc}. To obtain a more precise impression of the convergence, we compute the norm of the difference between the open probability of the wild type case and the open probability of the solution of the system (6.5)–(6.7) as a function of k_{bc} using the norm defined by (2.40) on page 46. The result is shown in Fig. 6.3 and we again observe that, when k_{bc} becomes sufficiently large, the effect of the mutation is repaired completely.

6.3 An Open State Drug

The reaction scheme of an open state blocker for a mutant is

$$C \underset{\mu k_{co}}{\overset{k_{oc}}{\leftrightarrows}} O \underset{k_{ob}}{\overset{k_{bo}}{\leftrightarrows}} B.$$

We learned above that we had limited success in using the equilibrium solution to derive an optimal characterization of the open state drug. We will therefore directly optimize the two parameters k_{bo} and k_{ob}.

6.3.1 Probability Density Model for Open State Blockers in 2D

The probability density model in the presence of an open state drug is

$$\frac{\partial}{\partial x}\left(a_o^x \rho_o\right) + \frac{\partial}{\partial y}\left(a_o^y \rho_o\right) = \mu k_{co}\rho_c - (k_{oc} + k_{ob})\rho_o + k_{bo}\rho_b, \tag{6.8}$$

$$\frac{\partial}{\partial x}\left(a_c^x \rho_c\right) + \frac{\partial}{\partial y}\left(a_c^y \rho_c\right) = k_{oc}\rho_o - \mu k_{co}\rho_c, \tag{6.9}$$

$$\frac{\partial}{\partial x}\left(a_c^x \rho_b\right) + \frac{\partial}{\partial y}\left(a_c^y \rho_b\right) = k_{ob}\rho_o - k_{bo}\rho_b. \tag{6.10}$$

In Fig. 6.4, we show the cost function defined by the norm (see (2.40) on page 46) of the difference between the open probability density function of the wild type (solution of (6.1) and (6.2) with $\mu = 1$) and the open probability density function of the solution of the system (6.8)–(6.10) with $\mu = 3$. By minimizing the cost function, using Matlab's *Fminsearch* with default parameters and $k_{ob} = k_{bo} = 1$ as an initial guess, we find that an optimal open state blocker is given by

$$k_{ob} = 0.3225\ \text{ms}^{-1},\ k_{bo} = 0.3346\ \text{ms}^{-1}. \tag{6.11}$$

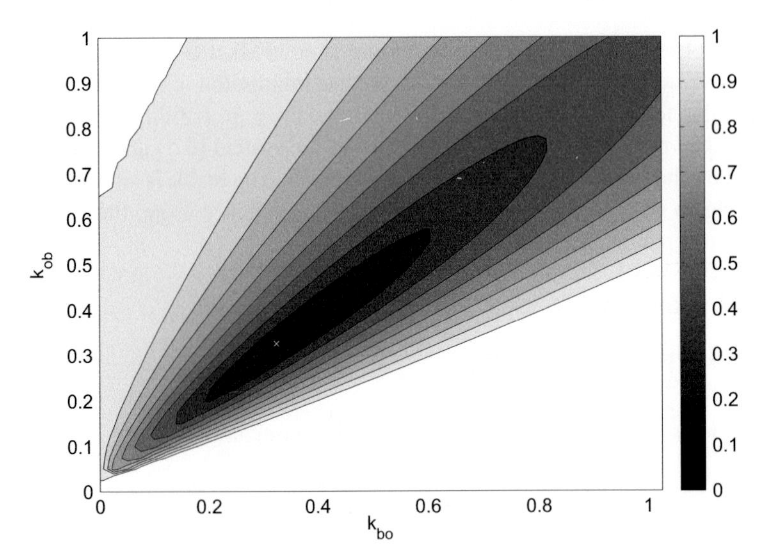

Fig. 6.4 Relative difference between the wild type and the mutant with an open state blocker for the case $\mu = 3$. There is a minimum around $(k_{bo}, k_{ob}) \approx (0.3, 0.3)\ \text{ms}^{-1}$ marked by a small $\times$

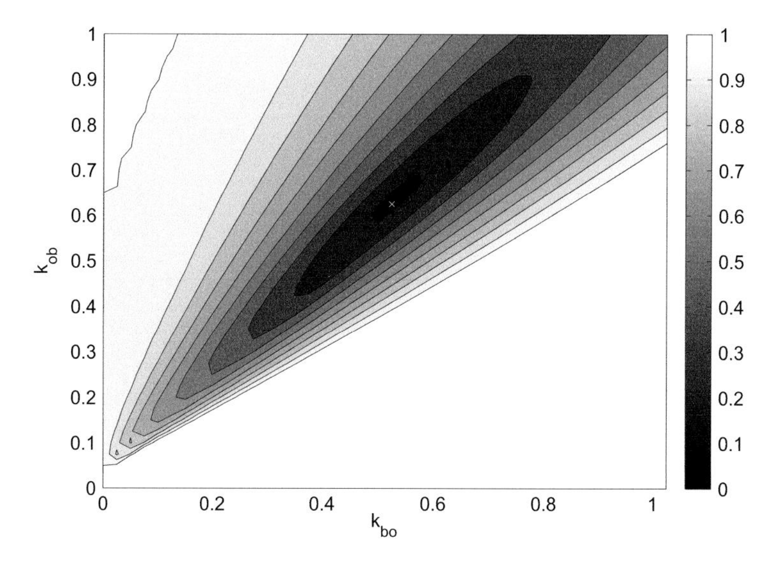

Fig. 6.5 Relative difference between the wild type and the mutant with an open state blocker for the case $\mu = 10$. There is a minimum around $(k_{bo}, k_{ob}) = (0.53, 0.63)$ ms^{-1}

6.3.1.1 Does the Optimal Theoretical Drug Change with the Severity of the Mutation?

One issue here is to see if the drug changes with the mutation severity index. Numerical experiments show that the optimal drug does change. In Fig. 6.5, we show the case in which $\mu = 10$ and the optimum has shifted compared to Fig. 6.4.

6.4 Statistical Properties of the Open and Closed State Blockers in 2D

We introduced statistical properties of probability density functions in Sect. 4.2 (see page 72). In Sect. 4.6 (page 88), we observed that, for the 1D release problem, the closed state blocker completely repaired the statistical properties of the open state probability density functions. In addition, an optimized version of an open state blocker gave good results, but it was unable to repair the standard deviation of the open state probability density functions for the particular CO-mutations we considered.

The statistical properties of the solutions for 2D release are summarized in Table 6.3. The results are quite similar to the 1D case. Again, for the CO-mutations, the closed state blocker improves as the value of k_{bc} increases and the optimized version of the open state blocker also provides good results.

Table 6.3 Statistical properties of the open probability density function in the mutant case when a blocker is applied. For the mutant case, we use $\mu = 3$

Case	π_o	E_{x_o}	E_{y_o}	σ_{x_o}	σ_{y_o}
Closed blocker, k_{bc}= 0.01	0.547	10.55	144.2	4.726	58.93
Closed blocker, k_{bc}=0.1	0.465	13.60	188.9	5.890	73.66
Closed blocker, k_{bc}=1	0.422	13.69	205.7	5.231	53.08
Closed blocker, k_{bc}=10	0.428	12.80	203.2	5.014	47.15
Open blocker, k_{bo}=0.33, k_{ob}=0.32	0.484	13.04	187.5	4.724	48.34
Wild type	0.430	12.63	202.4	4.948	46.27
Mutant, no drug	0.743	9.64	131.7	2.419	18.90

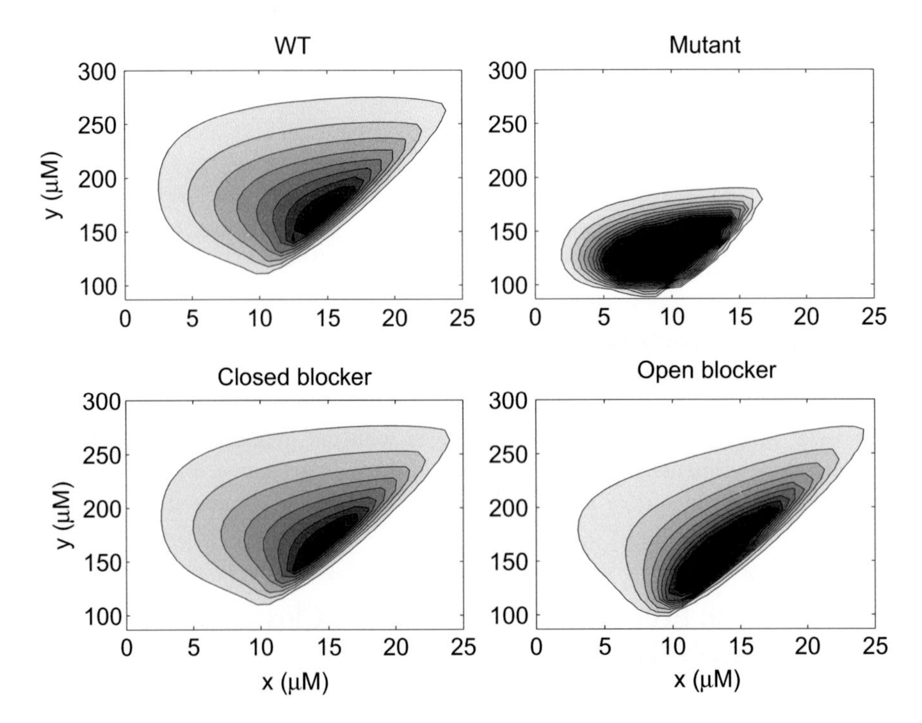

Fig. 6.6 Open probability density function for the wild type, the mutant ($\mu = 3$), the mutant plus the closed state blocker, and the mutant plus the open state blocker. We compute the stationary solution by solving the time-dependent equations until $T = 100$ ms. In the computation we use $\Delta t = 0.001$ ms, $\Delta x = 0.92$ μM, and $\Delta y = 9.3$ μM. The model parameters are specified in Table 6.1

6.5 Numerical Comparison of Optimal Open and Closed State Blockers

In the 1D case, we saw that for CO-mutations the closed state blocker was able to completely remove the effect of the mutation, whereas the open state blocker was less efficient. This result also holds in the 2D case. In Fig. 6.6, we compare the open probability density function of the steady state solution of the wild type (solution of (6.1) and (6.2) with $\mu = 1$), the mutant (solution of (6.1) and (6.2) with $\mu = 3$), the optimal closed state blocker (solution of (6.5)–(6.7) using $\mu = 3$ and $k_{bc} = 10\ \text{ms}^{-1}$) and the optimal open state blocker (solution of (6.8)–(6.10) with $\mu = 3, k_{ob} = 0.3225\ \text{ms}^{-1}$, $k_{bo} = 0.3346\ \text{ms}^{-1}$). We observe that it is hard to see any difference between the open probability density function of the wild type and the mutant when the closed state blocker is applied. In addition, the optimal open state blocker improves the solution, but not as much as the closed state blocker does.

6.6 Stochastic Simulations in 2D Using Optimal Drugs

We have used the probability density approach to find an optimal closed state blocker. In Fig. 6.7 we show how the closed state blocker works in a dynamic

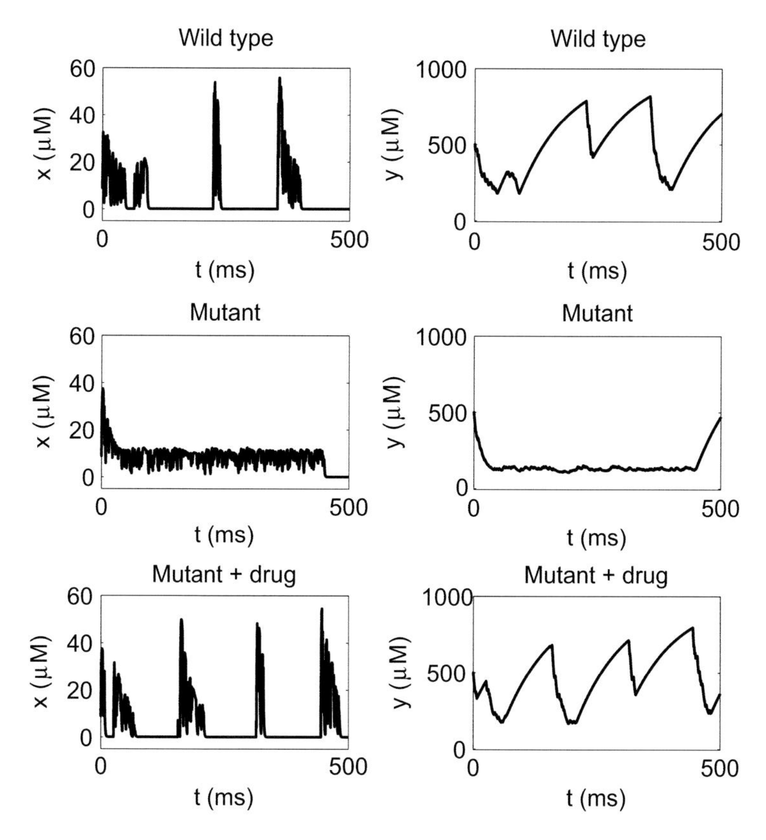

Fig. 6.7 Stochastic simulation of dyad concentrations (*left*, $x = x(t)$) and JSR concentrations (*right*, $y = y(t)$) for the wild type (*upper*), the mutant ($\mu = 3$, *middle*), and the mutant where the closed state drug is applied (*lower*, $k_{bc} = 10\ \text{ms}^{-1}$). Here we use $\Delta t = 0.01$ ms. The model parameters are specified in Table 6.1, and the initial conditions are given by $x(0) = c_0$ and $y(0) = c_1$ with the channel being closed

simulation based on the scheme (5.11) and (5.12). We plot the concentrations of the wild type, the mutant ($\mu = 3$), and the mutant when the closed state blocker is applied ($k_{bc} = 10\ \text{ms}^{-1}$, $k_{cb} = (\mu - 1)k_{bc}$). The dyad concentrations ($x = x(t)$) are on the left-hand side and the JSR concentrations ($y = y(t)$) are on the right-hand side. As for the 1D simulations, we observe that the mutations significantly reduce the variability of the solutions and that this effect is basically completely repaired by the closed state blocker.

6.7 Notes

1. The 2D stochastic differential equation and the associated probability density system is taken from Huertas and Smith [35].

Chapter 7
Generalized Systems Governing Probability Density Functions

So far we have considered one-dimensional and two-dimensional release processes. When the channel can take on two states—open or closed—we have seen that the associated probability density functions are governed by 2×2 systems of partial differential equations. When a drug is added to the Markov model, an extra state is introduced associated with either the open or the closed state and we obtain a model for the probability density functions phrased in terms of 3×3 systems of partial differential equations. In subsequent chapters, we will study situations involving many states and, to do so without drowning in cumbersome notation, we need mathematical formalism to present such models compactly. The compact form we use here is taken from Huertas and Smith [35]. We will introduce the more compact notation simply by providing a couple of examples. These will, hopefully, clarify how to formulate rather complex models in an expedient manner.

7.1 Two-Dimensional Calcium Release Revisited

Let us start by recalling that the two-dimensional process of calcium release illustrated in Fig. 5.2 on page 92 can be modeled as

$$\bar{x}'(t) = \bar{\gamma}(t)v_r(\bar{y} - \bar{x}) + v_d(c_0 - \bar{x}), \tag{7.1}$$

$$\bar{y}'(t) = \bar{\gamma}(t)v_r(\bar{x} - \bar{y}) + v_s(c_1 - \bar{y}), \tag{7.2}$$

where $\bar{\gamma} = \bar{\gamma}(t)$ is a stochastic variable governed by a Markov model represented by a reaction scheme of the form

$$C \underset{k_{co}}{\overset{k_{oc}}{\leftrightarrows}} O.$$

A. Tveito, G.T. Lines, *Computing Characterizations of Drugs for Ion Channels and Receptors Using Markov Models*, Lecture Notes in Computational Science and Engineering 111, DOI 10.1007/978-3-319-30030-6_7

We have seen (see, e.g., page 102) that the probability density functions of the open state (ρ_o) and the closed state (ρ_c) are governed by the system

$$\frac{\partial \rho_o}{\partial t} + \frac{\partial}{\partial x}\left(a_o^x \rho_o\right) + \frac{\partial}{\partial y}\left(a_o^y \rho_o\right) = k_{co}\rho_c - k_{oc}\rho_o, \tag{7.3}$$

$$\frac{\partial \rho_c}{\partial t} + \frac{\partial}{\partial x}\left(a_c^x \rho_c\right) + \frac{\partial}{\partial y}\left(a_c^y \rho_c\right) = k_{oc}\rho_o - k_{co}\rho_c, \tag{7.4}$$

where

$$\begin{aligned} a_o^x &= v_r\,(y-x) + v_d\,(c_0 - x)\,, \\ a_o^y &= v_r\,(x-y) + v_s\,(c_1 - y)\,, \\ a_c^x &= v_d\,(c_0 - x)\,, \\ a_c^y &= v_s\,(c_1 - y)\,. \end{aligned} \tag{7.5}$$

To prepare ourselves for more complex systems, we number the states in this simple system with $i = 1, 2$, where $i = 1$ is for the open state and $i = 2$ is for the closed state. The system can now be written in the form

$$\frac{\partial \rho_i}{\partial t} + \frac{\partial}{\partial x}\left(a_i^x \rho_i\right) + \frac{\partial}{\partial y}\left(a_i^y \rho_i\right) = (K\rho)_i\,,$$

where $(K\rho)_i$ denotes the ith component of the matrix vector product $K\rho$. Here the vector ρ is given by

$$\rho = \begin{pmatrix} \rho_1 \\ \rho_2 \end{pmatrix} = \begin{pmatrix} \rho_o \\ \rho_c \end{pmatrix}$$

and the matrix is given by

$$K = \begin{pmatrix} -k_{12} & k_{21} \\ k_{12} & -k_{21} \end{pmatrix} = \begin{pmatrix} -k_{oc} & k_{co} \\ k_{oc} & -k_{co} \end{pmatrix}.$$

Furthermore, we introduce the functions

$$\begin{aligned} a_i^x &= \gamma_i v_r\,(y-x) + v_d\,(c_0 - x)\,, \\ a_i^y &= \gamma_i v_r\,(x-y) + v_s\,(c_1 - y)\,, \end{aligned}$$

where γ_i is one for the open state (i.e., $i = 1$) and zero for the closed state (i.e., $i = 2$).

7.2 Four-State Model

It useful to illustrate this compact notation for a slightly more complex model based on four states. Suppose that the Markov model governing the stochastic variable $\bar{\gamma}$ in model (7.1) and (7.2) is based on four states: two open states O_1 and O_2 and two closed states C_1 and C_2, as shown in Fig. 7.1.

The probability density system associated with the model (7.1) and (7.2) when the Markov model is given by Fig. 7.1 can now be written in the form

$$
\begin{aligned}
\frac{\partial \rho_{o_1}}{\partial t} + \frac{\partial}{\partial x}\left(a_o^x \rho_{o_1}\right) + \frac{\partial}{\partial y}\left(a_o^y \rho_{o_1}\right) &= k_{c_1 o_1}\rho_{c_1} - \left(k_{o_1 c_1} + k_{o_1 o_2}\right)\rho_{o_1} + k_{o_2 o_1}\rho_{o_2}, \\
\frac{\partial \rho_{o_2}}{\partial t} + \frac{\partial}{\partial x}\left(a_o^x \rho_{o_2}\right) + \frac{\partial}{\partial y}\left(a_o^y \rho_{o_2}\right) &= k_{c_2 o_2}\rho_{c_2} - \left(k_{o_2 c_2} + k_{o_2 o_1}\right)\rho_{o_2} + k_{o_1 o_2}\rho_{o_1}, \\
\frac{\partial \rho_{c_1}}{\partial t} + \frac{\partial}{\partial x}\left(a_c^x \rho_{c_1}\right) + \frac{\partial}{\partial y}\left(a_c^y \rho_{c_1}\right) &= k_{o_1 c_1}\rho_{o_1} - \left(k_{c_1 o_1} + k_{c_1 c_2}\right)\rho_{c_1} + k_{c_2 c_1}\rho_{c_2}, \\
\frac{\partial \rho_{c_2}}{\partial t} + \frac{\partial}{\partial x}\left(a_c^x \rho_{c_2}\right) + \frac{\partial}{\partial y}\left(a_c^y \rho_{c_2}\right) &= k_{c_1 c_2}\rho_{c_1} - \left(k_{c_2 c_1} + k_{c_2 o_2}\right)\rho_{c_2} + k_{o_2 c_2}\rho_{o_2},
\end{aligned}
\tag{7.6}
$$

where

$$
\begin{aligned}
a_o^x &= v_r\,(y - x) + v_d\,(c_0 - x), \\
a_o^y &= v_r\,(x - y) + v_s\,(c_1 - y), \\
a_c^x &= v_d\,(c_0 - x), \\
a_c^y &= v_s\,(c_1 - y).
\end{aligned}
\tag{7.7}
$$

By defining the states O_1, O_2, C_1, and C_2 to be the states 1, 2, 3, and 4, respectively, we can write the system (7.6) in the more compact form

$$
\frac{\partial \rho_i}{\partial t} + \frac{\partial}{\partial x}\left(a_i^x \rho_i\right) + \frac{\partial}{\partial y}\left(a_i^y \rho_i\right) = (K\rho)_i \tag{7.8}
$$

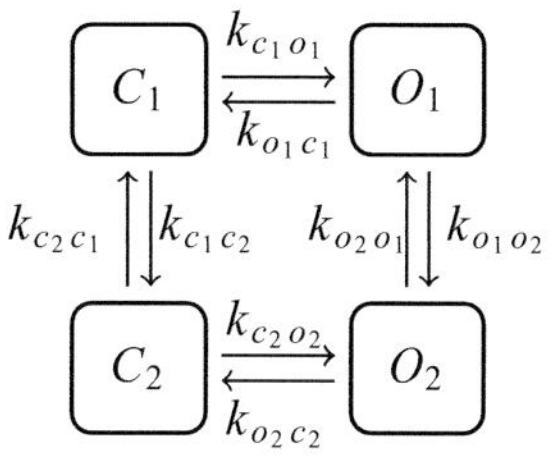

Fig. 7.1 Markov model including four possible states: two open states, O_1 and O_2, and two closed states, C_1 and C_2

for $i = 1, 2, 3, 4$, where

$$a_i^x = \gamma_i v_r (y - x) + v_d (c_0 - x),$$
$$a_i^y = \gamma_i v_r (x - y) + v_s (c_1 - y),$$

and $\rho = (\rho_1, \rho_2, \rho_3, \rho_4)^T$. Here γ_i is one for the open states (i.e., $i = 1$ and $i = 2$) and zero for the closed states (i.e., $i = 3$ and $i = 4$). Furthermore, the matrix is given by

$$K = \begin{pmatrix} -(k_{o_1c_1} + k_{o_1o_2}) & k_{o_2o_1} & k_{c_1o_1} & 0 \\ k_{o_1o_2} & -(k_{o_2c_2} + k_{o_2o_1}) & 0 & k_{c_2o_2} \\ k_{o_1c_1} & 0 & -(k_{c_1o_1} + k_{c_1c_2}) & k_{c_2c_1} \\ 0 & k_{o_2c_2} & k_{c_1c_2} & -(k_{c_2c_1} + k_{c_2o_2}) \end{pmatrix},$$

which in compact notation is

$$K = \begin{pmatrix} -(k_{13} + k_{12}) & k_{21} & k_{31} & 0 \\ k_{12} & -(k_{24} + k_{21}) & 0 & k_{42} \\ k_{13} & 0 & -(k_{31} + k_{34}) & k_{43} \\ 0 & k_{24} & k_{34} & -(k_{43} + k_{42}) \end{pmatrix}.$$

7.3 Nine-State Model

We have seen how to formulate probability density systems for two-state and four-state Markov models. For even larger Markov models, it is useful to introduce two-dimensional numbering. This will be illustrated using the nine-state model given in Fig. 7.2. Here S_{ij}, $i,j = 1,2,3$, denotes the states of the Markov model and K_{ij}^{mn}

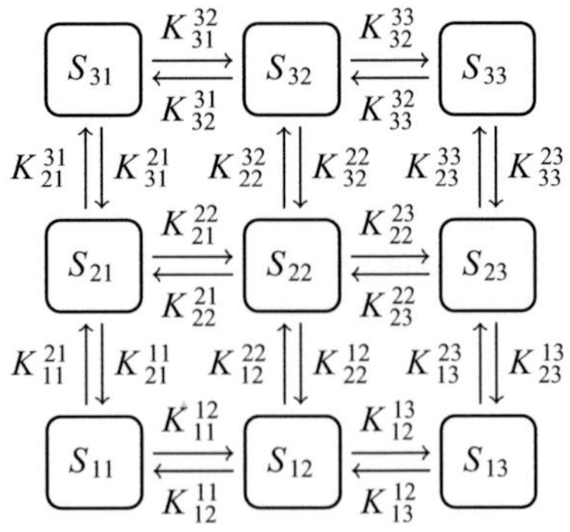

Fig. 7.2 Markov model including nine possible states

denotes[1] the reaction rate from the state S_{ij} to the state S_{mn}. The system governing the probability density functions of these states can be written in the form

$$\frac{\partial \rho_{ij}}{\partial t} + \frac{\partial}{\partial x}\left(a_{ij}^{x}\rho_{ij}\right) + \frac{\partial}{\partial y}\left(a_{ij}^{y}\rho_{ij}\right) = R_{ij}, \tag{7.9}$$

where

$$\begin{aligned} R_{ij} = {} & K_{i,j+1}^{i,j}\rho_{i,j+1} + K_{i+1,j}^{i,j}\rho_{i+1,j} + K_{i,j-1}^{i,j}\rho_{i,j-1} + K_{i-1,j}^{i,j}\rho_{i-1,j} \\ & - \left(K_{i,j}^{i,j+1} + K_{i,j}^{i+1,j} + K_{i,j}^{i,j-1} + K_{i,j}^{i-1,j}\right)\rho_{i,j}. \end{aligned}$$

Here ρ_{ij} denotes the probability density function of the state S_{ij} and we use the convention that $K_{ij}^{mn} = 0$ for $i, j, m, n \notin \{1, 2, 3\}$. We also have

$$\begin{aligned} a_{ij}^{x} &= \gamma_{ij} v_r (y - x) + v_d (c_0 - x), \\ a_{ij}^{y} &= \gamma_{ij} v_r (x - y) + v_s (c_1 - y), \end{aligned}$$

where $\gamma_{ij} = 1$ when the state S_{ij} represents an open state and $\gamma_{ij} = 0$ when S_{ij} represents a closed state.

[1] We use K_{ij} as shorthand for $K_{i,j}$, but we use the comma when an index of the form $j+1$ is needed, that is we write $K_{i,j+1}$.

Chapter 8
Calcium-Induced Calcium Release

We started in Chap. 2 by assuming that the concentrations of the junctional sarcoplasmic reticulum (JSR) and the network sarcoplasmic reticulum (NSR) are identical and that the L-type current can be ignored and thus we studied a one-dimensional problem where the calcium concentration of the dyad was the only variable of interest. The model is illustrated in Figs. 2.1 and 2.2. Then, in Chap. 5, we extended the model to account for the varying concentrations in the dyad and the JSR, but we still ignored the effect of the voltage-gated L-type channels and kept the concentration of the cytosol and the NSR constant. The two-dimensional model is illustrated in Figs. 5.1 and 5.2. Our aim is now to include the effect of L-type channels. The L-type channels open and close depending on the transmembrane potential V, so the model will therefore be parameterized by V. The model is illustrated in Figs. 8.1 and 8.2.

It should be noted that we are still interested in the dynamics related to the dyad and not to the whole cell. We therefore keep the concentration of the cytosol and NSR constant and assume that the concentration of the extracellular space (c_e) only affects the concentration of the dyad through the voltage-gated L-type calcium channels (LCCs). In a whole-cell model, this would be different in many ways, but we shall not consider that topic here.

The state of a voltage-gated channel is governed by a Markov model where the transitions depend on the transmembrane potential (or voltage for short). If the electrical potential in the dyad is given by V_i (intracellular potential) and the extracellular potential is given by V_e, we define the transmembrane potential to be

$$V = V_i - V_e.$$

As a notational convention, we use the subscript r to indicate that $\bar{\gamma}_r$ models the open or closed state of the ryanodine receptor (RyR) and the subscript l in the term $\bar{\gamma}_l J_l$ is used to indicate that this is the flux through the LCC.

A. Tveito, G.T. Lines, *Computing Characterizations of Drugs for Ion Channels and Receptors Using Markov Models*, Lecture Notes in Computational Science and Engineering 111, DOI 10.1007/978-3-319-30030-6_8

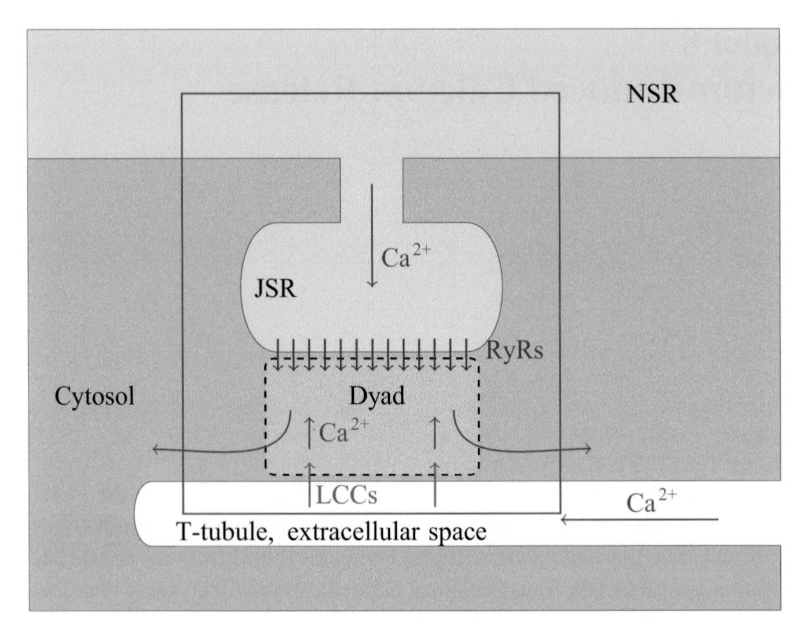

Fig. 8.1 The figure is a modified version of Figure 1 (panel A) of Winslow et al. [105] and illustrates the components involved in calcium-induced calcium release (CICR). In this chapter, we concentrate on the dynamics in the box surrounded by a *thin red line*. We assume that the concentrations of the cytosol, the NSR, and the extracellular domain represented by the T-tubule are kept constant and that inflow of calcium through the LCCs is governed by a voltage-dependent Markov model

	Extracellular, c_e		
Cytosol, c_0	Dyad, $\bar{x}(t)$	JSR, $\bar{y}(t)$	NSR, c_1

Fig. 8.2 Sketch of a release unit. The cytosolic (c_0), NSR (c_1), and extracellular (c_e) calcium concentrations are assumed to be constant, while the concentrations of the dyad and JSR are given by $\bar{x} = \bar{x}(t)$ and $\bar{y} = \bar{y}(t)$, respectively. Furthermore, we assume that the flux of calcium from the extracellular space to the dyad is voltage gated. Recall that $c_0 \ll c_1$

8.1 Stochastic Release Model Parameterized by the Transmembrane Potential

In the models we have studied so far, a very basic building block has been that, if x_0 denotes the concentration of a large reservoir of calcium and $x = x(t)$ denotes the concentration of a small space connected to the reservoir, then the concentration x

Table 8.1 Values of parameters used in simulations in this chapter

v_d	1 ms^{-1}
v_r	0.1 ms^{-1}
v_s	0.01 ms^{-1}
c_0	0.1 μM
c_1	1,000 μM
c_e	1,800 μM

evolves according to the model

$$x'(t) = v\left(x_0 - x(t)\right), \tag{8.1}$$

where v denotes the speed of diffusion between the two spaces. Here we assume that the concentration of the large reservoir, x_0, can be kept constant. This model can be extended to the case where the channel between the spaces can be either closed or open:

$$\bar{x}'(t) = \bar{\gamma}(t)v\left(x_0 - \bar{x}(t)\right), \tag{8.2}$$

where $\bar{\gamma}$ is a random variable taking on two possible values, one (open) and zero (closed). The stochastic release models studied above are derived by gluing together pieces of models of exactly this type.

In this chapter, one additional effect is added: We now allow calcium to flow into the dyad through the LCCs. This flow depends on both the gradient of the concentration and of the electrical potential across the membrane dividing the extracellular space and the dyad.

The process illustrated in Fig. 8.2 can be modeled as follows

$$\bar{x}' = \bar{\gamma}_r v_r\left(\bar{y} - \bar{x}\right) + v_d\left(c_0 - \bar{x}\right) - \bar{\gamma}_l J_l, \tag{8.3}$$

$$\bar{y}' = \bar{\gamma}_r v_r\left(\bar{x} - \bar{y}\right) + v_s\left(c_1 - \bar{y}\right). \tag{8.4}$$

This model is almost the same as the one we analyzed above (see (5.1) and (5.2) on page 92). The new term is given by $-\bar{\gamma}_l J_l$ and it models the inflow of calcium through the LCCs. The function $\bar{\gamma}_l$ is governed by a Markov model and, as usual, it takes on two values: zero (closed) and one (open). The Markov model governing $\bar{\gamma}_l$ depends on the transmembrane potential V and the flux depends on V, the extracellular calcium concentration c_e and the dyad concentration $x = x(t)$. As above, v_r denotes the rate of release from the JSR to the dyad, v_d denotes the speed of calcium diffusion from the dyad to the cytosol, and v_s denotes the speed of calcium diffusion from the NSR to the JSR. The model parameters are given in Table 8.1.

The Markov model governing $\bar{\gamma}_r$ will be the same as above, but we need to introduce a Markov model governing $\bar{\gamma}_l$. We will also combine these Markov models to simplify the introduction of a probability density formulation. Furthermore, we need to describe the electrochemical flux J_l.

8.1.1 Electrochemical Goldman–Hodgkin–Katz (GHK) Flux

Consider Fig. 8.1 and suppose that the membrane between the T-tubule and the dyad has thickness L. If the electrical field is constant through the channel, the flux is given by

$$J_l = \frac{D}{L}\frac{2F}{RT}\frac{x - c_e e^{-\frac{2FV}{RT}}}{1 - e^{-\frac{2FV}{RT}}}V, \tag{8.5}$$

which is referred to as the GHK flux (see Keener and Sneyd [42]). Here D is Fick's diffusion constant, F is Faraday's constant, R is the gas constant, and T is the absolute temperature. By defining

$$V_0 = \frac{RT}{2F},$$

we have

$$J_l = \frac{D}{L}\frac{x - c_e e^{-\frac{V}{V_0}}}{1 - e^{-\frac{V}{V_0}}}\frac{V}{V_0}, \tag{8.6}$$

where F, R, T, and V_0 are given in Table 8.2.

8.1.2 Assumptions

As for the model in Chap. 5, we will make the following assumptions for the parameters involved:

$$c_1 \gg c_0 \text{ and } v_r, v_d, v_s > 0, \tag{8.7}$$

$$v_d v_s \geq v_r^2. \tag{8.8}$$

Table 8.2 Parameters in (8.5)

F	96485.3 C mol^{-1}
R	8.3145 J mol^{-1}K^{-1}
T	310 K
V_0	13.357 mV
$\frac{D}{L}$	0.02 ms^{-1}

8.1.3 Equilibrium Potential

The electrochemical equilibrium over the membrane separating the extracellular space and the dyad is characterized by

$$J_l = 0.$$

In equilibrium, we must have

$$x = c_e e^{-\frac{V}{V_0}},$$

so the equilibrium transmembrane potential is given by

$$V_{eq} = V_0 \ln \frac{c_e}{x}. \tag{8.9}$$

For this value of the transmembrane potential V, the driving force $-\bar{\gamma}_l J_l$ in the system (8.3) and (8.4) is zero even if the channel is open. It should also be noted that the equilibrium transmembrane potential depends on the concentration x of the dyad and will therefore be a dynamic quantity. Here it is useful to recall that we regard V as a parameter input to the system and not a part of the dynamics.

8.1.4 Linear Version of the Flux

We mentioned above that our modeling so far has been based on very simple linear fluxes of the form given in (8.1). In the case we are considering now, the flux depends on both the difference in concentration and the electrical potential over the membrane; see (8.6). A Taylor series expansion of the GHK flux can be written as

$$J_l = \frac{D}{L}(x - c_e) + \frac{D}{2L}(x + c_e)\frac{V}{V_0} + O\left((V/V_0)^2\right) \tag{8.10}$$

and, therefore, if $V = 0$, the flux is given by

$$J_l = \frac{D}{L}(x - c_e)$$

so the term $-\bar{\gamma}_l J_l$ has the form we used in (8.2). This means that the electrochemical flux given by (8.6) reduces to a purely concentration-based flux when there is no difference in electrical potential across the membrane.

8.1.5 Markov Models for CICR

As discussed above, two Markov processes are involved in the CICR. We have seen that the gating of the release of calcium from the sarcoplasmic reticulum to the dyad is given by the stochastic variable $\bar{\gamma}_r = \bar{\gamma}_r(t)$, which is governed by the reaction scheme

$$C_r \underset{k_{co}^r}{\overset{k_{oc}^r}{\leftrightarrows}} O_r. \tag{8.11}$$

We recall here that r is used to indicate the relation to the RyR channels. Similarly, the Markov model for the LCC is given by

$$C_l \underset{k_{co}^l}{\overset{k_{oc}^l}{\leftrightarrows}} O_l, \tag{8.12}$$

where l is used to indicate the relation to the LCCs. This Markov model governs the stochastic variable $\bar{\gamma}_l = \bar{\gamma}_l(t)$.

It is convenient to combine these two Markov models into one reaction scheme of the form illustrated in Fig. 8.3.The states of this combined Markov model are given by C_lC_r (both closed), C_lO_r (LCC closed, RyR open), O_lO_r (both open), and O_lC_r (LCC open, RyR closed). In our computations, we use the rates shown in Table 8.3.

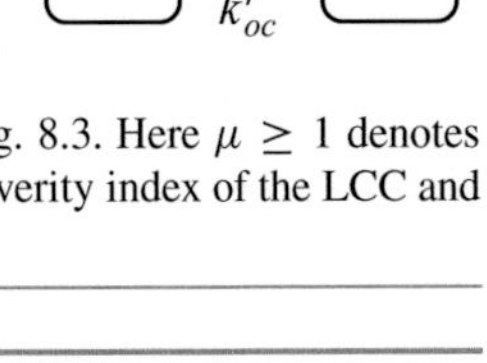

Fig. 8.3 Markov model including four possible states: C_lC_r (both closed), C_lO_r (LCC closed, RyR open), O_lO_r (both open), and O_lC_r (LCC open, RyR closed)

Table 8.3 Reaction rates used in the Markov model illustrated in Fig. 8.3. Here $\mu \geq 1$ denotes the mutation severity index of the RyR, $\eta \geq 1$ denotes the mutation severity index of the LCC and $\mu = \nu = 1$ represents the wild type case

RyR	LCC
$k_{co}^r = \mu \frac{x^4}{K(y)^4 + x^4}$ ms^{-1}	$k_{co}^l = \eta\, l_\infty(V)/\tau_l$
$k_{oc}^r = 1$ ms^{-1}	$k_{oc}^l = (1 - l_\infty(V))/\tau_l$
$K(y) = K_{max} - y/1000$	$l_\infty(V) = 0.01 \exp(-(V-5)^2/500)$
$K_{max} = 7.4\ \mu$M	$\tau_l = 1$ ms

8.1.6 *Numerical Scheme for the Stochastic CICR Model*

A numerical scheme for running simulations based on the CICR model (8.3) and (8.4) is given by

$$x_{n+1} = x_n + \Delta t \left(\gamma_n^r v_r (y_n - x_n) + v_d (c_0 - x_n)\right) - \Delta t \gamma_n^l J_l(x_n, V), \tag{8.13}$$

$$y_{n+1} = y_n + \Delta t \left(\gamma_n^r v_r (x_n - y_n) + v_s (c_1 - y_n)\right), \tag{8.14}$$

where γ_n^r and γ_n^l are computed according to the Markov model illustrated in Fig. 8.3.

8.1.7 *Monte Carlo Simulations of CICR*

In Fig. 8.4, we show the results of stochastic simulations using the model (8.3) and (8.4). The computations are based on the numerical scheme (8.13) and (8.14) with the parameters given in Table 8.1 and $\Delta t = 0.01$ ms. As initial conditions we have used $x(0) = c_0$ and $y(0) = c_1$ with both gates closed. From top to bottom, the transmembrane potential is given by $V = 20, 0, -20$, and -40 mV.

The associated calcium concentrations of the dyad given by $x = x(t)$ are graphed in the left panels and the calcium concentrations of the JSR given by $y = y(t)$ are graphed in the right panels. In all cases, we show the solution for a time interval ranging from 0 ms to 1000 ms. The calcium concentration clearly depends on the transmembrane potential and we observe in particular that there is no activity for $V = -40$ mV, since the LCC is inactivated at that voltage.

In Fig. 8.5, we show a detailed view of the case of $V = 0$ mV. In the upper part of the graph we show the state of the RyR (upper) and the LCCs (lower). The CICR mechanism is illustrated in the first part of the graph: The LCC opens at $t \approx 5$ ms, but the release is too short-lived to trigger an RyR opening and we therefore observe just a minor increase in the dyad calcium concentration given by x. Next time, at $t \approx 9$ ms, there is a new opening and now the channel is open for a longer time; there is an increase in x leading to opening of the RyR channel and then the concentration increases dramatically.

8.2 Invariant Region for the CICR Model

We have seen in both the one- and two-dimensional models above that we can derive invariant regions for the stochastic models and that these regions define the computational domain for the probability density system. Our aim is now to derive

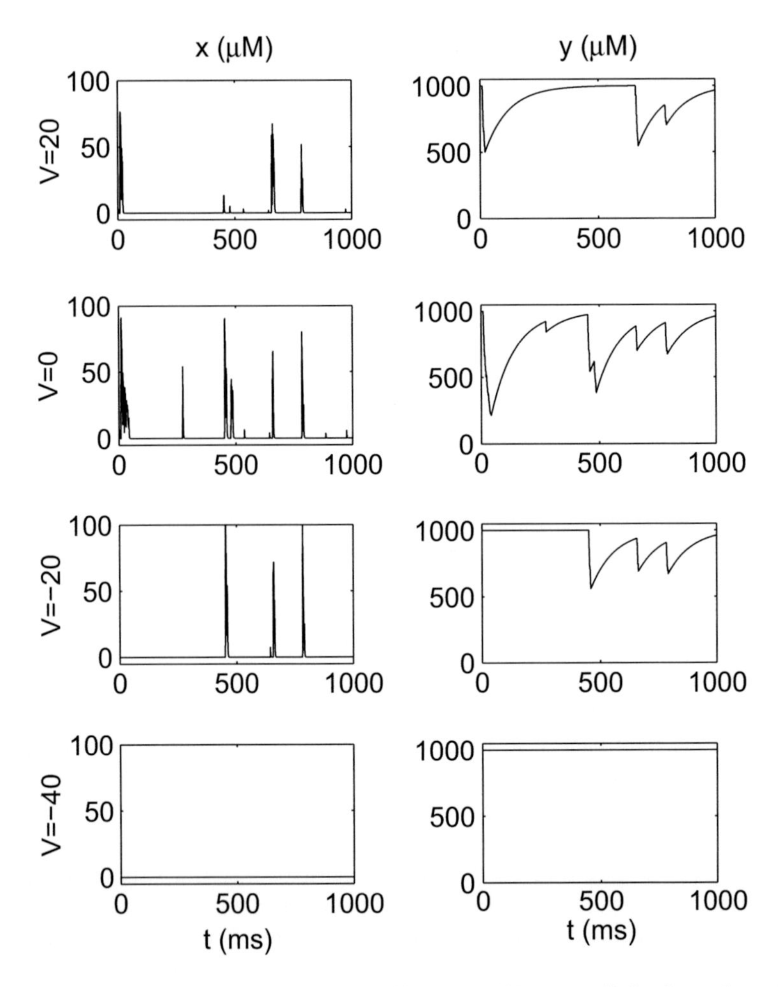

Fig. 8.4 Calcium dynamics of the dyad $x = x(t)$ and the JSR $y = y(t)$ for four values of the transmembrane potential V

an invariant region for the CICR model given by

$$\bar{x}' = \bar{\gamma}_r v_r (\bar{y} - \bar{x}) + v_d (c_0 - \bar{x}) - \bar{\gamma}_l J_l, \tag{8.15}$$

$$\bar{y}' = \bar{\gamma}_r v_r (\bar{x} - \bar{y}) + v_s (c_1 - \bar{y}). \tag{8.16}$$

Here it is convenient to write the GHK flux in the form

$$J_l(x) = a_0(x - x_0),$$

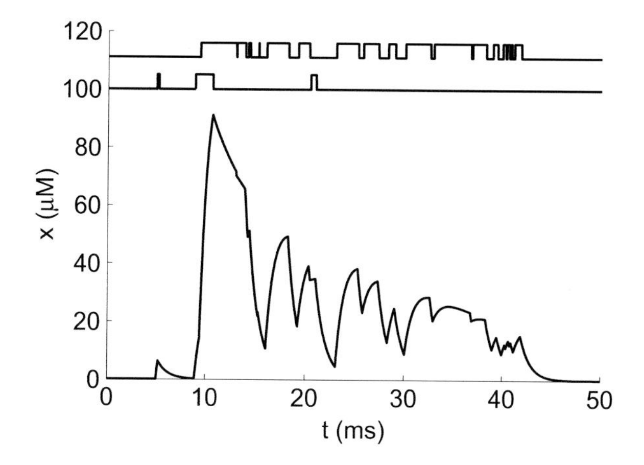

Fig. 8.5 A detailed view of the case of $V = 0$ mV taken from Fig. 8.4. In addition, we show the state of the RyR channel (*upper panel*) and the LCC (*lower panel*). The first spike at 5 ms in the LCC is very short and does not trigger an RyR release. The next one, at 9 ms, does trigger an RyR release

where

$$a_0 = \frac{D}{L}\frac{1}{1-e^{-\frac{V}{V_0}}}\frac{V}{V_0}$$

and

$$x_0 = c_e e^{-\frac{V}{V_0}},$$

so the system takes the form

$$\bar{x}' = \bar{\gamma}_r v_r\,(\bar{y}-\bar{x}) + v_d\,(c_0-\bar{x}) + \bar{\gamma}_l a_0(x_0-\bar{x}), \tag{8.17}$$

$$\bar{y}' = \bar{\gamma}_r v_r\,(\bar{x}-\bar{y}) + v_s\,(c_1-\bar{y})\,. \tag{8.18}$$

8.2.1 A Numerical Scheme

Let us consider the numerical scheme (8.13, 8.14),

$$x_{n+1} = x_n + \Delta t\left(\gamma_n^r v_r\,(y-x) + v_d\,(c_0-x) + \gamma_n^l a_0(x_0-x)\right), \tag{8.19}$$

$$y_{n+1} = y_n + \Delta t\left(\gamma_n^r v_r\,(x-y) + v_s\,(c_1-y)\right). \tag{8.20}$$

Here γ_n^r and γ_n^l simply denotes constants that take on the value zero or one and their values will be specified in order to study the dynamics of the system when the associated channels are open or closed. The numerical scheme can be written in the form

$$x_{n+1} = F(x_n, y_n), \tag{8.21}$$

$$y_{n+1} = G(x_n, y_n), \tag{8.22}$$

with

$$F(x,y) = x + \Delta t\left(\gamma_r v_r (y-x) + v_d (c_0 - x) + \gamma_l a_0 (x_0 - x)\right),$$
$$G(x,y) = y + \Delta t\left(\gamma_r v_r (x-y) + v_s (c_1 - y)\right).$$

Here we assume that

$$\Delta t \leqslant \min\left(\frac{1}{v_d + a_0 + v_r}, \frac{1}{v_s + v_r}\right). \tag{8.23}$$

Under this condition, we observe that

$$\frac{\partial F}{\partial x} = 1 - \Delta t\left(v_d + \gamma_l a_0 + \gamma_r v_r\right) \geqslant 0$$

for any choice of γ_l and γ_r. We also have

$$\frac{\partial F}{\partial y} = \Delta t \gamma_r v_r \geqslant 0.$$

Similarly, we find that

$$\frac{\partial G}{\partial x} = \Delta t \gamma_r v_r \geqslant 0 \tag{8.24}$$

and

$$\frac{\partial G}{\partial y} = 1 - \Delta t\left(v_s + \gamma_r v_r\right) \geqslant 0. \tag{8.25}$$

Assume that

$$0 \leqslant x_n, y_n \leqslant M, \tag{8.26}$$

where

$$M = \max\left(c_1, \frac{c_0 v_d + a_0 x_0}{a_0 + v_d}\right).$$

Since

$$\frac{\partial F}{\partial x}, \frac{\partial F}{\partial y}, \frac{\partial G}{\partial x}, \frac{\partial G}{\partial y} \geqslant 0,$$

we have

$$x_{n+1} = F(x_n, y_n) \leqslant F(M, M) = M + \Delta t \left(v_d \left(c_0 - M\right) + \gamma_l a_0 (x_0 - M)\right) \leqslant M$$

and

$$y_{n+1} = G(x_n, y_n) \leqslant G(M, M) = M + \Delta t \left(v_s \left(c_1 - M\right)\right) \leqslant M.$$

Furthermore, we have

$$x_{n+1} = F(x_n, y_n) \geqslant F(0, 0) = \Delta t \left(v_d c_0 + \gamma_l a_0 x_0\right) \geqslant 0$$

and

$$y_{n+1} = G(x_n, y_n) \geqslant G(0, 0) = \Delta t v_s c_1 \geqslant 0.$$

So, by induction, the invariant region (8.26) holds for all $n \geqslant 0$.

8.3 Probability Density Model Parameterized by the Transmembrane Potential

The probability density formulation of the system (8.3) and (8.4) is given by the system of partial differential equations

$$\frac{\partial \rho_{oo}}{\partial t} + \frac{\partial}{\partial x}\left(a^x_{oo}\rho_{oo}\right) + \frac{\partial}{\partial y}\left(a^y_{oo}\rho_{oo}\right) = k^l_{co}\rho_{co} - \left(k^l_{oc} + k^r_{oc}\right)\rho_{oo} + k^r_{co}\rho_{oc}, \tag{8.27}$$

$$\frac{\partial \rho_{oc}}{\partial t} + \frac{\partial}{\partial x}\left(a^x_{oc}\rho_{oc}\right) + \frac{\partial}{\partial y}\left(a^y_{oc}\rho_{oc}\right) = k^l_{co}\rho_{cc} - \left(k^l_{oc} + k^r_{co}\right)\rho_{oc} + k^r_{oc}\rho_{oo}, \tag{8.28}$$

$$\frac{\partial \rho_{cc}}{\partial t} + \frac{\partial}{\partial x}\left(a^x_{cc}\rho_{cc}\right) + \frac{\partial}{\partial y}\left(a^y_{cc}\rho_{cc}\right) = k^l_{oc}\rho_{oc} - \left(k^l_{co} + k^r_{co}\right)\rho_{cc} + k^r_{oc}\rho_{co}, \tag{8.29}$$

$$\frac{\partial \rho_{co}}{\partial t} + \frac{\partial}{\partial x}\left(a^x_{co}\rho_{co}\right) + \frac{\partial}{\partial y}\left(a^y_{co}\rho_{co}\right) = k^l_{oc}\rho_{oo} - \left(k^l_{co} + k^r_{oc}\right)\rho_{oc} + k^r_{co}\rho_{cc}, \tag{8.30}$$

where $\rho_{oo}, \rho_{oc}, \rho_{cc}$, and ρ_{co} represent the probability densities of the states denoted O_lO_r, O_lC_r, C_lC_r, and C_lO_r, respectively. The terms of the fluxes are given by

$$\begin{aligned}
a^x_{oo} &= v_r\,(y-x) + v_d\,(c_0 - x) - J_l(x,V), & a^y_{oo} &= v_r\,(x-y) + v_s\,(c_1 - y)\,,\\
a^x_{oc} &= v_d\,(c_0 - x) - J_l(x,V), & a^y_{oc} &= v_s\,(c_1 - y)\,,\\
a^x_{cc} &= v_d\,(c_0 - x)\,, & a^y_{cc} &= v_s\,(c_1 - y)\,,\\
a^x_{co} &= v_r\,(y-x) + v_d\,(c_0 - x)\,, & a^y_{co} &= v_r\,(x-y) + v_s\,(c_1 - y)\,,
\end{aligned}$$

where we use the convention that in the expression $a^x_{\alpha\beta}$, the index α indicates whether the LCC is open ($\alpha = o$) or closed ($\alpha = c$) and the index β plays the same role for the RyR channel. Similar notation is used for the flux terms represented by $a^y_{\alpha\beta}$. As usual, the sum of total probabilities is one:

$$\int_{\Omega} (\rho_{oo} + \rho_{oc} + \rho_{cc} + \rho_{co})\, dx\, dy = 1. \tag{8.31}$$

8.4 Computing Probability Density Representations of CICR

In Fig. 8.6, we show solutions of the system (8.15) and (8.16) defined in the computational domain $\Omega = \Omega(V)$ for four values of the transmembrane potential: $V = 20, 0, -20$, and -40 mV. In all computations, the parameters are given in Table 8.1 and the Markov model is illustrated in Fig. 8.3. All distributions are initially set to zero, except that $\rho_{cc}(c_0, c_1) = 1/(\Delta x \Delta y)$. Hence the initial discrete probability densities integrates to one;

$$\Delta x \Delta y \sum_{i,j} \rho_{i,j} = 1, \tag{8.32}$$

which is a discrete version of (8.31) with $\rho = \rho_{oo} + \rho_{oc} + \rho_{co} + \rho_{cc}$.

The simulation results are shown in Fig. 8.6 and summarized in Table 8.4. We observe that the transmembrane potential V significantly influences the probability density functions. In Table 8.4, we observe that the probability of the LCC being in the open state is highest for $V = 0$ mV and it is almost zero for $V = -40$ mV. In the computations, we use $\Delta t = 0.001$ ms, $\Delta x = 1.02$, 1.23, 1.54 and 1.95 µM (the domain size varies with V), and $\Delta y = 9.3$ µM. Note that the scale of the plots varies (see Fig. 8.6).

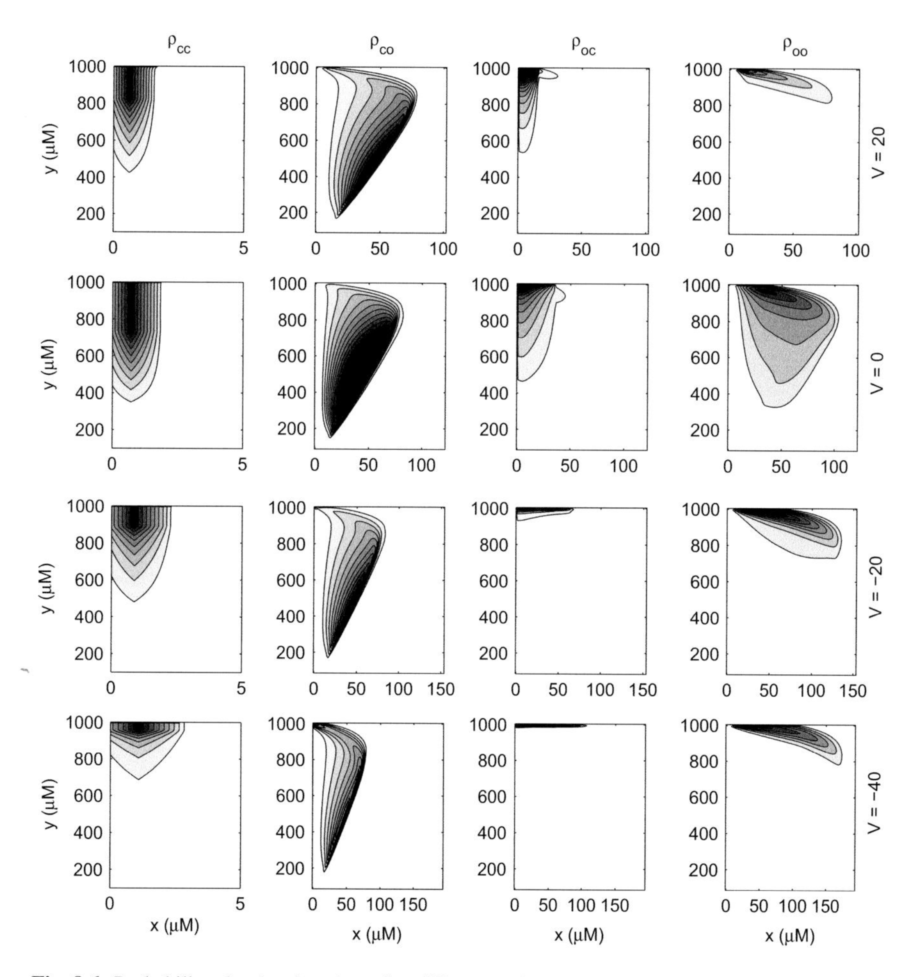

Fig. 8.6 Probability density functions for different voltages. The LCC is more prone to being open (last two columns) when the voltage is close to $V = 5$ mV, that is, where $l_{\infty}(V)$ is close to its maximum. Black corresponds to 10^{-3} for ρ_{cc} and to 10^{-6} for the other three distributions

Table 8.4 Probability of being in the four states for different voltages. Recall that the probabilities are computed using (4.7) at page 72 where the probability density functions are numerical solutions of the system (8.27)–(8.30)

V	π_{cc}	π_{co}	π_{oc}	π_{oo}
20	0.978	0.015	0.005	0.001
0	0.959	0.032	0.007	0.003
−20	0.982	0.015	0.002	0.001
−40	0.993	0.006	0.000	0.000

8.5 Effects of LCC and RyR Mutations

We are now in a position to study the effect of both LCC and RyR mutations. We assume that both the LCC and RyR mutations lead to leaky channels that can be represented by increasing the reaction rate from closed to open. So we again consider CO-mutations.

The reaction scheme in the presence of mutations is illustrated in Fig. 8.7. Here $\mu \geq 1$ denotes the strength of the RyR mutations and $\eta \geq 1$ denotes the strength of the LCC mutations. Note that $\mu = 1$ and $\eta = 1$ represent the wild type.

8.5.1 *Effect of Mutations Measured in a Norm*

To measure the effect of the mutations, we introduce the norm

$$\|\rho^{\eta,\mu} - \rho^{1,1}\| = \frac{1}{6}\sum_{V}\sum_{z}\frac{\|\rho_z^{\eta,\mu} - \rho_z^{1,1}\|_{L^2(\Omega)}}{\|\rho_z^{\eta,\mu}\|_{L^2(\Omega)} + \|\rho_z^{1,1}\|_{L^2(\Omega)}}, \tag{8.33}$$

where ρ_z represents $\rho_{oo}, \rho_{oc}, \rho_{co}$, or ρ_{cc} and V represents summation over the following values of the transmembrane potential: −80, −60, −40, −20, 0, and 20 mV. Furthermore,

$$\|\rho\|_{L^2(\Omega)} = \left(\int_{\Omega}\rho^2 d\Omega\right)^{1/2}. \tag{8.34}$$

The difference between the wild type solution and the solution based on mutated reaction rates is depicted in Fig. 8.8. The figure shows the difference as a function of the two mutation severity indices μ and η.

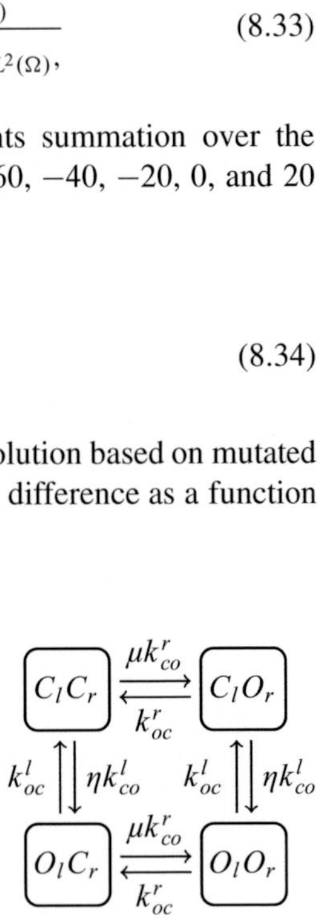

$$\begin{array}{ccc} C_lC_r & \underset{k^r_{oc}}{\overset{\mu k^r_{co}}{\rightleftarrows}} & C_lO_r \\ k^l_{oc}\uparrow\downarrow\eta k^l_{co} & & k^l_{oc}\uparrow\downarrow\eta k^l_{co} \\ O_lC_r & \underset{k^r_{oc}}{\overset{\mu k^r_{co}}{\rightleftarrows}} & O_lO_r \end{array}$$

Fig. 8.7 Mutant version of the Markov model given in Fig. 8.3 including four possible states: C_lC_r (both closed), C_lO_r (LCC closed, RyR open), O_lO_r (both open), and O_lC_r (LCC open, RyR closed)

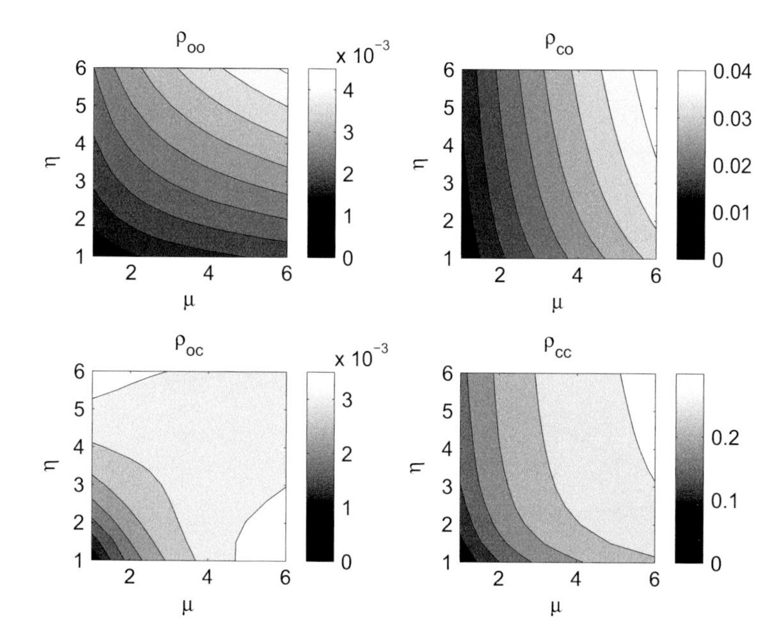

Fig. 8.8 Difference between wild type solutions and mutated solutions, defined in terms of the norm given by (8.33). The wild type solution is represented by $\mu = \eta = 1$

8.5.2 *Mutations Increase the Open Probability of Both the LCC and RyR Channels*

In Sect. 4.2 (page 72), we introduced statistical measures for the probability density functions. We will now consider how the LCC and RyR mutations affect the statistical properties of the associated probability density functions. Let us first consider how the mutations affect the total probability of being in the different states. In Fig. 8.9, we show the total probability of being in the states OO, CO, OC, and CC, where, as above, the first letter denotes the state of the LCC and the second letter indicates the state of the RyR channel. Here the value of the transmembrane potential is $V = 0$ mV. In Fig. 8.10, we show similar results in the case of $V = -80$ mV; the probability of the LCC being open is very small and the LCC mutation must be extremely severe to change this. Basically, at $V = -80$ mV, the LCC is closed independent of the mutations. This observation certainly depends heavily on the particular reaction rates used in these computations (see Table 8.3 on page 130).

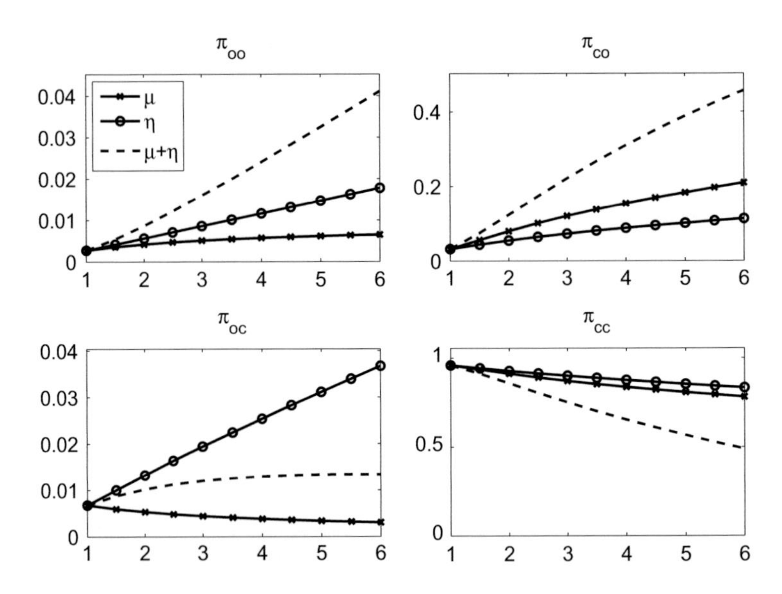

Fig. 8.9 Probability of being in the state OO, CO, OC, or CC at $V = 0$ mV as a function of the mutation severity index of the LCC, represented by η, and the mutation severity index of the RyR channel, represented by μ. Here $\eta = \mu = 1$ represents the wild type

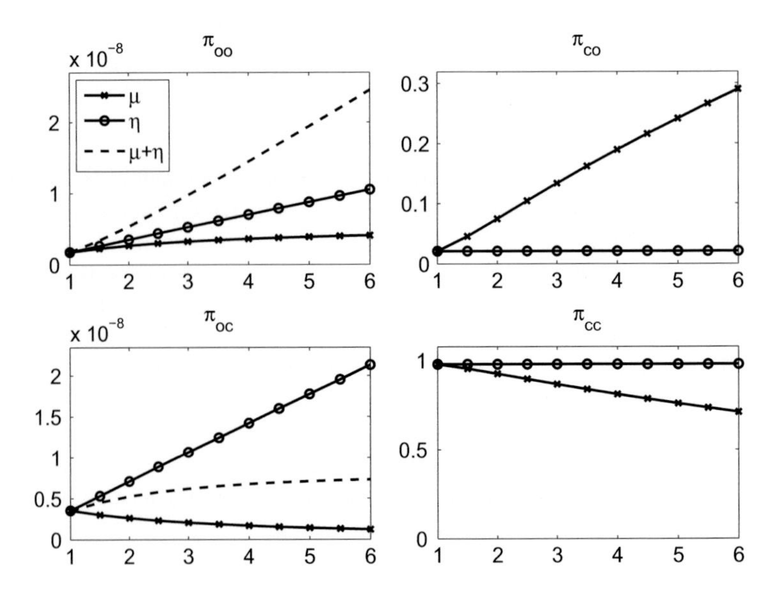

Fig. 8.10 Probability of being in the state OO, CO, OC, or CC at $V = -80$ mV as a function of the mutation severity index of the LCC, represented by η, and the mutation severity index of the RyR channel, represented by μ. Here $\eta = \mu = 1$ represents the wild type. Note the scale of the axis in the plots on the left-hand side

8.5.3 Mutations Change the Expected Values of Concentrations

Figures 8.11 and 8.12 show the development of the expected concentration for varying strengths of mutations. In Fig. 8.11, we set $V = 0$ mV and see that the mutations change the expected concentrations significantly. More specifically, both mutations lead to lower expected JSR concentrations. In Fig. 8.12, we set $V = -80$ mV and observe that the expected concentrations are not altered by the LCC mutation. As for the total probabilities discussed above, the reason for this is that, at this value of V, the probability of going from closed to open is practically zero and the mutation must be orders of magnitude larger to open the LCC at this voltage. Again, this observation is based on the particular form of the reaction rates given in Table 8.3.

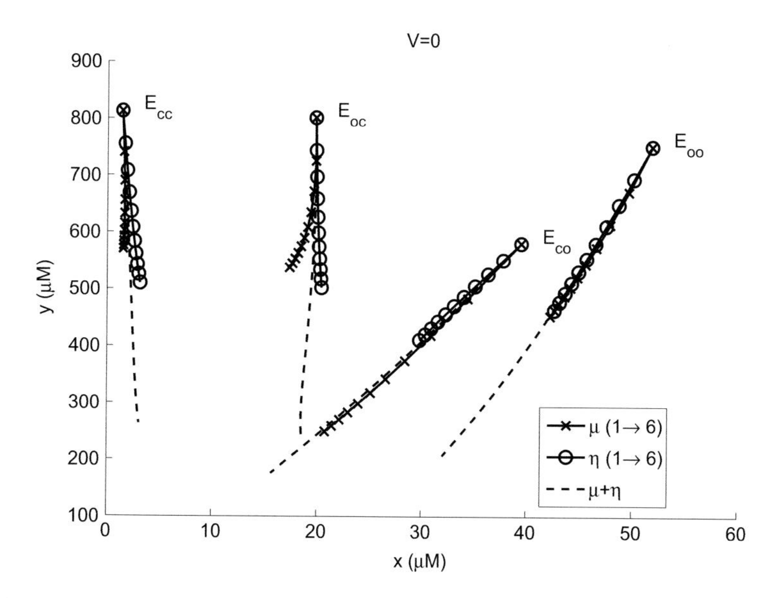

Fig. 8.11 This figure shows how the expected concentrations of the dyad (given by x) and the JSR (given by y) change as functions of the mutation severity indices. The curve denoted by E_{cc} starts at the circle that represents the expected values of x and y in the case of both the LCC and RyR being closed. The starting point represents the wild type and the curves represent the two mutations (or combinations of them) and similarly for the curves starting at the circles next to E_{oc}, E_{co}, and E_{oo}. All curves are computed using $V = 0$ mV

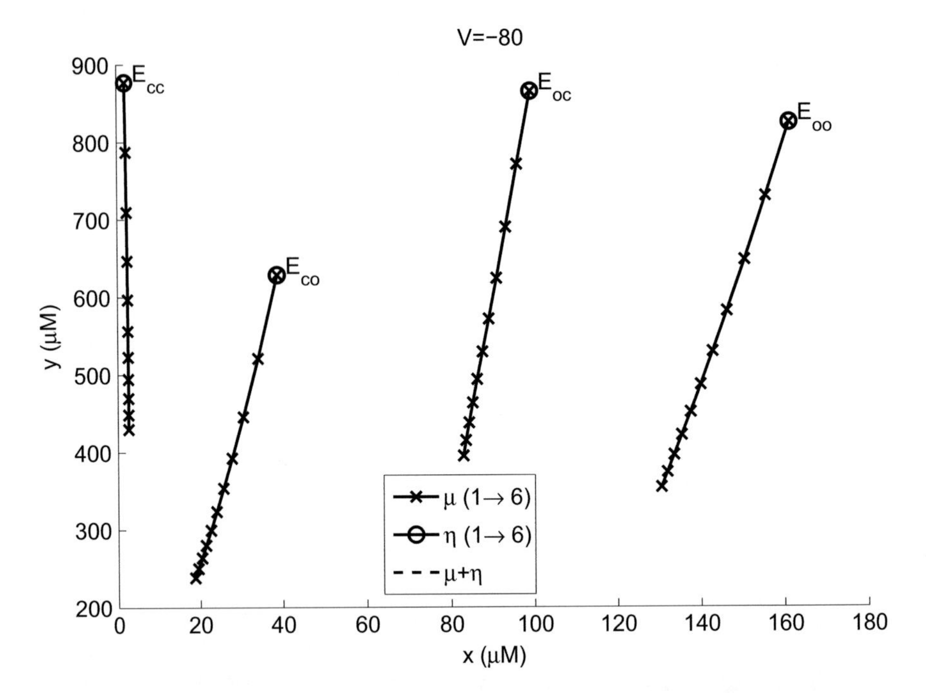

Fig. 8.12 This figure shows how the expected concentrations of the dyad (given by x) and the JSR (given by y) change as functions of the mutation severity indices. The curve denoted by E_{cc} starts at the circle that represents the expected values of x and y in the case of both LCC and RyR being closed. The starting point represents the wild type and the curves represent the two mutations (or combinations of them) and similarly for the curves starting at the circles next to E_{oc}, E_{co}, and E_{oo}. All curves are computed using $V = -80$ mV

8.6 Notes

1. The Markov model (including parameters) given in Fig. 8.3 and the probability density system (8.27)–(8.30) are taken from Williams et al. [102].
2. The functions given in Table 8.3 are motivated by the models of Stern et al. [89].

Chapter 9
Numerical Drugs for Calcium-Induced Calcium Release

In the previous chapter, we developed models of calcium-induced calcium release (CICR) in terms of both a stochastic release model and a model of the probability density functions of the states involved in the stochastic release model. The models incorporated the effects of mutations in both the ryanodine receptors (RyRs) and the L-type calcium channels (LCCs). The purpose of the present chapter is to introduce theoretical drugs aimed at repairing the effect of mutations of both the LCCs and RyR channels. Model parameters used throughout this chapter are given in Table 9.1.

We have seen in previous chapters that, if we ignore the effect of the LCC, we can completely repair the effect of an RyR mutation using a closed state blocker if the mutation is of the CO type. In this chapter, we want to see if this result also holds when the effect of the LCCs is taken into account. Since the transmembrane potential V enters the model as a parameter, it is sufficient to control the effect of the LCCs for a number of different values of V. The next issue we want to address is how to repair the effect of LCC mutations. We will find optimal open and closed state blockers.

9.1 Markov Models for CICR, Including Drugs

We consider a situation where the RyR or the LCC may be affected by CO-mutations. Both effects are modeled by Markov models and in this section we introduce theoretical drugs in terms of open and closed state blockers for both the RyR and the LCC.

A. Tveito, G.T. Lines, *Computing Characterizations of Drugs for Ion Channels and Receptors Using Markov Models*, Lecture Notes in Computational Science and Engineering 111, DOI 10.1007/978-3-319-30030-6_9

Table 9.1 Values of parameters used in simulations in this chapter

v_d	$1\ \text{ms}^{-1}$
v_r	$0.1\ \text{ms}^{-1}$
v_s	$0.01\ \text{ms}^{-1}$
c_0	$0.1\ \mu\text{M}$
c_1	$1{,}000\ \mu\text{M}$

9.1.1 Theoretical Blockers for the RyR

As discussed above, the gating of the release of calcium from the sarcoplasmic reticulum to the dyad is given by the stochastic variable $\bar{\gamma}_r = \bar{\gamma}_r(t)$ governed by the reaction scheme

$$C_r \underset{\mu k_{co}^r}{\overset{k_{oc}^r}{\leftrightarrows}} O_r. \tag{9.1}$$

Here μ is the mutation severity index, which is one in the wild type case. We have seen that open and closed state blockers can be added to the reaction as

$$B_c^r \underset{k_{bc}^r}{\overset{k_{cb}^r}{\leftrightarrows}} C_r \underset{\mu k_{co}^r}{\overset{k_{oc}^r}{\leftrightarrows}} O_r \underset{k_{ob}^r}{\overset{k_{bo}^r}{\leftrightarrows}} B_o^r, \tag{9.2}$$

where B_c^r and B_o^r denote the blocked states associated with the closed and open states, respectively. The characteristics of the drugs are given by the constants k_{cb}^r and k_{bc}^r (for the closed state blocker) and k_{ob}^r and k_{bo}^r (for the open state blocker).

9.1.2 Theoretical Blockers for the LCC

The Markov model governing the stochastic variable $\bar{\gamma}_l = \bar{\gamma}_l(t)$ of the LCC is given by

$$C_l \underset{\eta k_{co}^l}{\overset{k_{oc}^l}{\leftrightarrows}} O_l, \tag{9.3}$$

where we have introduced the parameter η to indicate a mutation of the LCC. The wild type case is again represented by $\eta = 1$ and any $\eta > 1$ denotes a leaky LCC. We introduce a theoretical representation of a drug as for the RyR channels:

$$B_c^l \underset{k_{bc}^l}{\overset{k_{cb}^l}{\leftrightarrows}} C_l \underset{\eta k_{co}^l}{\overset{k_{oc}^l}{\leftrightarrows}} O_l, \underset{k_{ob}^l}{\overset{k_{bo}^l}{\leftrightarrows}} B_o^l, \tag{9.4}$$

where, in line with the RyR case, B_c^l and B_o^l denote the blocked states associated with the closed and open states, respectively, and the characteristics of the LCC drugs are given by the constants k_{cb}^l and k_{bc}^l (for the closed state blocker) and k_{ob}^l and k_{bo}^l (for the open state blocker).

9.1.3 *Combined Theoretical Blockers for the LCC and the RyR*

To use the probability density formalism, it is convenient to rewrite the two Markov models as one combined model of the form illustrated in Fig. 9.1.This model consists of 16 separate states given by

$$\begin{array}{llll} B_c^l B_c^r & B_c^l C_r & B_c^l O_r & B_c^l B_o^r \\ C_l B_c^r & C_l C_r & C_l O_r & C_l B_o^r \\ O_l B_c^r & O_l C_r & O_l O_r & O_l B_o^r \\ B_o^l B_c^r & B_o^l C_r & B_o^l O_r & B_o^l B_o^r \end{array} \tag{9.5}$$

and the combined LCC and RyR drug is fully specified by

$$k_{cb}^r, k_{bc}^r, k_{bo}^r, k_{ob}^r, k_{cb}^l, k_{bc}^l, k_{bo}^l, \text{ and } k_{ob}^l. \tag{9.6}$$

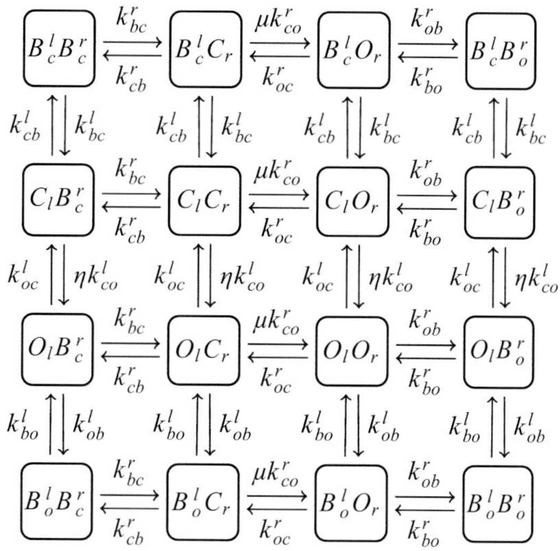

Fig. 9.1 The Markov model represented in Fig. 8.3 extended to account for blockers for the LCC and the RyR

9.2 Probability Density Functions Associated with the 16-State Model

As mentioned in Chap. 7 (see page 119), it is convenient to use a more compact notation to represent the system of partial differential equations governing the probability density functions when the Markov model consists of numerous states. By using the notation introduced in Chap. 7 , we can write the probability density system associated with the Markov model in Fig. 9.1 in the form

$$\frac{\partial \rho_{ij}}{\partial t} + \frac{\partial}{\partial x}\left(a_{ij}^{x}\rho_{ij}\right) + \frac{\partial}{\partial y}\left(a_{ij}^{y}\rho_{ij}\right) = R_{ij}, \tag{9.7}$$

where

$$R_{ij} = K_{i,j+1}^{i,j}\rho_{i,j+1} + K_{i+1,j}^{i,j}\rho_{i+1,j} + K_{i,j-1}^{i,j}\rho_{i,j-1} + K_{i-1,j}^{i,j}\rho_{i-1,j}$$
$$- \left(K_{i,j}^{i,j+1} + K_{i,j}^{i+1,j} + K_{i,j}^{i,j-1} + K_{i,j}^{i-1,j}\right)\rho_{i,j}.$$

The flux terms are given by

$$a_{ij}^{x} = \gamma_i^r v_r\,(y-x) + v_d\,(c_0 - x) - \gamma_j^l J_l,$$
$$a_{ij}^{y} = \gamma_i^r v_r\,(x-y) + v_s\,(c_1 - y),$$

where $\gamma_i^r = 1$ when the RyR state is open and $\gamma_i^r = 0$ when the RyR state is closed and similarly for γ^l and the LCC.

9.3 RyR Mutations Under a Varying Transmembrane Potential

In this section, we assume that a mutation affects the RyR such that the mutation severity index is increased. This problem has been discussed several times above, but here we also need to take into account that the value of the transmembrane potential may change. In our computations, we use $\mu = 3$ and we try to repair the effect of the mutation by adding a closed state blocker to the Markov model of the RyR channel. The Markov model is shown in Fig. 9.2.

The closed state drug applied to the RyR channel is represented by the two parameters k_{cb}^r and k_{bc}^r. We have seen above that for closed state blockers of the RyR it is reasonable to define

$$k_{cb}^r = (\mu - 1)\,k_{bc}^r,$$

where the value of k_{bc}^r remains to be decided.

$$
\begin{array}{ccccc}
C_l B_c^r & \underset{k_{cb}^r}{\overset{k_{bc}^r}{\rightleftarrows}} & C_l C_r & \underset{k_{oc}^r}{\overset{\mu k_{co}^r}{\rightleftarrows}} & C_l O_r \\
k_{oc}^l \uparrow\downarrow k_{co}^l & & k_{oc}^l \uparrow\downarrow k_{co}^l & & k_{oc}^l \uparrow\downarrow k_{co}^l \\
O_l B_c^r & \underset{k_{cb}^r}{\overset{k_{bc}^r}{\rightleftarrows}} & O_l C_r & \underset{k_{oc}^r}{\overset{\mu k_{co}^r}{\rightleftarrows}} & O_l O_r
\end{array}
$$

Fig. 9.2 The Markov model represented in Fig. 8.3 extended to include an RyR mutation and a closed state blocker for the RyR

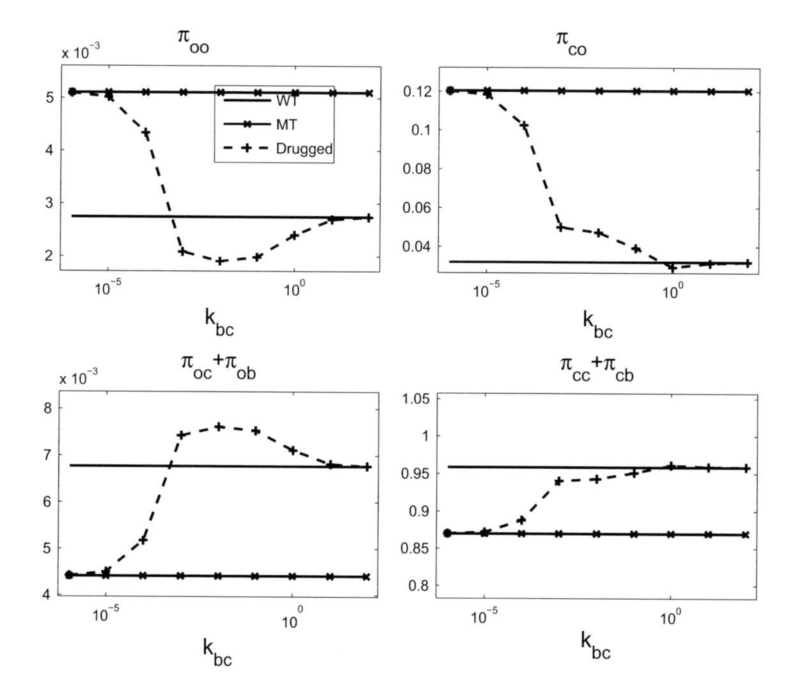

Fig. 9.3 Total probabilities based on the model for the probability density functions associated with the Markov model in Fig. 9.2. A closed state blocker is applied, the mutation severity index is $\mu = 3$, and the transmembrane potential is $V = 0$ mV. The *plots* show the total probability of being in the state OO, (OC+OB), CO, or (CC+CB) as a function of k_{bc}^r. In the *upper left plot*, the total probability of being in the OO state is higher for the mutant than for the wild type. This is repaired by the closed state drug. Similar results are shown for the other states

9.3.1 Theoretical Closed State Blocker Repairs the Open Probabilities of the RyR CO-Mutation

Numerical results using the closed state drug shown in Fig. 9.2 are given in Fig. 9.3. Note that we aim to repair the probability of being in the open state and are not

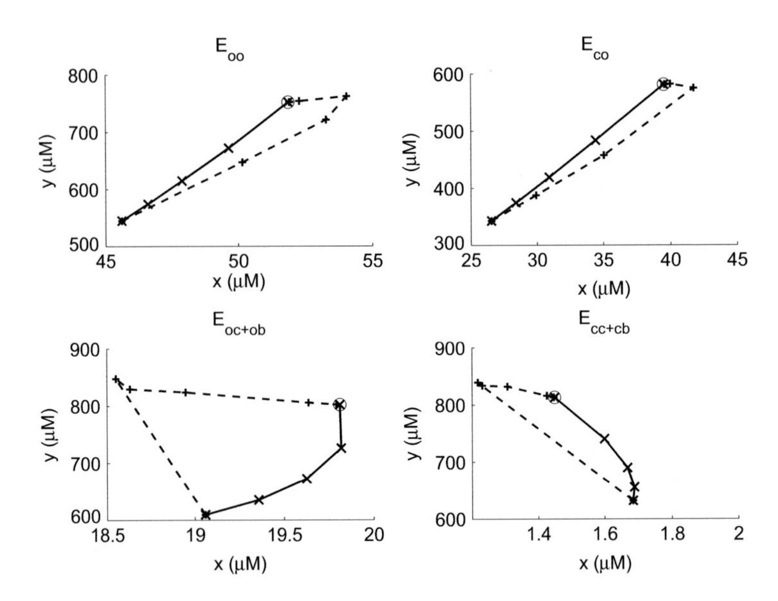

Fig. 9.4 Based on the probability density functions of the states OO, (OC+OB), CO, and (CC+CB), we can compute the expected concentrations of the dyad (x) and the JSR (y). The wild type is denoted by ∘ and the RyR mutation index μ increases from one to three along the *solid line*. In the *dashed line*, we keep $\mu = 3$ and increase the value of k_{bc}^r from 0 to 100 ms^{-1}. We observe that as k_{bc}^r increases, the expected concentrations are completely repaired. The experiment is carried out for the case of $V = 0$ mV

interested in whether the channel is in a blocked state or in a closed state. The probability of being in a closed or blocked state is therefore added in the graphs. We observe from the graphs that the mutant channel is completely repaired by the closed state blocker.

In Fig. 9.4, we show the development of the expected concentrations of the dyad (x) and the junctional sarcoplasmic reticulum (JSR) (y) and observe that the expected concentrations are repaired by a sufficiently strong version of the blocker associated with the closed state of the RyR channel.

9.3.2 *The Open State Blocker Does Not Work as Well as the Closed State Blocker for CO-Mutations in RyR*

In Table 9.2, we report on the performance of the open and closed state blockers for the RyR mutation. Recall that the probability π_{oo}, the expected dyad concentration (E_{oo}^x), and the expected JSR concentration (E_{oo}^y) are defined on page 72. The closed blocker clearly is best suited to repair this mutation.

Table 9.2 Properties of the probability density function (ρ_{oo}) of being in the state OO with $\mu = 3$ (and $\eta = 1$). The closed state blocker works fine in the sense that it is well suited for repairing a CO-mutation of the RyR. The open state blocker is unable to completely repair the effect of the mutation. The open state blocker is found using Matlab's *Fminsearch*, with a cost function defined to minimize the difference between the wild type and the mutation when the drug is applied. In this table, WT and MT mean wild type and mutant, respectively, and $V = 0$ mV is used in the simulations

	WT	MT	Optimal closed blocker	Optimal open blocker
$10^3 \times \pi_{oo}$	2.75	5.11	2.74	0.81
E^x_{oo}	51.87	45.62	51.92	52.46
E^y_{oo}	751.76	544.30	751.99	713.89

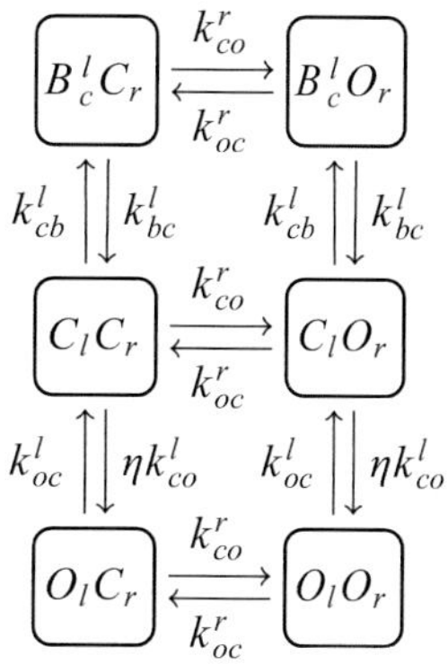

Fig. 9.5 The Markov model represented in Fig. 8.3 extended to include an LCC mutation and a closed state blocker for the LCC

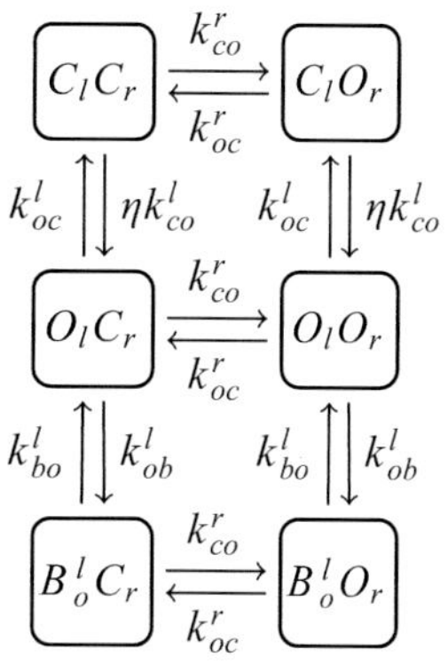

Fig. 9.6 The Markov model represented in Fig. 8.3 extended to include an LCC mutation and an open state blocker for the LCC

9.4 LCC Mutations Under a Varying Transmembrane Potential

Next, we address the problem of defining a theoretical drug for LCC mutations. We consider closed state LCC blockers of the form given in Fig. 9.5 and open state blockers of the form given in Fig. 9.6.

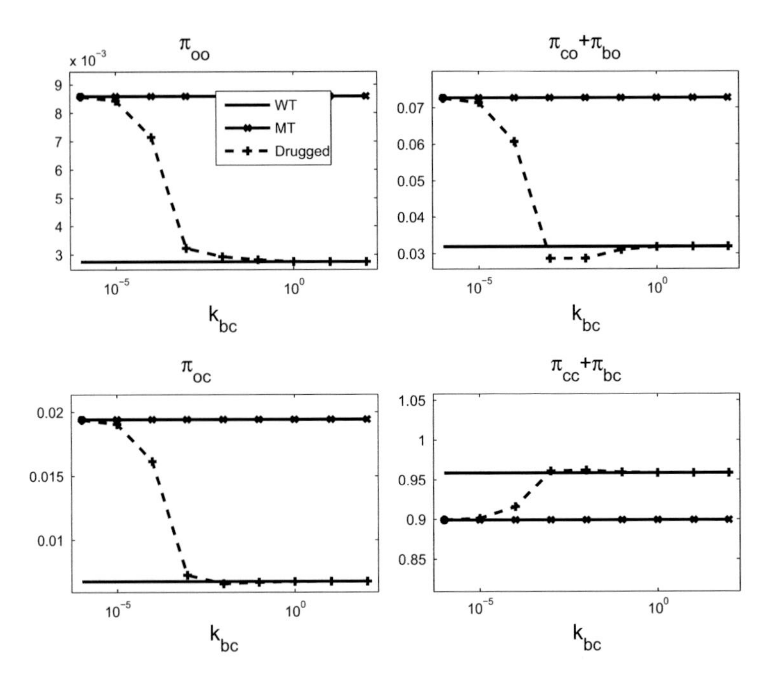

Fig. 9.7 Total probabilities based on the model for the probability density functions associated with the Markov model in Fig. 9.5, where an LCC-type closed state blocker is included. The LCC mutation severity index is $\eta = 3$ and the transmembrane potential is $V = 0$ mV. The *plots* show the total probability of being in the state OO, OC, (CO+BO), or (CC+BC) as a function of k^l_{bc}. In the *upper left plot*, the total probability of being in the OO state is higher for the mutant than for the wild type. This is repaired by the closed state drug. Similar results are shown for the other states

For the closed state blockers, we need to determine the two parameters k^l_{bc} and k^l_{cb} and for the open state blockers we must determine k^l_{bo} and k^l_{ob}. For the closed state blockers we define

$$k^l_{cb} = (\eta - 1)\, k^l_{bc}$$

and we consider various values of k^l_{bc}.

9.4.1 The Closed State Blocker Repairs the Open Probabilities of the LCC Mutant

The results of applying the theoretical closed state blocker associated with the closed state (see Fig. 9.5) of the LCC are given in Figs. 9.7, 9.8, and 9.9. In the first figure, we show how the closed state blocker repairs the total probabilities and in the

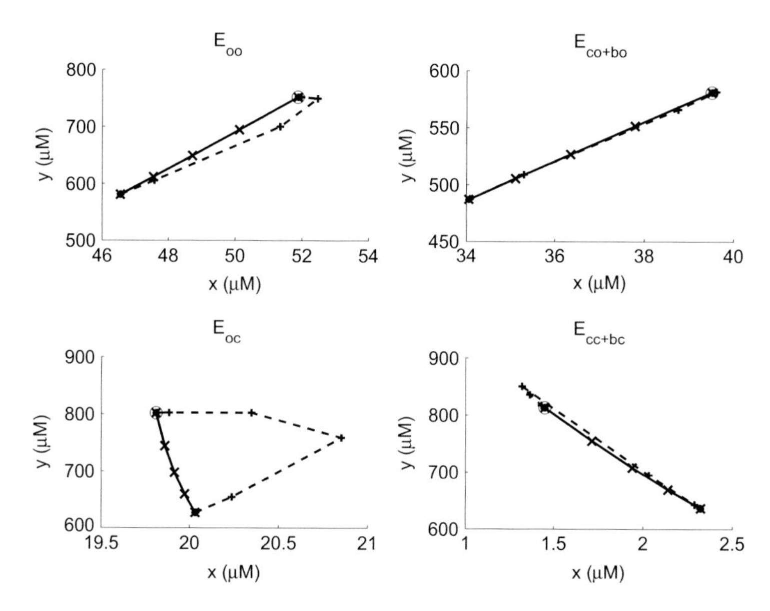

Fig. 9.8 Using the probability density functions of the states OO, OC, (CO+BO), and (CC+BC), we compute the expected concentrations of the dyad (x) and the JSR (y). The wild type is denoted by ◦ and the LCC mutation index η increases from one to three along the *solid line*. In the *dashed line*, we keep $\eta = 3$ and increase the value of k_{bc}^{l} from 0 to 100 ms^{-1}. We observe that as k_{bc}^{l} increases, the expected concentrations are completely repaired. The simulations are performed using $V = 0$ mV

second figure we consider the expected concentrations. In Fig. 9.9, we show how the expected concentrations are repaired for six values of the transmembrane potential.

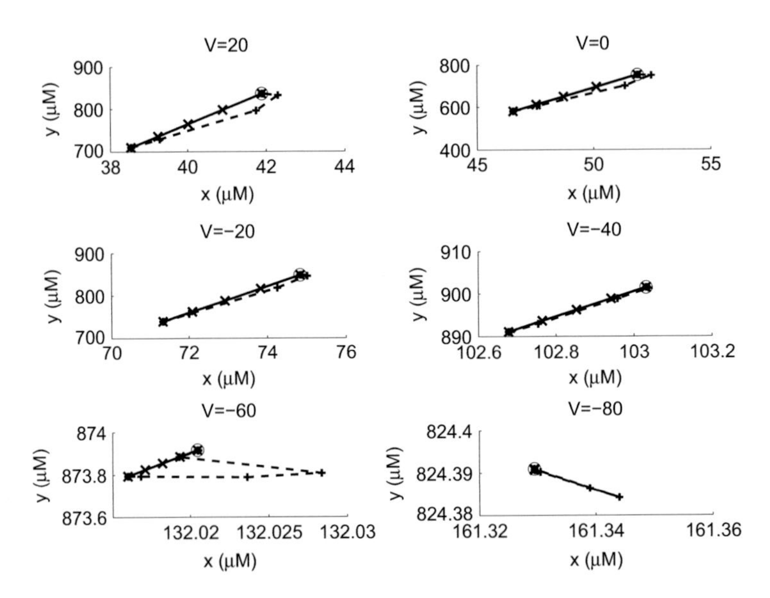

Fig. 9.9 The expected concentration of the dyad (x) and the JSR (y) for the OO state for the transmembrane potential changing from −80 to 20 mV. The wild type is denoted by ∘ and the LCC mutation index η increases from one to three along the *solid line*. In the *dashed line*, we keep $\eta = 3$ and increase the value of k_{bc}^{l} from 0 to 100 ms^{-1}. In all cases, the closed state blocker repairs the effect of the mutation

Chapter 10
A Prototypical Model of an Ion Channel

So far we have been concerned with calcium-induced calcium release (CICR) as illustrated in Fig. 8.2 (page 126). To study CICR, we started by studying the development of the concentration of calcium ions in the dyad and kept everything else constant. The interesting part was then to see how the release mechanism of the ryanodine receptor RyR changes the dynamics of the dyad concentration. In particular, we were interested in RyR mutations and their theoretical effect on the dyad concentration through changes in the open probability of the RyR channel. We saw how theoretical blockers could be defined in order to repair the effect of the mutations, in the sense that we were able to restore essential properties of the process. We also introduced the effect of allowing the concentration of the junctional sarcoplasmic reticulum to change and we studied how the overall processes were affected by introducing the transmembrane potential and allowing the L-type calcium channel (LCC) to open and close.

Now we leave the RyR and Markov models based on concentrations of calcium ions and focus on voltage-gated channels. We touched upon this topic earlier, since the LCC is voltage gated, but now we will dynamically update the voltage and focus solely on how voltage develops and how it affects the transitions of the Markov model.

We will start by studying a very simple channel to explain the basics steps as carefully as possible. This channel does not have a name and probably does not exist in nature, but it provides a good example to get a handle on the steps involved in understanding much more complex (and more realistic) ion channels.

In the study of CICR, we examined what was going on in a very small part of the cell based on the tacit assumption that if we can repair what is going on in every tiny part of the cell, we will probably also do a decent job in repairing all of the cell. We will follow the same strategy in studying voltage-gated channels: We will study a single channel and see how mutations may affect the function of the channel and thereby how the transmembrane potential is changed. Again, we will

A. Tveito, G.T. Lines, *Computing Characterizations of Drugs for Ion Channels and Receptors Using Markov Models*, Lecture Notes in Computational Science and Engineering 111, DOI 10.1007/978-3-319-30030-6_10

derive theoretical drugs and see how they should be defined in order to repair the effect of the mutations. However, the assumption that small domains can be studied independently is less reliable for voltage-gated channels than for the CICR process in the vicinity of the dyad. The reason for this is that electrical diffusion waves travel much faster than concentration waves.

10.1 Stochastic Model of the Transmembrane Potential

The transmembrane potential is defined to be the difference between the intracellular potential v_i and the extracellular potential v_e:

$$v = v_i - v_e. \tag{10.1}$$

Let us consider a membrane consisting of a leakage current with conductance given by g_L and an ion channel with conductance given by g_i. The transmembrane potential of such a membrane is governed by the differential equation

$$Cv' = -g_L (v - V_L) - g_i(v - V_i), \tag{10.2}$$

where C is the capacitance of the membrane, V_L is the resting potential of the leakage current, and V_i is the resting potential of the ion channel. In our computations, we will consider an example[1] with the parameters listed in Table 10.1. We assume that the ion channel can be either open (O), with $g_i = 1$ mS/cm^2, or closed (C), with $g_i = 0$ mS/cm^2. The state of the stochastic ion channel is governed by a Markov model of the form

$$C \underset{k_{co}}{\overset{k_{oc}}{\leftrightarrows}} O, \tag{10.3}$$

Table 10.1 Values of the parameters used in the model (10.2)

C	1 μF/cm^2
g_L	1/10 mS/cm^2
V_L	0 mV
V_i	11/10 mV

[1] Here, the choice of the parameter V_i may seem a bit strange, but we will see below that it will lead to a very simple computational domain for the probability density functions.

where the reactions rates will be specified below. With these definitions, the stochastic equation takes the form

$$v' = -\frac{1}{10}v - \gamma\left(v - \frac{11}{10}\right), \tag{10.4}$$

where γ is zero (closed) or one (open) depending on the state of the Markov model (10.3).

10.1.1 A Numerical Scheme

We compute numerical solutions of the model (10.4) using the scheme

$$v_{n+1} = v_n - \Delta t\left(\frac{1}{10}v_n + \gamma_n\left(v_n - \frac{11}{10}\right)\right), \tag{10.5}$$

where Δt denotes the time step and γ_n takes on values based on the state of the Markov model. Based on the Markov model, the value of γ_n is computed as described on page 28. We assume that the time step (in ms) satisfies the condition

$$\Delta t < \frac{10}{11}. \tag{10.6}$$

10.1.2 An Invariant Region

We discussed above that it is useful to derive an invariant region for the stochastic model since such a region can be used to define the computational domain of the probability density equation. We claim that, under the condition (10.6) for the time step, the solutions generated by scheme (10.5) will always remain in the interval given by

$$\Omega = (0, 1),$$

provided that the initial condition is in this region. To show that Ω is an invariant region for solutions generated by scheme (10.5), we write the scheme in the form

$$v_{n+1} = H(v_n, \gamma_n),$$

where

$$H(v, \gamma) = v - \Delta t\left(\frac{1}{10}v + \gamma\left(v - \frac{11}{10}\right)\right).$$

Since

$$\frac{\partial H(v,\gamma)}{\partial v} = 1 - \Delta t\left(\frac{1}{10} + \gamma\right) > 0$$

because of (10.6) and

$$\frac{\partial H(v,\gamma)}{\partial \gamma} = \Delta t\left(\frac{11}{10} - v\right) > 0$$

for any $v \in \Omega$, we have

$$v_{n+1} = H(v_n, \gamma_n) \leqslant H(1,1) = 1$$

and

$$v_{n+1} = H(v_n, \gamma_n) \geqslant H(0,0) = 0.$$

So, by induction, we have $v_n \in \Omega$ for all n.

10.2 Probability Density Functions for the Voltage-Gated Channel

We can now follow exactly the same steps as in Sect. 2.2 (see page 30) to derive a model of the probability density functions of the open state and the closed state. The probability of the channel being in the open state for voltages between v and $v + \Delta v$ is given by

$$P_o\{v < V(t) < v + \Delta v\} = \int_v^{v+\Delta v} \rho_o(w,t)dw,$$

where ρ_o is the probability density function of the open state. Similarly, we have

$$P_c\{v < V(t) < v + \Delta v\} = \int_v^{v+\Delta v} \rho_c(w,t)dw$$

where ρ_c is the probability density function of the closed state. By the arguments given in Sect. 2.2, we find that the probability density functions must be solutions of the system

$$\frac{\partial \rho_o}{\partial t} + \frac{\partial}{\partial v}(a_o\rho_o) = k_{co}\rho_c - k_{oc}\rho_o, \tag{10.7}$$
$$\frac{\partial \rho_c}{\partial t} + \frac{\partial}{\partial v}(a_c\rho_c) = k_{oc}\rho_o - k_{co}\rho_c,$$

where the flux terms are given by

$$a_o = -g_L(v - V_L) - (v - V_i) = \frac{11}{10}(1 - v), \tag{10.8}$$
$$a_c = -g_L(v - V_L) = -\frac{1}{10}v$$

As usual, the boundary conditions are set up to avoid a probability leak across the boundary. Hence we need the fluxes $a_o\rho_o$ and $a_c\rho_c$ to be zero for $v = 0$ and $v = 1$. Note that $a_o(1) = a_c(0) = 0$; so we require $\rho_o(0) = 0$ and $\rho_c(1) = 0$. In the numerical simulations presented below, we use the scheme described in Sect. 2.3. Stationary solutions of the numerical scheme are computed as described on page 44.

10.3 Analytical Solution of the Stationary Case

We showed in Sect. 2.6 how an analytical solution can be derived for a stationary system of the form (10.7). Here we shall repeat this derivation for a voltage-gated channel. For simplicity we shall consider a channel where the reaction scheme of the Markov model is independent of the voltage; we choose

$$k_{oc} = 1 \text{ ms}^{-1} \text{ and } k_{co} = \mu \text{ ms}^{-1}.$$

So, we will again focus on CO-mutations. Here μ, referred to as the mutation severity index, will be specified in the computations below. In all computations, $\mu = 1$ will be referred to as the wild type case. Increased values of k_{co} will increase the open probability of the ion channel in (10.2) and therefore bring the transmembrane potential closer to the maximum value (given by $V_+ = 1$ mV).

The first step in the derivation of the analytical solution is to observe that, in the steady state, the sum of the equations of (10.7) results in the equation

$$\frac{\partial}{\partial v}(a_o\rho_o + a_c\rho_c) = 0.$$

The second step is to observe that the boundary conditions imply that

$$a_o\rho_o + a_c\rho_c = 0.$$

Therefore, for the present model, we find that

$$\rho_c = -\frac{a_o}{a_c}\rho_o = \frac{11}{v}(1-v)\,\rho_o$$

and, from (10.7), we have

$$\frac{\partial}{\partial v}(a_o\rho_o) = \mu\rho_c - \rho_o = \left(11\mu\frac{1-v}{v} - 1\right)\rho_o.$$

By differentiation, we obtain

$$a_o\frac{\partial}{\partial v}\rho_o = \left(11\mu\frac{1-v}{v} - 1 - \frac{\partial}{\partial v}a_o\right)\rho_o$$

and thus

$$\rho_o' = a(v)\rho_o, \tag{10.9}$$

where

$$a(v) = \left(\frac{10\mu}{v} + \frac{1}{11(1-v)}\right).$$

The solution of (10.9) is given by

$$\rho_o = c\frac{v^{10\mu}}{(1-v)^{1/11}} \tag{10.10}$$

and then

$$\rho_c = 11c\,(1-v)^{10/11}\,v^{10\mu-1}.$$

Here the constant c must be chosen such that

$$\int_\Omega (\rho_o + \rho_c)\,dv = 1.$$

It is interesting to note here that, even if both ρ_o and ρ_c depend heavily on the mutation severity index μ, the relation between these functions is independent of μ since

$$\frac{\rho_o}{\rho_c} = \frac{v}{11(1-v)}.$$

10.4 Comparison of Monte Carlo Simulations and Probability Density Functions

In previous chapters we gave many examples showing that the probability density functions faithfully represent the frequency distributions that can be computed using Monte Carlo simulations. We will briefly show that this also holds for the ion channel model considered here. In Fig. 10.1, we compare the open probability density function given by (10.10) and a histogram computed using Monte Carlo simulations based on the numerical scheme given by (10.5). We observe again—and by now we are starting to get used to it—that the probability density functions more or less coincide with the histograms computed using Monte Carlo simulations.[2]

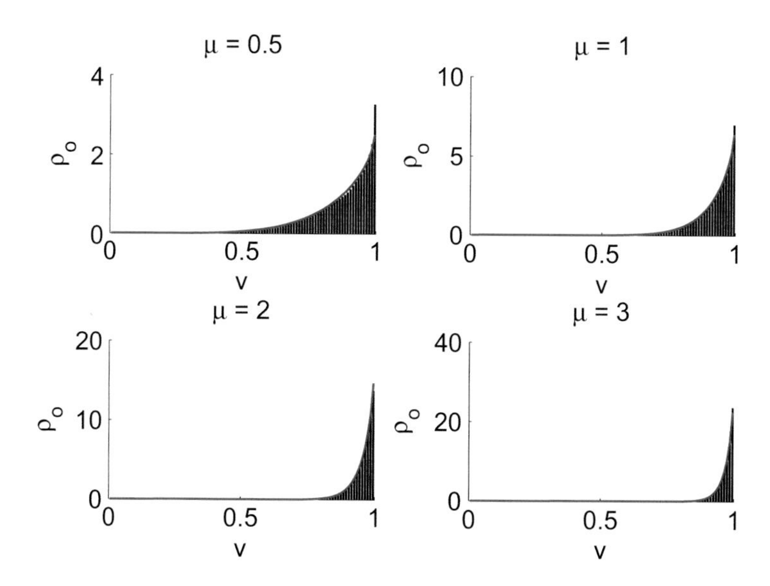

Fig. 10.1 Comparison of the results of Monte Carlo simulations (histogram) and analytical solutions of the system governing the probability density functions for four values of the mutation severity index μ. The unit interval is divided into 100 sub-intervals where the number of occurrences is counted in the Monte Carlo simulations. The analytical solutions are evaluated in the center of these sub-intervals. Each case was simulated for 10 s, with $\Delta t = 0.01$ ms

[2] At this point it feels appropriate to remind the reader of one of the many great quotes by John von Neumann: "In mathematics you don't understand things. You just get used to them."

10.5 Mutations and Theoretical Drugs

In our analysis of the RyR, we studied the effect of mutations increasing the open probability of the channel. In addition, for voltage-gated ion channels, mutations may affect the open probability of the channel and thereby change the dynamics of the transmembrane potential. We will study specific examples of this below, where we present actual mutations and their effect on actual ion channels, such as the sodium channel. However, for the time being, we will stick to our not so realistic but rather cute model. We will assume that the stochastic dynamics of the transmembrane potential are governed by (10.2), that the probability density functions are governed by (10.7), and that the Markov model is given by

$$C \underset{k_{co}}{\overset{k_{oc}}{\leftrightarrows}} O, \tag{10.11}$$

where $k_{oc} = 1\ \text{ms}^{-1}$ and $k_{co} = \mu\ \text{ms}^{-1}$. As usual, μ is the mutation severity index and $\mu = 1$ denotes the wild type case. Motivated by the results for the RyR mutations, we will try to repair the effect of the mutation using an open or a closed state blocker. This will prove to be quite efficient, since we are dealing with a CO-mutation.

10.5.1 *Theoretical Open State Blocker*

The Markov model of the theoretical open state blocker is

$$C \underset{k_{co}}{\overset{k_{oc}}{\leftrightarrows}} O \underset{k_{ob}}{\overset{k_{bo}}{\leftrightarrows}} B, \tag{10.12}$$

where the parameters k_{bo} and k_{ob} need to be determined. The associated steady state version of the probability density system is given by

$$\begin{aligned} \frac{\partial}{\partial v}(a_o\rho_o) &= k_{co}\rho_c - (k_{oc} + k_{ob})\,\rho_o + k_{bo}\rho_b, \\ \frac{\partial}{\partial v}(a_c\rho_c) &= k_{oc}\rho_o - k_{co}\rho_c, \\ \frac{\partial}{\partial v}(a_c\rho_b) &= k_{ob}\rho_o - k_{bo}\rho_b, \end{aligned} \tag{10.13}$$

where ρ_o, ρ_c, and ρ_b denote the probability density functions of the open (O), closed (C), and blocked (B) states, respectively. We compute optimal values of the parameters k_{bo} and k_{ob} using the *Fminsearch* function in Matlab applied to the difference between the open probability density function computed by solving (10.13) and the wild type solution given by system (10.7), with $\mu = 1$. The function used in the minimization is given by

$$\frac{\sqrt{\int |\rho_{o,\mathrm{mt+d}} - \rho_{o,\mathrm{wt}}|^2 dv}}{\sqrt{\int \rho_{o,\mathrm{wt}}^2 dv}},$$

where $\rho_{o,\mathrm{wt}}$ is the wild type open probability density function and $\rho_{o,\mathrm{mt+d}}$ is the mutant open probability density function where the theoretical drug is applied.

10.5.2 Theoretical Closed State Blocker

The Markov model of the theoretical closed state blocker is

$$B \underset{k_{bc}}{\overset{k_{cb}}{\leftrightarrows}} C \underset{k_{co}}{\overset{k_{oc}}{\leftrightarrows}} O, \tag{10.14}$$

where the parameters k_{cb} and k_{bc} must be computed. Following the arguments on page 58, we find that these parameters must be related as

$$k_{cb} = (\mu - 1)\, k_{bc} \tag{10.15}$$

and thus we are left with the task of finding a proper value for only one parameter: k_{bc}. Of course, based on what we learned for the RyR channel, we suspect that k_{bc} should be as large as possible. The computations reported below will verify this suspicion.

The steady state version of the probability density system associated with the Markov model (10.14) is given by

$$\begin{aligned}
\frac{\partial}{\partial v}(a_o\rho_o) &= k_{co}\rho_c - k_{oc}\rho_o, \\
\frac{\partial}{\partial v}(a_c\rho_c) &= k_{oc}\rho_o - (k_{co} + (\mu - 1)\, k_{bc})\, \rho_c + k_{bc}\rho_b, \\
\frac{\partial}{\partial v}(a_c\rho_b) &= (\mu - 1)\, k_{bc}\rho_c - k_{bc}\rho_b,
\end{aligned} \tag{10.16}$$

where, again, ρ_o, ρ_c, and ρ_b denote the probability density functions of the open (O), closed (C), and blocked (B) states, respectively. Here, the value of k_{bc} characterizing the drug remains to be determined and will be discussed below.

10.5.3 Numerical Computations Using the Theoretical Blockers

Let us start by showing that the closed state blocker is improved by increasing values of k_{bc}. In Fig. 10.2, we show the numerical solutions of system (10.16) with increasing values of k_{bc} for four values of the mutation severity index μ. We observe, as expected, that the drug is improved as k_{bc} is increased.

In Fig. 10.3, we compare a good theoretical closed state blocker (using $k_{bc} = 100\ \text{ms}^{-1}$) and the best open state blocker for four values of the mutation severity index μ. This figure does not reveal much difference between the two alternative blockers, but we will see below that the statistical properties of the solutions show that there is a significant difference.

10.5.4 Statistical Properties of the Theoretical Drugs

To further compare the properties of the drugs, it is useful to use the statistical properties introduced above. We recall that the probability of being in state i is

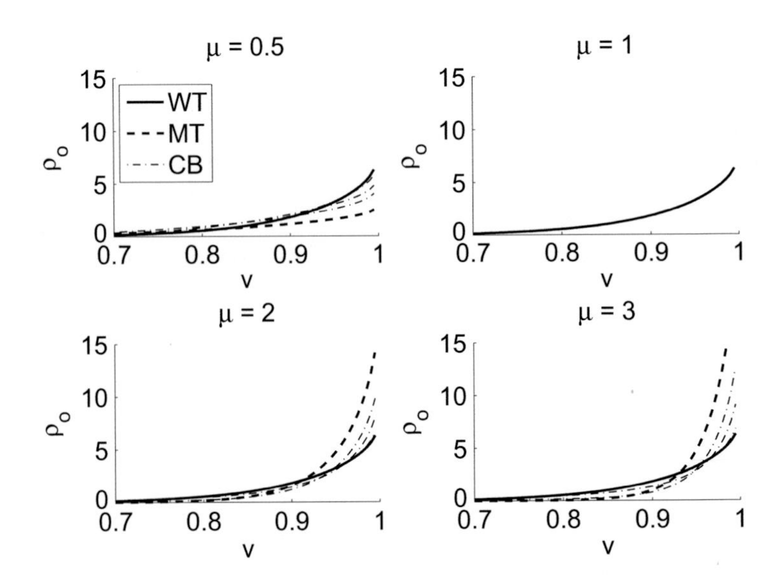

Fig. 10.2 The open probability density functions of the wild type (WT), mutants (MT) and mutants in the presence of the closed state blocker (CB) for four values of the mutation severity index μ. We use $k_{bc} = 0.1,\ 1,\ 10,\ 100\ \text{ms}^{-1}$ and observe that, for the largest value of k_{bc}, the drugged solutions are virtually indistinguishable from the wild type solution

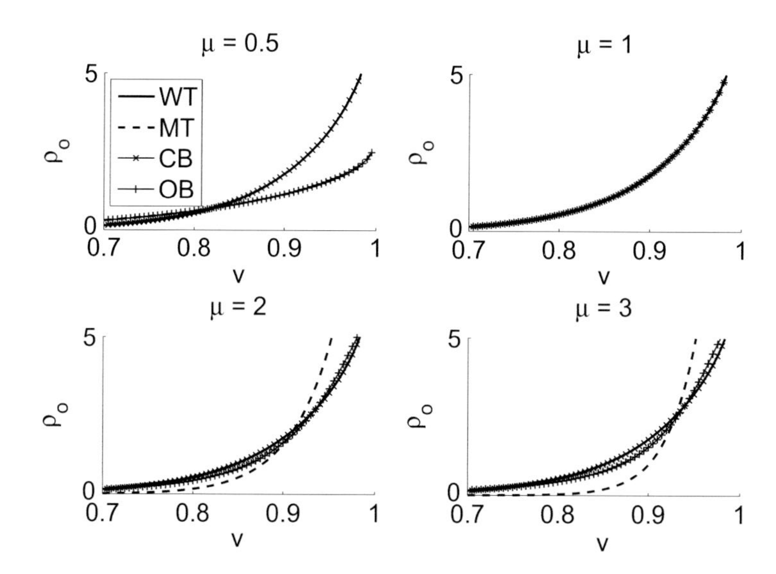

Fig. 10.3 Comparison of the best closed and open state blockers for four values of the mutation severity index. For the case $\mu = 0.5$ the optimization did not find any open state blockers that helped (the solution for the mutant in the presence of the open state blocker (OB) is superimposed on the solution for the mutant (MT) in the lower trace.) We found the following specifications of the open state blockers to be optimal: For $\mu = 2$, we used $k_{bo} = 0.37\ \mathrm{ms}^{-1}$ and $k_{ob} = 0.21\ \mathrm{ms}^{-1}$ and, for $\mu = 3$, we used $k_{bo} = 0.45\ \mathrm{ms}^{-1}$ and $k_{ob} = 0.35\ \mathrm{ms}^{-1}$. In all cases, we used the closed state blocker characterized by $k_{bc} = 100\ \mathrm{ms}^{-1}$ and $k_{cb} = (\mu - 1)\, k_{bc}$

given by

$$\pi_i = \int_\Omega \rho_i dv,$$

where $i = o, c$, or b for the open, closed, or blocked state, respectively. The expected value of the transmembrane potential under the condition that the channel is open, closed, or blocked is given by

$$E_i = \frac{1}{\pi_i} \int_\Omega v \rho_i dv,$$

for $i = o, c$, or b, respectively. Finally, for $i = o, c$, or b, the standard deviations are given by

$$\sigma_i^2 = \frac{1}{\pi_i} \int_\Omega v^2 \rho_i dv - E_i^2.$$

Table 10.2 Statistics of the open probability density functions in the case of $\mu = 3$. The closed state blocker is given by $k_{bc} = 100\ \text{ms}^{-1}$ and $k_{cb} = (\mu - 1)\, k_{bc}$ and the open state blocker is given by $k_{bo} = 0.45\ \text{ms}^{-1}$ and $k_{ob} = 0.35\ \text{ms}^{-1}$

	WT	MT	CB	OB
π_o	0.500	0.750	0.500	0.478
E_o	0.922	0.969	0.922	0.919
σ_o	0.076	0.031	0.076	0.088

In Table 10.2, we compare the statistical properties of the solutions based on different theoretical blockers. We see that the mutation significantly increases the open probability but leaves the expected value of the transmembrane potential more or less unchanged. The standard deviation, however, is significantly reduced by the mutation.

Both the open and closed state blockers are able to significantly reduce the effect of the mutations, as illustrated in Fig. 10.3. However, the closed state blocker is slightly better at this than the optimal open state blocker.

10.6 Notes

1. The equation

$$Cv' = -g_L\,(v - V_L) - g_i(v - V_i) \tag{10.17}$$

(see (10.2)) underpins this chapter and most of the rest of these lecture notes. It is a classical equation and derivations are found in numerous places. A thorough discussion is given in the classical text by Plonsey and Barr [66]. The basic idea of the derivation is to equate the flux of ions through the membrane with the associated change of the charge in the extracellular and intracellular domains.

Chapter 11
Inactivated Ion Channels: Extending the Prototype Model

Experimental evidence suggests that some ion channels can take on three main states: open (O), closed (C), or inactivated (I). Here both C and I mean that the channel is non-conducting, but when the channel is inactivated, it is harder to open again than when the channel is in the closed state. This feature is useful in modeling an action potential. In the action potential of a cardiac cell, the upstroke is driven mainly by the sodium current. When the upstroke is completed, the sodium channels are inactivated to avoid spurious new upstrokes before the cell has undergone a restitution period. Certain mutations impair the ability of the channel to deactivate, which may lead to arrhythmias. We will return to this topic below. Here, it suffices to state that we need to introduce an inactivated state in the prototype model discussed above.

The stochastic model considered in this chapter is the same as in Chap. 10

$$Cv' = -g_L (v - V_L) - g_i(v - V_i), \tag{11.1}$$

with the parameters given in Table 10.1 on page 154.

11.1 Three-State Markov Model

The reaction scheme of an ion channel taking on the three states O, C, and I is given in Fig. 11.1. To model the properties of the action potential in the way we described above, we need to introduce reaction rates that depend on the transmembrane potential v. At this point, we just want to derive a prototypical model and we

A. Tveito, G.T. Lines, *Computing Characterizations of Drugs for Ion Channels and Receptors Using Markov Models*, Lecture Notes in Computational Science and Engineering 111, DOI 10.1007/978-3-319-30030-6_11

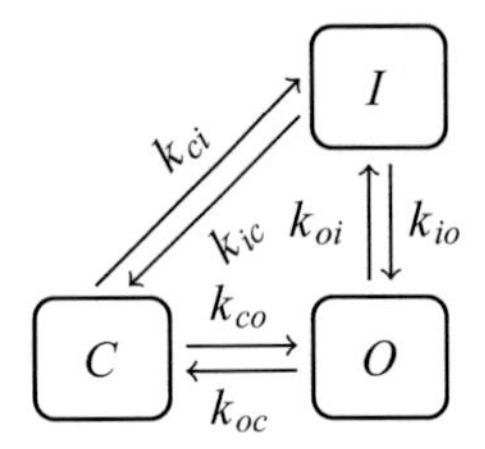

Fig. 11.1 Markov model including three possible states: open (O), closed (C), and inactivated (I)

therefore, admittedly somewhat arbitrarily, define the following rates:

$$\begin{aligned} k_{co} &= \frac{k_{co}^{\infty}}{\tau_{co}}, \quad k_{oc} = \frac{1-k_{co}^{\infty}}{\tau_{co}}, \\ k_{oi} &= 1, \qquad k_{io} = \frac{k_{co}k_{oi}k_{ic}}{k_{oc}k_{ci}}, \\ k_{ic} &= e^{-30v}, \; k_{ci} = \frac{1}{100}, \end{aligned} \tag{11.2}$$

where

$$k_{co}^{\infty} = \frac{1}{1+e^{6-16v}}$$

and

$$\tau_{co} = \frac{1}{10}.$$

By the definition of k_{io}, these rates satisfy the principle of detailed balance (see page 10 and the notes of Chap. 1).

11.1.1 Equilibrium Probabilities

We saw above (see page 8) that the equilibrium state of the reaction shown in Fig. 11.1 is given by

$$\begin{aligned} o &= \frac{1}{1+\frac{k_{oc}}{k_{co}}+\frac{k_{oi}}{k_{io}}}, \\ c &= \frac{\frac{k_{oc}}{k_{co}}}{1+\frac{k_{oc}}{k_{co}}+\frac{k_{oi}}{k_{io}}}, \\ i &= \frac{\frac{k_{oi}}{k_{io}}}{1+\frac{k_{oc}}{k_{co}}+\frac{k_{oi}}{k_{io}}}. \end{aligned}$$

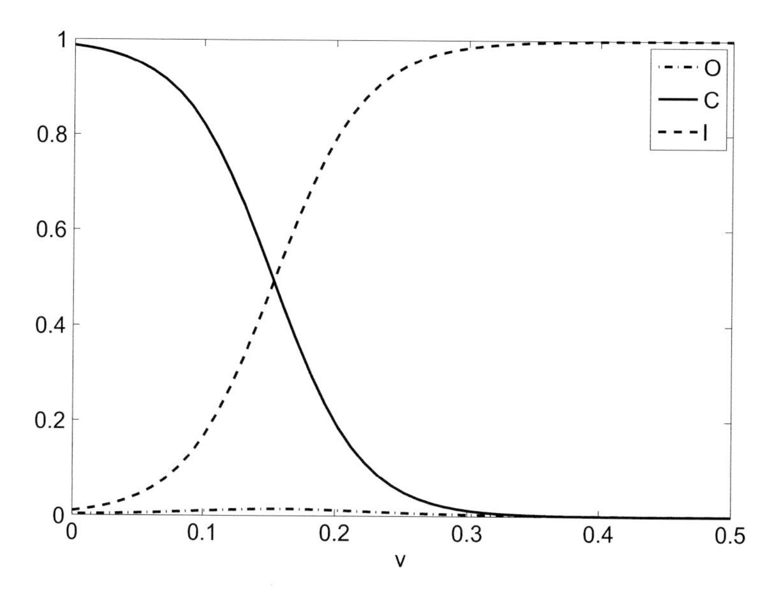

Fig. 11.2 Equilibrium probabilities of the open, closed, and inactivated states as functions of the transmembrane potential v

These probabilities are graphed as functions of the transmembrane potential in Fig. 11.2. Note that the open probability in equilibrium is quite small; the channel is basically closed for v close to zero and it is inactivated for large values of v.

11.2 Probability Density Functions in the Presence of the Inactivated State

When the inactivated state is included in the model, as indicated in Fig. 11.1, the system governing the associated probability density functions is given by

$$\frac{\partial \rho_o}{\partial t} + \frac{\partial}{\partial v}(a_o \rho_o) = k_{co}\rho_c - (k_{oc} + k_{oi})\rho_o + k_{io}\rho_i, \tag{11.3}$$

$$\frac{\partial \rho_c}{\partial t} + \frac{\partial}{\partial v}(a_c \rho_c) = k_{oc}\rho_o - (k_{co} + k_{ci})\rho_c + k_{ic}\rho_i, \tag{11.4}$$

$$\frac{\partial \rho_i}{\partial t} + \frac{\partial}{\partial v}(a_c \rho_i) = k_{oi}\rho_o - (k_{io} + k_{ic})\rho_i + k_{ci}\rho_c, \tag{11.5}$$

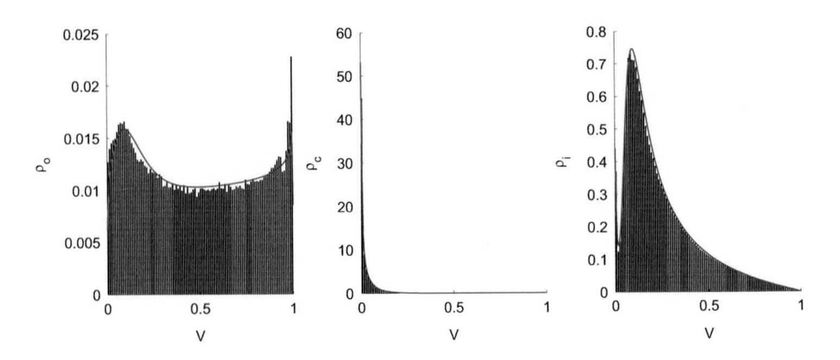

Fig. 11.3 Probability density functions of the open, closed, and inactivated states (*red lines*) computed as numerical solutions of the system (11.3)–(11.5) and histograms based on Monte Carlo simulations using the stochastic differential equation (11.1)

where

$$a_o = -g_L(v - V_L) - (v - V_i) = \frac{11}{10}(1 - v), \tag{11.6}$$

$$a_c = -g_L(v - V_L) = -\frac{1}{10}v.$$

11.2.1 Numerical Simulations

Again, we want to compare the solution computed by Monte Carlo simulations based on the stochastic differential equation given in (11.1) and the probability density functions defined by the system (11.3)–(11.5). The numerical results are given in their usual form in Fig. 11.3. As expected, the histograms computed using Monte Carlo simulations and the numerical solution of the system (11.3)–(11.5) are quite similar. In these computations, the stochastic simulation ran for 100 s, with $\Delta t = 0.01$ ms, and we used the mesh size $\Delta v = 0.01$ in the numerical solution of the system (11.3)–(11.5). It is particularly interesting to see that the tiny boundary layer close to $v = 0$ for the probability density function of the inactivated state is captured using both the Monte Carlo and the probability density function approaches.

11.3 Mutations Affecting the Inactivated State of the Ion Channel

Certain mutations of the sodium channel are known to impair the channel's ability to deactivate. We introduce a mutation severity index μ and assume that the reaction rates of the mutant are changed such that both the probabilities of moving from

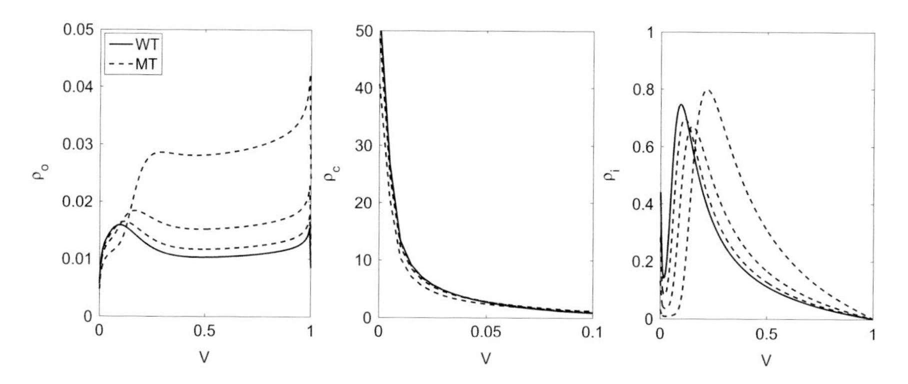

Fig. 11.4 Probability density functions of the open, closed, and inactivated states for the wild type and for three values of the mutation severity index: $\mu = 1.5, 3, 10$. Larger values of μ give solutions farther away from the wild type solution (*solid line*). The probability density of the closed state is only shown for v between 0 and 0.1 to magnify very small differences

the inactivated to the closed state and from the inactivated to the open state are increased. The effect of these changes will clearly be to lower the probability of the channel being in the inactivated state.

In mathematical terms, we define

$$\bar{k}_{ic} = \mu k_{ic}, \tag{11.7}$$
$$\bar{k}_{io} = \mu k_{io},$$

where $\mu \geqslant 1$ and where k_{ic} and k_{io} are the wild type reaction rates given by (11.2). It should be noted that the new reaction rates still satisfy the principle of detailed balance. In Fig. 11.4, we show the equilibrium probability density functions of the open, closed, and inactivated states for the wild type and for three values of the mutation severity index μ.

11.4 A Theoretical Drug for Mutations Affecting the Inactivation

We want to derive a theoretical drug repairing the effect of the mutation described in (11.7). In the Markov model illustrated in Fig. 11.5, we have introduced a blocked state associated with the open, closed, and inactivated state and we now want to figure out what the best choice might be. The equilibrium solution of the reaction

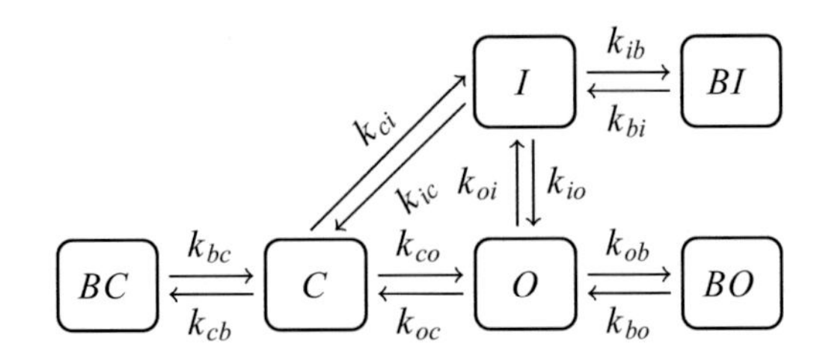

Fig. 11.5 The model represented in Fig. 11.1 extended to account for blockers associated with the closed state (BC), the open state (BO), and inactivated state (BI)

represented in Fig. 11.5 is characterized by the equations

$$k_{co}c = k_{oc}o,\ k_{ci}c = k_{ic}i,$$
$$k_{oi}o = k_{io}i,\ k_{bc}b_c = k_{cb}c,$$
$$k_{bo}b_o = k_{ob}o,\ k_{bi}b_i = k_{ib}i.$$

It is useful to define

$$r_{xy} = \frac{k_{xy}}{k_{yx}}$$

and to note that

$$r_{xy} = \frac{1}{r_{yx}}.$$

With this notation, the principle of detailed balance stating that

$$\frac{k_{co}k_{oi}k_{ic}}{k_{oc}k_{io}k_{ci}} = 1$$

can be written as

$$r_{co}r_{oi}r_{ic} = r_{oc}r_{io}r_{ci} = 1.$$

The equations above can now be written as

$$c = r_{oc}o,\ c = r_{ic}i,$$
$$o = r_{io}i,\ b_c = r_{cb}c,$$
$$b_o = r_{ob}o,\ b_i = r_{ib}i.$$

It is convenient to express all probabilities in terms of the open probability:

$$
\begin{aligned}
c &= r_{oc} o, \\
i &= r_{oi} o, \\
b_c &= r_{cb} c = r_{cb} r_{oc} o, \\
b_o &= r_{ob} o, \\
b_i &= r_{ib} i = r_{ib} r_{oi} o.
\end{aligned}
$$

Since $c + i + o + b_c + b_o + b_i = 1$, we have

$$o = p^{-1},$$

where

$$p = 1 + r_{oc}\left(1 + r_{cb}\right) + r_{oi}\left(1 + r_{ib}\right) + r_{ob}.$$

We refer to p as the inverse open probability and we note that for the wild type it is given by

$$p = 1 + r_{oc} + r_{oi}.$$

11.4.1 Open Probability in the Mutant Case

As discussed above, we are interested in understanding how to define a theoretical drug for mutations affecting the inactivation of the ion channel. We assume that the mutation affects the inactivation in a way that reduces the probability of being in the inactivated state. As mentioned above, this can be modeled by increasing the reaction rates from the inactivated state to both the closed and the open states. We assume that

$$\bar{k}_{ic} = \mu k_{ic}, \; \bar{k}_{io} = \mu k_{io},$$

where $\mu \geqslant 1$ is the mutation severity index. This gives

$$\bar{r}_{ic} = \frac{\bar{k}_{ic}}{k_{ci}} = \mu r_{ic}$$

and

$$\bar{r}_{io} = \frac{\bar{k}_{io}}{k_{oi}} = \mu r_{io}.$$

We assume that the reaction rates between the closed and open states are unaffected by the mutation and therefore

$$\bar{r}_{oc} = r_{oc}.$$

Detailed balance dictates that we should have

$$(\mu k_{ic})k_{co}k_{oi} = (\mu k_{io})k_{oc}k_{ci},$$

which holds regardless of the choice of μ, since the wild type rates satisfy the principle of detailed balance.

The inverse open probability in the presence of the mutations is given by

$$\bar{p} = 1 + r_{oc} + \bar{r}_{oi} = 1 + r_{oc} + 1/\bar{r}_{io} = 1 + r_{oc} + \frac{1}{\mu r_{io}} = 1 + r_{oc} + \frac{r_{oi}}{\mu}.$$

11.4.2 The Open Probability in the Presence of the Theoretical Drug

When the drug given in Fig. 11.5 is applied, the inverse open probability is

$$p_b = 1 + r_{oc}\left(1 + r_{cb}\right) + \frac{r_{oi}}{\mu}\left(1 + r_{ib}\right) + r_{ob}$$

where r_{cb}, r_{ib}, and r_{ob} are used to characterize the drug. Our aim is to now use these parameters to tune the drug such that

$$p_b \approx p,$$

where p is the inverse open probability of the wild type. More precisely, we want to determine the constants r_{cb}, r_{ib}, and r_{ob} such that

$$1 + r_{oc}\left(1 + r_{cb}\right) + \frac{r_{oi}}{\mu}\left(1 + r_{ib}\right) + r_{ob} \approx 1 + r_{oc} + r_{oi}$$

holds for all relevant values of the transmembrane potential v. We observe that if we put $r_{cb} = r_{ob} = 0$, we obtain the condition

$$\frac{r_{oi}}{\mu}\left(1 + r_{ib}\right) \approx r_{oi}$$

and therefore we set

$$r_{ib} = \mu - 1.$$

We conclude that we can repair the equilibrium state of the mutation completely by applying a drug consisting of a blocker of the inactivated state, provided that the reaction rates of the drug satisfy

$$\frac{k_{ib}}{k_{bi}} = \mu - 1,$$

where μ is the severity index of the mutation. This means that we have reduced the problem of finding a drug to a single parameter given by k_{bi}. This remaining degree of freedom will be addressed below.

11.5 Probability Density Functions Using the Blocker of the Inactivated State

In Sect. 11.2 above, we derived a system governing the probability density functions of the open, closed, and inactivated states. Here, we want to extend the system to account for the theoretical drug represented by a blocker of the inactivated state. The Markov model of the drug is given in Fig. 11.6. The drug will completely repair the equilibrium state of the Markov model, provided that

$$k_{ib} = (\mu - 1)\, k_{bi}, \tag{11.8}$$

where μ is the mutation severity index of the mutation (see (11.7)). The stationary probability density functions of the states in the Markov model of Fig. 11.6 are governed by the system

$$\frac{\partial}{\partial v}(a_o \rho_o) = k_{co}\rho_c - (k_{oc} + k_{oi})\,\rho_o + \mu k_{io}\rho_i, \tag{11.9}$$

$$\frac{\partial}{\partial v}(a_c \rho_c) = k_{oc}\rho_o - (k_{co} + k_{ci})\,\rho_c + \mu k_{ic}\rho_i, \tag{11.10}$$

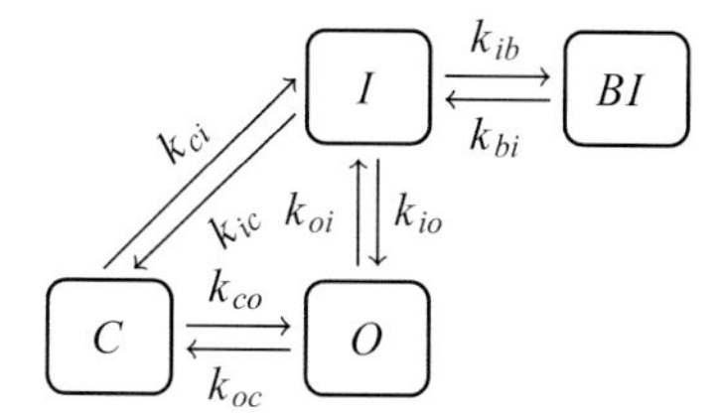

Fig. 11.6 Markov model of the prototype ion channel with a blocker associated with the inactivated state

$$\frac{\partial}{\partial v}(a_c \rho_i) = k_{oi}\rho_o - (\mu k_{io} + \mu k_{ic} + (\mu - 1) k_{bi})\rho_i + k_{ci}\rho_c + k_{bi}\rho_b, \tag{11.11}$$

$$\frac{\partial}{\partial v}(a_c \rho_b) = (\mu - 1) k_{bi}\rho_i - k_{bi}\rho_b, \tag{11.12}$$

where ρ_o, ρ_c, ρ_i, and ρ_b denote the probability density functions of the open, closed, inactivated, and blocked states, respectively, and where the flux terms are given by

$$a_o = -g_L(v - V_L) - (v - V_i) = \frac{11}{10}(1 - v),$$

$$a_c = -g_L(v - V_L) = -\frac{1}{10}v.$$

The associated model of the wild type is given by

$$\frac{\partial}{\partial v}(a_o \rho_o) = k_{co}\rho_c - (k_{oc} + k_{oi})\rho_o + k_{io}\rho_i, \tag{11.13}$$

$$\frac{\partial}{\partial v}(a_c \rho_c) = k_{oc}\rho_o - (k_{co} + k_{ci})\rho_c + k_{ic}\rho_i, \tag{11.14}$$

$$\frac{\partial}{\partial v}(a_c \rho_i) = k_{oi}\rho_o - (k_{io} + k_{ic})\rho_i + k_{ci}\rho_c. \tag{11.15}$$

All the reactions rates used in the computations are given in (11.2); the computational domain is given by $\Omega = [0, 1]$ and we used 201 mesh points. In Fig. 11.7, we show the difference between the open state probability density function of the wild type, denoted by ρ_o, computed by solving the system (11.13)–(11.15), and the mutant where the drug is applied, computed by solving (11.9)–(11.12), denoted by ρ_o^*. The difference is defined by the norm

$$\|\rho_o - \rho_o^*\| = \frac{\|\rho_o - \rho_o^*\|_{L^2(\Omega)}}{\|\rho_o\|_{L^2(\Omega)} + \|\rho_o^*\|_{L^2(\Omega)}}, \tag{11.16}$$

where, as usual,

$$\|\rho\|_{L^2(\Omega)} = \left(\int_\Omega \rho^2 dv\right)^{1/2}.$$

We observe that, as k_{bi} increases, the drug defined by (11.8) completely repairs the effect of the mutation.

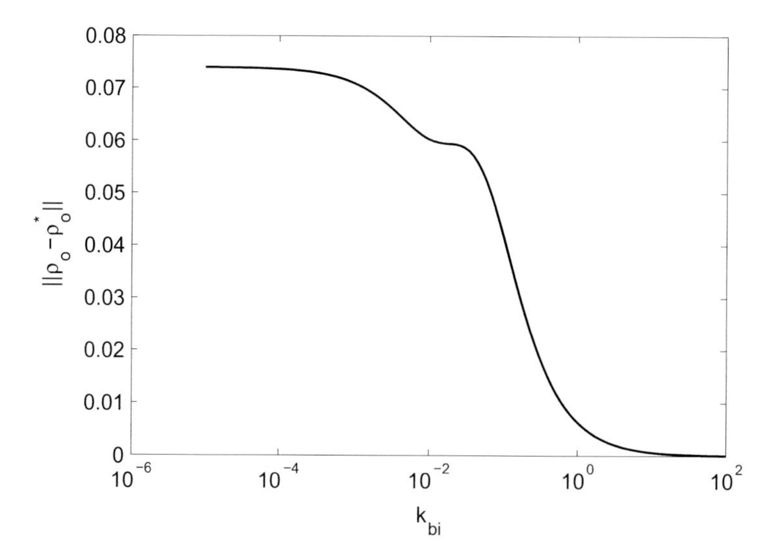

Fig. 11.7 The difference between the open probability density function of the wild type (ρ) and the open probability density function (ρ^*) of the mutant using the drug defined by (11.8), measured by the norm $\|\rho_o - \rho_o^*\|$ defined in (11.16). The difference goes to zero as the parameter k_{bi} is increased

Chapter 12
A Simple Model of the Sodium Channel

In the previous two chapters, we studied a prototypical model of an ion channel. The model consisted of a differential equation involving a gating mechanism that could be either open or closed. A Markov model governed the gating and we derived a system giving the probability density functions of the states involved in the Markov model. We used the probability density approach to compute optimal theoretical drugs and noted that a mutation leading to an increase in the closed to open reaction rate could be completely repaired by an optimal closed state drug.

Next, we extended the prototypical model to also include an inactivated state. The inactivated state can also be affected by mutations and we studied the particular case in which the rates from inactivated to open and from inactivated to closed were increased by a factor μ referred to as the mutation severity index. In this case, we observed that an optimal drug was represented by a blocker associated with the inactivated state. We were again able to completely repair the effect of the mutation using the theoretical drug.

In this chapter, we shall move closer to realistic Markov models of sodium channels. These models tend to be somewhat more intricate than the prototypical model we have studied so far. Providing Markov models of the sodium channels has been a very active field of research for decades and a series of models are available. We have chosen to study models that seem to capture the basic structure applied in many models but are manageable from a mathematical point of view. We choose this approach for clarity of presentation and not for its ability to represent specific data. It is, hopefully, quite clear that the method we use to analyze the models is applicable to many other models.

Mutations of the sodium channel can lead to impaired inactivation. This may lead to leakage of the sodium current, which can again trigger arrhythmias. Here we will consider a model of the ΔKPQ mutation of the SCN5A gene. This mutation may lead to an arrhythmogenic disorder referred to as the long-QT syndrome, which can lead to sudden cardiac death in the worst case. There are several models representing

A. Tveito, G.T. Lines, *Computing Characterizations of Drugs for Ion Channels and Receptors Using Markov Models*, Lecture Notes in Computational Science and Engineering 111, DOI 10.1007/978-3-319-30030-6_12

the effect of the ΔKPQ mutation. One that is well known is provided by Clancy and Rudy [14]. Their approach to model the impaired inactivation is to introduce a burst mode in the model where no inactivation state is available. We will consider two ways of modeling the effect of the mutation.

In the first approach, we will use the method utilized above. We will simply increase the reaction rate from the inactivated to the closed state and from the inactivated to the open state by a factor $\mu \geq 1$, referred to as the mutation severity index. This change will clearly reduce the probability of being in the inactivated state. It is therefore a model of impaired inactivation.

The second approach is to introduce a burst mode in the model. When the channel is in the burst mode, there is no inactivated state. This model will be parameterized such that it is highly unlikely that the channel will enter the burst mode for the wild type case, but the probability of entering the burst mode is considerably higher in the mutant case.

12.1 Markov Model of a Wild Type Sodium Channel

Markov models have turned out to be a powerful tool in representing the physics of the sodium channel and a series of alternatives have been proposed by various authors. Since this is still a very active field of research, it is hard to claim one particular model as the definitive model. We shall therefore focus on a kind of model that has a structure that seems to be more or less agreed upon but, as usual, we attack this problem with simplicity in mind. This also holds true for the way we introduce the effect of a mutation.

We start by considering a simple model of the sodium channel, illustrated in Fig. 12.1. The actual functions used in our computations will be given below. However, we should note that the functions will always be chosen such that they satisfy the principle of detailed balance, which, for the model given in Fig. 12.1, means that the following relation holds:

$$k_{io}k_{oc}k_{ci} = k_{oi}k_{ic}k_{co}. \tag{12.1}$$

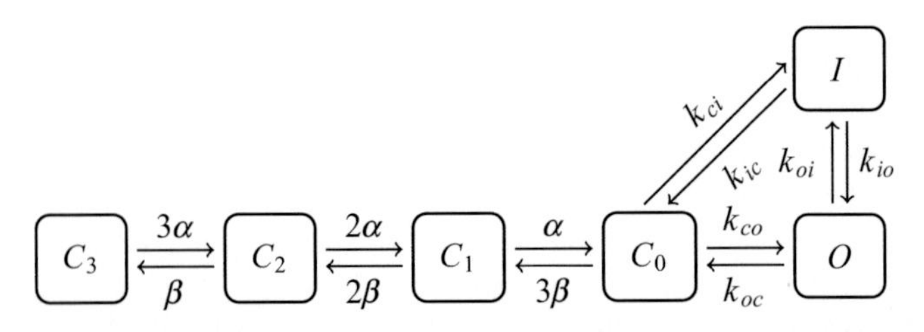

Fig. 12.1 Markov model of a wild type sodium channel consisting of an open state (O), an inactivated state (I), and four closed states (C_0, C_1, C_2, C_3)

The model of the closed states deserves a comment or two. Let us assume that a sodium channel consists of three subunits and these subunits may exist in two states: closed or permissible. The whole channel is in the state C_0 if all three units are in the permissible state. Over a brief period given by Δt, the channel can change from the state C_0 to the open state and the probability of this event is $\Delta t k_{co}$ or it can change to the inactivated state with probability $\Delta t k_{ci}$. However, the channel can also go from the permissible state C_0 to the state C_1 and the probability of doing this is $3\Delta t\beta$. The reason for the factor of three here is that it is sufficient that one of the three subunits closes. By assuming that the subunits act independently, we find that the probability is $3\Delta t\beta$. The same reasoning gives us the rest of the transitions between the different closed states.

12.1.1 The Equilibrium Solution

The equilibrium probabilities of the model given in Fig. 12.1 are characterized by the equations

$$\begin{aligned}
&k_{ci}c_0 = k_{ic}i, \quad k_{oi}o = k_{io}i, \quad k_{co}c_0 = k_{oc}o, \\
&3\beta c_0 = \alpha c_1,\ 2\alpha c_2 = 2\beta c_1,\ 3\alpha c_3 = \beta c_2,
\end{aligned}$$

where c_0 denotes the equilibrium probability of being in the state C_0. Similarly, the other variables are defined as the equilibrium probability of being in the states C_1, C_2, C_3, I, and O. We express all probabilities in terms of the open probability:

$$\begin{aligned}
i &= \frac{k_{oi}}{k_{io}}o,\ c_0 = \frac{k_{oc}}{k_{co}}o, \\
c_1 &= \frac{3\beta}{\alpha}\frac{k_{oc}}{k_{co}}o,\ c_2 = \frac{3\beta^2}{\alpha^2}\frac{k_{oc}}{k_{co}}o,\ c_3 = \frac{\beta^3}{\alpha^3}\frac{k_{oc}}{k_{co}}o.
\end{aligned}$$

Since $o+i+c_0+c_1+c_2+c_3 = 1$, we find the following equilibrium probabilities:

$$\begin{aligned}
o &= \frac{1}{q_w},\ i = \frac{k_{oi}/k_{io}}{q_w},\ c_0 = \frac{k_{oc}/k_{co}}{q_w}, \\
c_1 &= \frac{3\beta}{\alpha}\frac{k_{oc}/k_{co}}{q_w},\ c_2 = \frac{3\beta^2}{\alpha^2}\frac{k_{oc}/k_{co}}{q_w},\ c_3 = \frac{\beta^3}{\alpha^3}\frac{k_{oc}/k_{co}}{q_w},
\end{aligned} \tag{12.2}$$

where

$$q_w = 1 + \frac{k_{oi}}{k_{io}} + \frac{k_{oc}}{k_{co}}(1+\beta/\alpha)^3.$$

Here the subscript w is used to indicate that q_w represents the wild type case.

12.2 Modeling the Effect of a Mutation Impairing the Inactivated State

The mutation impairs the inactivated state of the channel. In Sect. 11.3 we modeled this by increasing the probability of moving from the inactivated state to the open state or to the closed state. This was done by increasing the rates k_{io} and k_{ic}. We use the same approach here and define

$$\bar{k}_{ic} = \mu k_{ic}, \tag{12.3}$$

$$\bar{k}_{io} = \mu k_{io}, \tag{12.4}$$

where, as usual, μ is the mutation severity index. From (12.1), we have

$$k_{io}k_{oc}k_{ci} = k_{ic}k_{co}k_{oi}$$

and therefore

$$(\mu k_{io})\, k_{oc}k_{ci} = (\mu k_{ic})\, k_{co}k_{oi};$$

so

$$\bar{k}_{io}k_{oc}k_{ci} = \bar{k}_{ic}k_{co}k_{oi}$$

and thus the principle of detailed balance also holds for the mutant case, in which the rates are given by (12.3) and (12.4).

12.2.1 *The Equilibrium Probabilities*

The reaction scheme of the mutant is illustrated in Fig. 12.2. In the mutant case, the equilibrium probabilities are given by

$$o = \frac{1}{q_m},\ i = \frac{k_{oi}/(\mu k_{io})}{q_m},\ c_0 = \frac{k_{oc}/k_{co}}{q_m}, \tag{12.5}$$
$$c_1 = \frac{3\beta}{\alpha}\frac{k_{oc}/k_{co}}{q_m},\ c_2 = \frac{3\beta^2}{\alpha^2}\frac{k_{oc}/k_{co}}{q_m},\ c_3 = \frac{\beta^3}{\alpha^3}\frac{k_{oc}/k_{co}}{q_m},$$

where

$$q_m = 1 + \frac{k_{oi}}{\mu k_{io}} + \frac{k_{oc}}{k_{co}}\left(1+\beta/\alpha\right)^3.$$

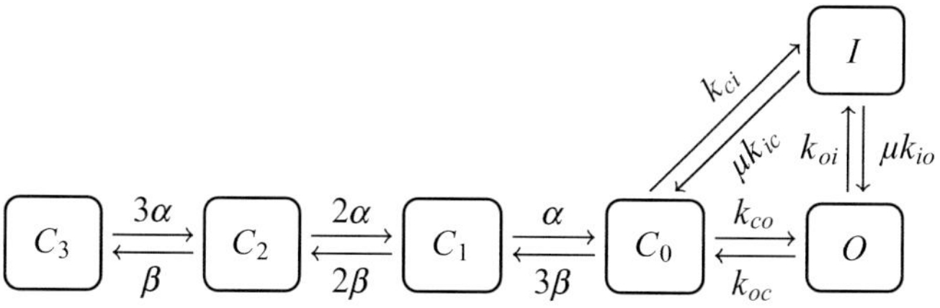

Fig. 12.2 Markov model of the mutant version of the sodium channel consisting of an open state (O), an inactivated state (I), and four closed states (C_0, C_1, C_2, C_3). Here μ is referred to as the mutation severity index

For the equilibrium state it is worth observing that, since

$$i = \frac{k_{oi}/k_{io}}{\frac{k_{oi}}{k_{io}} + \mu\left(1 + \frac{k_{oc}}{k_{co}}\left(1 + \beta/\alpha\right)^3\right)},$$

the probability of being in the inactivated state is reduced when μ is increased. Similarly, we observe that the associated open probability given by

$$o = \frac{1}{1 + \frac{k_{oi}}{\mu k_{io}} + \frac{k_{oc}}{k_{co}}\left(1 + \beta/\alpha\right)^3}$$

increases as μ increases. Although these calculations concern the equilibrium state, this is a pretty strong hint of an increased open probability in the dynamic case as well and an increased open probability is exactly the problem one observes when inactivation is impaired.

12.3 Stochastic Model of the Sodium Channel

We use the same model of the transmembrane potential as above (see (10.2) on page 154). Recall that the stochastic differential equation is given by

$$Cv' = -g_L(v - V_L) - \gamma g_{Na}(v - V_{Na}), \tag{12.6}$$

where C is the capacitance of the membrane, V_L is the resting potential of the leakage current, and V_{Na} is the resting potential of the sodium channel. The parameters are listed in Table 12.1.

The sodium channel can be either open (O), with $\gamma = 1$, or closed (C), with $\gamma = 0$, and, as usual, the state of the channel is determined by a Markov model.

Table 12.1 Values of the parameters used in model (12.6)

C	$1\,\mu\text{F/cm}^2$
g_L	$1/10\,\text{mS/cm}^2$
g_{Na}	$1\,\text{mS/cm}^2$
V_L	$-85\,\text{mV}$
V_{Na}	$45\,\text{mV}$

Since $C = 1$, we rewrite the equation in the more convenient form

$$v' = -g_L\,(v - V_L) - \gamma g_{Na}(v - V_{Na}), \tag{12.7}$$

where g_L and g_{Na} now have the unit[1] ms^{-1}.

12.3.1 A Numerical Scheme with an Invariant Region

A numerical scheme for the model (12.7) can be written in the form

$$v_{n+1} = v_n - \Delta t\,(g_L\,(v_n - V_L) + \gamma_n g_{Na}(v_n - V_{Na})), \tag{12.8}$$

where γ_n is either zero or one and where Δt denotes the time step. We assume that the condition

$$\Delta t < \frac{1}{g_L + g_{Na}} \tag{12.9}$$

holds and, under this condition, we will show that an invariant region for the solutions generated by the scheme (12.8) is given by

$$\Omega = (V_L, V_+)\,, \tag{12.10}$$

where

$$V_+ = \frac{g_L V_L + g_{Na} V_{Na}}{g_L + g_{Na}}$$

and, for the parameters we defined in (12.1), we have $V_+ \approx 33.18\,\text{mV}$.

To derive the invariant region, we proceed along the lines used on page 155 and thus start by defining

$$H(v,\gamma) = v - \Delta t\,(g_L\,(v - V_L) + \gamma g_{Na}(v - V_{Na})).$$

[1]The use of the odd units for g_L and g_{Na} stems from the fact that we have, for notational convenience, incorporated the capacitance of the membrane in these constants.

For values of v in the region Ω and for values of Δt satisfying condition (12.9), we have the properties

$$\frac{d}{dv}H(v,\gamma) = 1 - \Delta t\,(g_L + \gamma g_{Na}) \geqslant 1 - \Delta t\,(g_L + g_{Na}) > 0$$

and

$$\frac{d}{d\gamma}H(v,\gamma) = -\Delta t\,(g_{Na}(v - V_{Na})) > 0.$$

Using these observations, we obtain

$$v_{n+1} = H(v_n, \gamma_n) \leqslant H(V_+, 1) = V_+$$

and

$$v_{n+1} = H(v_n, \gamma_n) \geqslant H(V_L, 0) = V_L.$$

So, by induction, it holds that $\Omega = (V_L, V_+)$ is an invariant region for scheme (12.8).

12.4 Probability Density Functions for the Voltage-Gated Channel

The systems modeling the probability density functions in the wild type and mutant cases are of exactly the same form; the only difference is given by the mutation severity index. The probability density functions of the states of the Markov model given in Fig. 12.2 are given by

$$\begin{aligned}
\frac{\partial \rho_o}{\partial t} + \frac{\partial}{\partial v}(a_o\rho_o) &= k_{co}\rho_0 - (k_{oc} + k_{oi})\,\rho_o + \mu k_{io}\rho_i,\\
\frac{\partial \rho_i}{\partial t} + \frac{\partial}{\partial v}(a_c\rho_i) &= k_{oi}\rho_o - \mu\,(k_{io} + k_{ic})\,\rho_i + k_{ci}\rho_0,\\
\frac{\partial \rho_0}{\partial t} + \frac{\partial}{\partial v}(a_c\rho_0) &= k_{oc}\rho_o - (k_{ci} + k_{co} + 3\beta)\,\rho_0 + \mu k_{ic} i + \alpha\rho_1,\\
\frac{\partial \rho_1}{\partial t} + \frac{\partial}{\partial v}(a_c\rho_1) &= 2\alpha\rho_2 - (\alpha + 2\beta)\,\rho_1 + 3\beta\rho_0,\\
\frac{\partial \rho_2}{\partial t} + \frac{\partial}{\partial v}(a_c\rho_2) &= 3\alpha\rho_3 - (2\alpha + \beta)\,\rho_2 + 2\beta\rho_1,\\
\frac{\partial \rho_3}{\partial t} + \frac{\partial}{\partial v}(a_c\rho_3) &= -3\alpha\rho_3 + \beta\rho_2,
\end{aligned} \tag{12.11}$$

where

$$a_o = -g_L(v - V_L) - g_{Na}(v - V_{Na}), \tag{12.12}$$
$$a_c = -g_L(v - V_L),$$

with ρ_o denoting the probability density function of being in the open state, ρ_0 denoting the probability density function of being in the state C_0, and so on.

12.4.1 Model Parameterization

To carry out numerical computations comparing the properties of the wild type and the mutant sodium channel, we need to define the rates involved in the model described in Fig. 12.2. We use the rates

$$k_{ab}(v) = k_{ab}^{\infty}(v)/\tau_{ab}, \quad k_{ba}(v) = (1 - k_{ab}^{\infty}(v))/\tau_{ab},$$

with

$$k_{ab}^{\infty} = \frac{1}{1 + e^{s_{ab}(V_{ab} - v)}}.$$

Furthermore, the rates α and β in Fig. 12.2 are given by

$$\alpha = k_{cp}^{\infty}/\tau_{cp} \text{ and } \beta = (1 - k_{cp}^{\infty})/\tau_{cp}.$$

With this parameterization, the principle of detailed balance is satisfied, provided that

$$s_{co} + s_{ic} + s_{oi} = 0 \text{ and } s_{co}V_{co} + s_{oi}V_{oi} + s_{ic}V_{ic} = 0.$$

The parameters are given in Table 12.2 and we introduce the mutation as we did in the previous chapter: We increase the probability of going from the inactivated state to either the open or the closed state. More specifically, we define

$$\bar{k}_{ic} = \mu k_{ic} \text{ and } \bar{k}_{io} = \mu k_{io},$$

where, as usual, the wild type case is given by $\mu = 1$.

Table 12.2 Parameters of the Markov model illustrated in Figs. 12.1 and 12.2

ab	V_{ab} (mV)	s_{ab} (1/mV)	τ_{ab} (ms)
co	−60	0.1	0.01
oi	−120	0.05	3
ic	−80	−0.15	10
cp	−60	0.1	0.1

12.4.2 Numerical Experiments Comparing the Properties of the Wild Type and the Mutant Sodium Channel

In Fig. 12.3, we show the probability density functions of the open state, the inactivated state, and the sum of the closed states for the wild type case ($\mu = 1$) and two mutations ($\mu = 10$ and $\mu = 30$). The properties of the solutions are summarized in Table 12.3, which presents the expected values of the open state, the inactivated state, and the sum of the closed states.

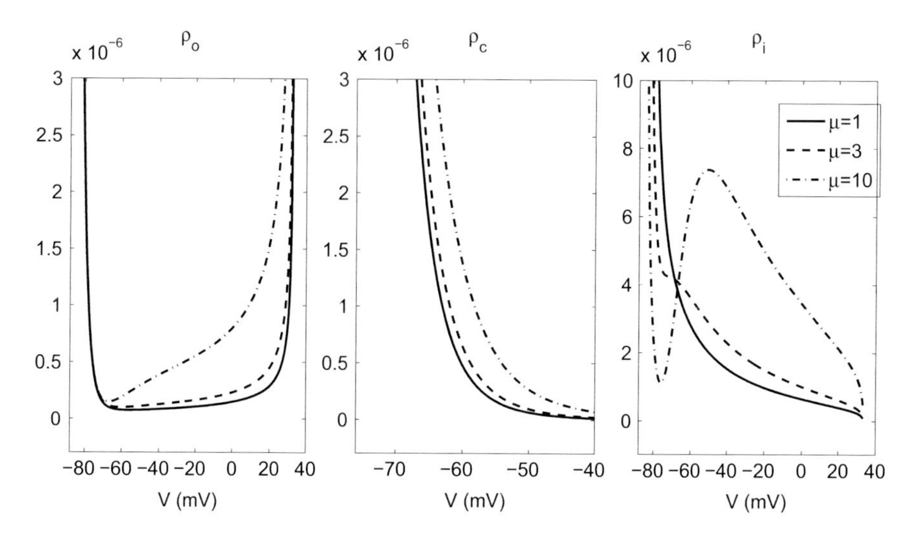

Fig. 12.3 The probability density functions of the open state (*left*), the sum of the closed states (*center*), and the inactivated state (*right*) for the wild type case (*solid line*) and two values of the mutation severity index: $\mu = 10$ and $\mu = 30$. The strongest mutation differs the most from the wild type solution

Table 12.3 Probability of being in the open, closed, or inactivated states and the expected value of the transmembrane potential, provided that the channel is open, closed, or inactivated

μ	$\pi_o \times 100$	π_c	$\pi_i \times 100$	E_o	E_c	E_i
1	0.0067	0.9951	0.4834	−50.8	−84.9	−83.5
3	0.0080	0.9982	0.1765	−41.1	−84.9	−79.6
10	0.0162	0.9989	0.0942	−13.4	−84.9	−57.0

12.4.3 Stochastic Simulations Illustrating the Late Sodium Current in the Mutant Case

Impaired inactivation of the sodium channel leads to a late sodium current, which is illustrated in Fig. 12.4. The figure also includes experimental data of the sodium current taken from Bennett et al. [2]. We observe that, by using $\mu = 30$, the model fits the experimental data fairly well.

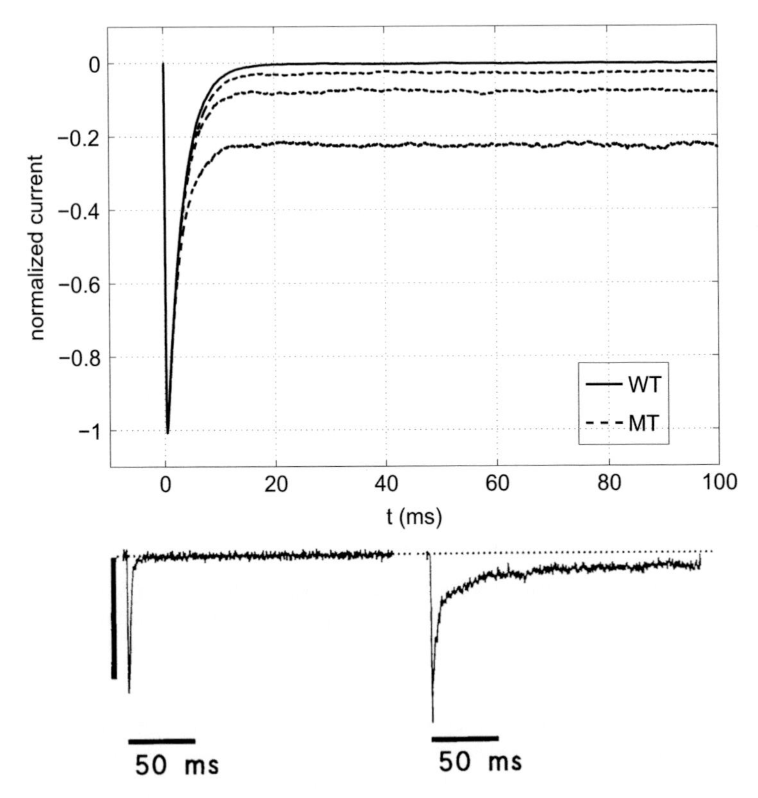

Fig. 12.4 Currents computed using the Markov model given in Fig. 12.2. *Top panel*: Currents based on numerical simulations for $\mu = 1, 10, 30, 100$. Each trace is an average of 10,000 Monte Carlo runs. The current is given by $I = g_{Na}P_o(v - V_{Na})$, with the transmembrane potential clamped at $v = 0$. The currents are normalized so that the wild type case peaks at -1. The parameters are given by $V_{Na} = 45$ and $g_{Na} = 1$ and P_o is the average ratio of open channels over 10,000 runs, computed at each time step. The lower graphs are from Bennett et al. [2], for the wild type case (*left*) and mutant case (*right*)

12.5 A Theoretical Drug Repairing the Sodium Channel Mutation

We introduce a theoretical drug for the sodium channel of the form given in Fig. 12.5. The equilibrium probabilities of the model are characterized by the equations

$$\begin{aligned}
&k_{ci}c_0 = \mu k_{ic}i, \ \ k_{oi}o = \mu k_{io}i, \ \ k_{co}c_0 = k_{oc}o, \\
&3\beta c_0 = \alpha c_1, \ \ 2\alpha c_2 = 2\beta c_1, \ \ 3\alpha c_3 = \beta c_2, \\
&k_{bc}b_0 = k_{cb}c_0, \ k_{bc}b_1 = k_{cb}c_1, \ k_{bc}b_2 = k_{cb}c_2, \\
&k_{bc}b_3 = k_{cb}c_3, \ \ k_{bi}b_i = k_{ib}i, \ \ k_{bo}b_o = k_{ob}o.
\end{aligned}$$

As usual, we express all probabilities in terms of the open state probability,

$$\begin{aligned}
i &= \frac{k_{oi}}{\mu k_{io}}o, \ c_0 = \frac{k_{oc}}{k_{co}}o, \\
c_1 &= \frac{3\beta}{\alpha}\frac{k_{oc}}{k_{co}}o, \ c_2 = \frac{3\beta^2}{\alpha^2}\frac{k_{oc}}{k_{co}}o, \ c_3 = \frac{\beta^3}{\alpha^3}\frac{k_{oc}}{k_{co}}o, \\
b_0 &= \delta_c\frac{k_{oc}}{k_{co}}o, \ b_1 = \delta_c\frac{3\beta}{\alpha}\frac{k_{oc}}{k_{co}}o, \ b_2 = \delta_c\frac{3\beta^2}{\alpha^2}\frac{k_{oc}}{k_{co}}o, \\
b_3 &= \delta_c\frac{\beta^3}{\alpha^3}\frac{k_{oc}}{k_{co}}o, \ b_i = \delta_i\frac{k_{oi}}{\mu k_{io}}o, \ b_o = \delta_o o,
\end{aligned}$$

where we have introduced the following parameters characterizing the drug:

$$\delta_o = \frac{k_{ob}}{k_{bo}}, \ \delta_i = \frac{k_{ib}}{k_{bi}}, \ \delta_c = \frac{k_{cb}}{k_{bc}}.$$

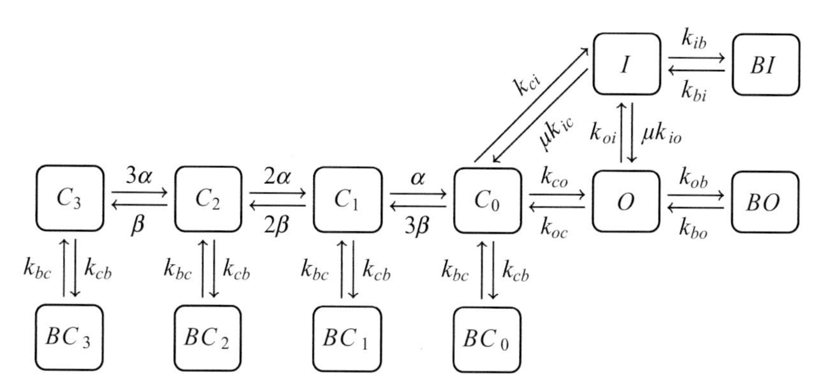

Fig. 12.5 Markov model for a theoretical drug of the sodium channel. The model consists of the usual states O, I, C_0, C_1, C_2, and C_3 and the blocked states BO, BI, BC_0, BC_1, BC_2, and BC_3

Since the sum of the probabilities is one, we obtain

$$o_{m,d} = \frac{1}{q_{m,d}},$$

where the subscript indicates the mutant case in the presence of a drug. Here,

$$q_{m,d} = 1 + \frac{k_{oi}}{\mu k_{io}} + \frac{k_{oc}}{k_{co}} (1 + \beta/\alpha)^3 (1 + \delta_c) + \delta_i \frac{k_{oi}}{\mu k_{io}} + \delta_o$$

and we recall that the wild type open probability is given by

$$o_w = \frac{1}{q_w},$$

where

$$q_w = 1 + \frac{k_{oi}}{k_{io}} + \frac{k_{oc}}{k_{co}} (1 + \beta/\alpha)^3 .$$

Obviously, we obtain $o_{m,d} \approx o_w$, provided that $q_{m,d} \approx q_w$. If we choose a drug characterized by

$$\delta_o = \delta_c = 0, \text{and } \delta_i = \mu - 1 \tag{12.13}$$

we find that

$$q_{m,d} = 1 + \frac{k_{oi}}{k_{io}} + \frac{k_{oc}}{k_{co}} (1 + \beta/\alpha)^3 = q_w$$

and therefore, with the drug specified by (12.13), we have $o_{m,d} = o_w$, so the open probability at equilibrium is repaired.

12.5.1 Numerical Experiments Using the Blocker of the Inactivated State

We have seen that a blocker of the inactivated state is a promising candidate for repairing the mutation described in Fig. 12.2. The drug is characterized by (12.13), so we have

$$k_{ib} = \delta_i k_{bi} = (\mu - 1)\, k_{bi} \tag{12.14}$$

and the parameter k_{bi} remains to be determined. In Table 12.4, we show that the blocker is more efficient the larger k_{bi} is. In fact, the blocker is able to repair all the

Table 12.4 The open probability, π_o, the expected value of the transmembrane potential, E_o, and the standard deviation, σ_o, for increasing values of k_{bi}. For large values of k_{bi}, the statistical properties of the mutant are completely repaired by the drug

k_{bi}	$\pi_o \times 10^3$	E_o	σ_o
WT	0.067	−50.794	46.828
MT	1.534	12.991	26.831
10^{-6}	1.341	12.940	26.913
10^{-5}	1.180	12.487	27.634
10^{-4}	0.556	8.240	33.343
10^{-3}	0.135	−16.903	49.326
0.01	0.070	−47.563	48.205
0.1	0.067	−50.729	46.869
1	0.067	−50.791	46.830

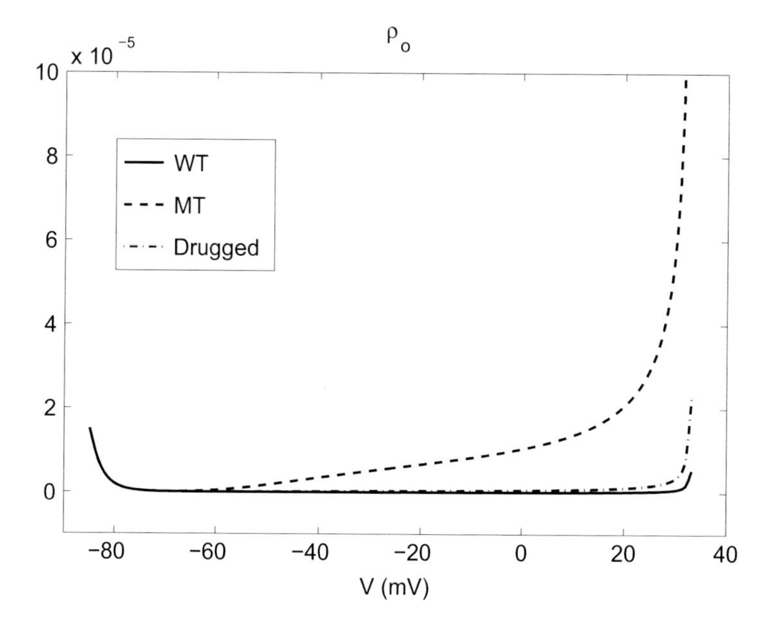

Fig. 12.6 The open probability density function for the wild type (WT) case and the mutant (MT) case using the mutation severity index $\mu = 30$ and, finally, the mutant case with the drug given by (12.14) with $k_{bi} = 0.001\ \text{ms}^{-1}$. A small value of k_{bi} was used to see a difference between the drugged case and the WT case

relevant statistical properties of the solution. The statistical properties presented in the table are introduced in Sect. 4.2 on page 72.

In Fig. 12.6, we show the open state probability density functions of the wild type, the mutant, and the drugged version of the mutant. Again, we see that the drug completely repairs the open state probability density function.

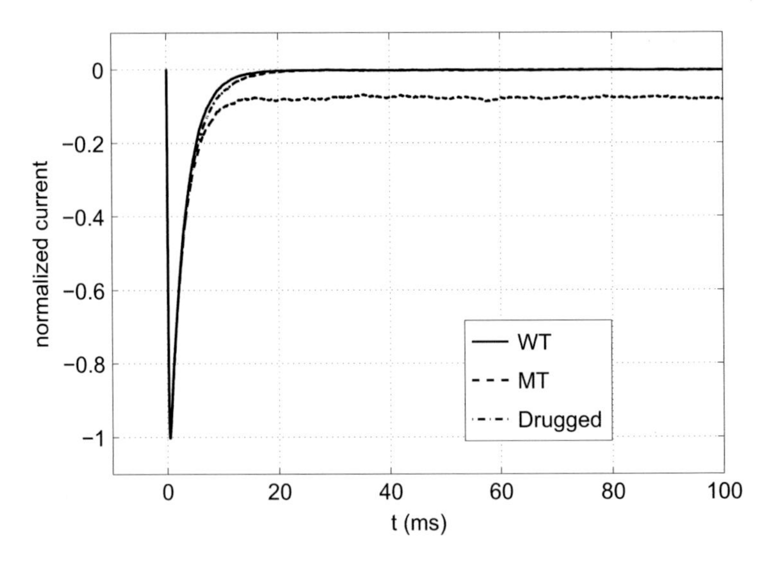

Fig. 12.7 The sodium current for the wild type (WT) and the mutant (MT) with the mutation severity index $\mu = 30$. The drug given by (12.14) with $k_{bi} = 0.01\ \mathrm{ms}^{-1}$ almost completely removes the late sodium current

12.5.2 The Late Sodium Current Is Removed by the Inactivated State Blocker

In Fig. 12.4 above, we demonstrated, using Monte Carlo simulations, that the mutation under consideration leads to a significant late sodium current comparable to the current observed in experiments. By using the drug described in (12.13) with $k_{bi} = 0.01\ \mathrm{ms}^{-1}$, we see that the late current more or less completely disappears (see Fig. 12.7).

12.6 Notes

1. The basic structure of the Markov model in Fig. 12.1 is taken from Patlak [65], who discusses and evaluates several possible models in relation to experimental data.
2. Modeling the effects of a drug on the sodium channel is motivated by the paper of Clancy et al. [16].

Chapter 13
Mutations Affecting the Mean Open Time

In the simplest case of Markov models of the form

$$C \underset{k_{co}}{\overset{k_{oc}}{\leftrightarrows}} O, \tag{13.1}$$

we have studied mutations leading to an increased open probability by increasing the rate from closed (C) to open (O), given by k_{co}. We refer to these as CO-mutations and for such mutations we have successfully derived closed state blockers represented as

$$B \underset{k_{bc}}{\overset{k_{cb}}{\leftrightarrows}} C \underset{\mu k_{co}}{\overset{k_{oc}}{\leftrightarrows}} O, \tag{13.2}$$

where $\mu \geqslant 1$ is the mutation severity index and $\mu = 1$ represents the wild type. These blockers can completely repair the equilibrium open probability of the mutant by adjusting the "on rate" divided by the "off rate" of the drug given by

$$\delta_c = \frac{k_{cb}}{k_{bc}}$$

(see, e.g., page 58). The remaining degree of freedom can be found using probability density systems and the resulting drugs have been proven to work exceptionally well in theoretical computations.

A. Tveito, G.T. Lines, *Computing Characterizations of Drugs for Ion Channels and Receptors Using Markov Models*, Lecture Notes in Computational Science and Engineering 111, DOI 10.1007/978-3-319-30030-6_13

There is, however, another way of modeling increased equilibrium open probability. Rather than increasing the rate from C to O, we can reduce the rate from O to C:

$$C \underset{k_{co}}{\overset{k_{oc}/\mu}{\leftrightarrows}} O, \tag{13.3}$$

where again $\mu \geqslant 1$ is referred to as the mutation severity index. This type of mutation is referred to as an OC-mutation and the equilibrium open probability for this Markov model is given by

$$o = \frac{1}{1 + \frac{k_{oc}/\mu}{k_{co}}},$$

which clearly increases for increasing values of μ. Formally, we can carry out the same math to devise a closed state drug that completely repairs the equilibrium open probability of the mutant; however, when this drug is put into the probability density system to determine the remaining degree of freedom of the drug, we quickly observe that the task is impossible and the theoretical drug does not provide significant improvement.

The core difficulty here is that a CO-mutation does not change the mean open time of the channel. A closed state blocker is therefore well suited because such a blocker does not affect the mean open time. However, for an OC-mutation, an increased mean open time is part of the problem and a closed state blocker is not the solution, simply because it cannot affect the mean open time. Rather, an open state blocker must be used.

In this chapter, we will explain the notion of mean open time and study mutations that lead to an increased open probability *and* an increased mean open time. We will show that open state blockers are optimal for such mutations.

13.1 The Mean Open Time

Let us briefly recall the interpretation of the Markov model

$$C \underset{k_{co}}{\overset{k_{oc}}{\leftrightarrows}} O.$$

This scheme means that if the channel is closed (C), the probability of changing the state from closed to open (O) in a small time interval Δt is given by $k_{co}\Delta t$. Clearly, this interpretation only holds for short time intervals, since the probability cannot exceed one. Note also that if the rate k_{co} increases, this leads to an increased probability of moving from C to O during the time step Δt. Similarly, $k_{oc}\Delta t$ denotes the probability of moving from the open state to the closed state in the time step Δt.

Suppose that the channel is open at time $t = 0$. The probability that the channel remains open after a short time step Δt is given by

$$p_1 = 1 - k_{oc}\Delta t.$$

If we take another time step, the probability that the channel is still open at time $t = 2\Delta t$ is given by

$$p_2 = p_1 (1 - k_{oc}\Delta t) = (1 - k_{oc}\Delta t)^2$$

and so on. At time $t = n\Delta t$, the probability of the channel still being open is given by

$$p_n = (1 - k_{oc}\Delta t)^n .$$

If we now introduce time given by

$$t = n\Delta t,$$

we have

$$(1 - k_{oc}\Delta t)^n = (1 - k_{oc}\Delta t)^{\frac{t}{\Delta t}} .$$

The probability of closing a channel that is in the open state during a time step is given by $\Delta t k_{oc}$ and therefore the probability of closing a channel that has remained open for n time steps is given by

$$\Delta t k_{oc} (1 - k_{oc}\Delta t)^{\frac{t}{\Delta t}} .$$

The expected open time is therefore given by

$$\sum_{n=1}^{\infty} n\Delta t (1 - k_{oc}\Delta t)^{\frac{t}{\Delta t}} \Delta t k_{oc}.$$

If we go to the limit of $\Delta t \to 0$ in this expression, we find that

$$\sum_{n=1}^{\infty} n\Delta t (1 - k_{oc}\Delta t)^{\frac{t}{\Delta t}} \Delta t k_{oc} \overset{\Delta t \to 0}{\longrightarrow} \int_0^{\infty} t k_{oc} e^{-k_{oc}t} dt = \frac{1}{k_{oc}}$$

and therefore we have found that the mean open time is given by

$$\tau_o = \frac{1}{k_{oc}}. \tag{13.4}$$

13.1.1 Mean Open Time for More Than One Open State

We have seen that the mean open time for a Markov model of the form

$$C \underset{k_{co}}{\overset{k_{oc}}{\leftrightarrows}} O$$

is given by

$$\tau_o = \frac{1}{k_{oc}}. \tag{13.5}$$

It is straightforward to extend the argument above to see that, for a Markov model of the form

$$C \underset{k_{co}}{\overset{k_{oc}}{\leftrightarrows}} O \underset{k_{ob}}{\overset{k_{bo}}{\leftrightarrows}} B,$$

the mean open time is given by

$$\tau_o = \frac{1}{k_{oc} + k_{ob}}. \tag{13.6}$$

But what happens if there is more than one open state? This situation will become relevant below, where we consider models including a burst mode. The models contain at least two open states. To understand the mean open time in the presence of more than one open state, we consider the generic extension illustrated in Fig. 13.1.

Assuming that the rates are set according to the principle of detailed balance, we have

$$k_{ul} o_u = k_{lu} o_l,$$

where o_u and o_l are the probabilities of being in the states O^u or O^l, respectively, and u and l represent the upper and lower states, respectively.

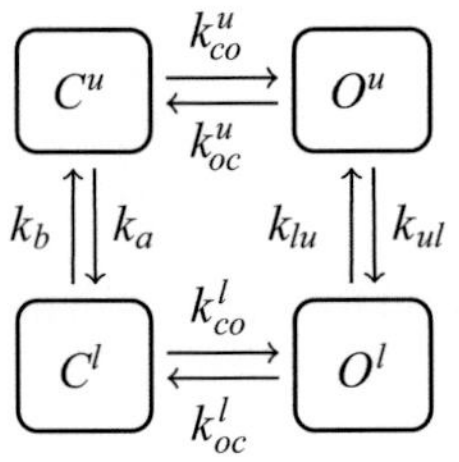

Fig. 13.1 Markov model with two open states (O^u, O^l) and two closed states (C^u, C^l)

As for the derivation above, we assume that the channel is open and our task is to figure out how long we can expect the channel to remain open. We know that, initially, the channel is either in the state O^u or O^l. Let us define q_u and q_l to be the conditional probabilities of being in the upper and lower open states, given that the channel is open. For the upper state we write

$$q_u = P(S = O_u | (S = O_u \text{ or } S = O_l)),$$

where $S = X$ means that the channel is in state X. Since

$$P(A|B) = P(A \text{ and } B)/P(B)$$

and, in our case, since (A and B) = A, we obtain

$$q_u = P(S = O_u)/P(S = O_u \text{ or } S = O_l) = \frac{o_u}{o_u + o_l}$$

and similarly for the lower state; with

$$q_l = P(S = O_l | (S = O_u \text{ or } S = O_l)),$$

we obtain

$$q_l = \frac{o_l}{o_u + o_l}.$$

It follows that $q_u + q_l = 1$ and that

$$q_u = \frac{k_{lu}}{k_{ul} + k_{lu}}$$

and

$$q_l = \frac{k_{ul}}{k_{ul} + k_{lu}}.$$

The probability of remaining in the open states in the first time step is now given by

$$\begin{aligned} p_1 &= \left(1 - \Delta t k_{oc}^u\right) q_u + \left(1 - \Delta t k_{oc}^l\right) q_l \\ &= 1 - \Delta t \left(\frac{k_{oc}^u k_{lu} + k_{oc}^l k_{ul}}{k_{ul} + k_{lu}} \right) \end{aligned}$$

and thus, by following the steps above, we find that

$$p_n = (1 - \Delta t K)^n,$$

where

$$K = \frac{k_{oc}^{u} k_{lu} + k_{oc}^{l} k_{ul}}{k_{ul} + k_{lu}}.$$

The probability of closing a channel that is in one of the open states during a time step is given by

$$\Delta t k_{oc}^{u} q_u + \Delta t k_{oc}^{l} q_l = \Delta t K$$

and, therefore, the probability of closing a channel in a time step that has remained open for n time steps is given by

$$\Delta t K \left(1 - \Delta t K\right)^{n}.$$

We find that the expected mean open time is given by

$$\tau_o = \frac{1}{K} = \frac{k_{ul} + k_{lu}}{k_{oc}^{u} k_{lu} + k_{oc}^{l} k_{ul}}. \tag{13.7}$$

13.1.1.1 Special Cases

It is interesting to consider the formula for the mean open time given by (13.7) in two special cases. First, we assume that $k_{oc}^{u} = k_{oc}^{l}$ and we let k_{oc} denote this common value. Then, by (13.7), we have

$$\tau_o = \frac{1}{k_{oc}}$$

which is the same as we found for the two-state scheme above. Next consider the case of $k_{ul} = k_{lu}$ (and $k_{oc}^{u} \neq k_{oc}^{l}$). By (13.7), we find

$$\tau_o = \frac{1}{(k_{oc}^{u} + k_{oc}^{u})/2}. \tag{13.8}$$

13.2 Numerical Experiments

It is useful to have a look at the mean open time computed in specific numerical experiments to determine how well it is represented by the theoretical value derived above. Similarly, it is useful to consider how well the theoretical equilibrium open probability represents the data we observe in actual computations. In this section, we will present experiments that hopefully clarify these matters.

13.2.1 Mean Open Time and Equilibrium Open Probability: Theoretical Values Versus Sample Mean Values

Let us illustrate the result above by a few numerical experiments. We start by considering the Markov model

$$C \underset{k_{co}}{\overset{k_{oc}}{\leftrightarrows}} O,$$

where we set $k_{co} = 1\ \mathrm{ms}^{-1}$ and we let

$$k_{oc} = \frac{1}{m}\mathrm{ms}^{-1}$$

for $m = 1, \ldots, 100$. For every value of k_{oc}, we run a simulation using the Markov model for $T = 10^4$ ms. The time instances when the channel changes state are stored in the sequence $\{t_i\}_{i=0}^{N}$ and the mean open time observed in the simulation is given by[1]

$$\tau_{o,s} = \frac{2}{N}\sum_i (t_i - t_{i-1})_o\,,$$

where

$$(t_i - t_{i-1})_o = \begin{cases} t_i - t_{i-1} & \text{if the channel is open in this interval,} \\ 0 & \text{if the channel is closed in this interval.} \end{cases}$$

With this notation we can also define the sample open probability by

$$o_s = \frac{1}{T}\sum_i (t_i - t_{i-1})_o\,.$$

In Fig. 13.2 (left panel), we plot the sample mean open time $\tau_{o,s}$ and the theoretical mean open time given by

$$\tau_o = \frac{1}{k_{oc}} \qquad (13.9)$$

[1]The index s here is used to indicate *sample*, since these are values for a specific computation and not the theoretical value computed above.

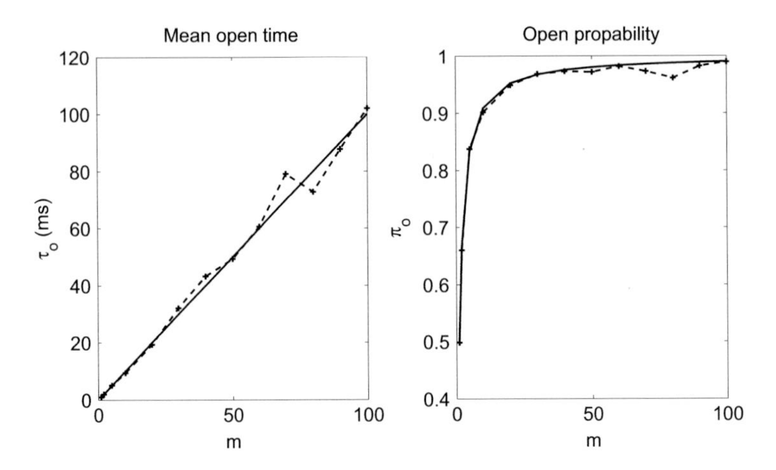

Fig. 13.2 Mean open time (*left*) and open probability (*right*), with $k_{oc} = 1/m$ ms^{-1} and $k_{co} = 1$ ms^{-1}. The sample values (*dashed lines*) correspond well with the theoretical values (*solid line*)

as functions of k_{oc}. We also plot (right panel) the sample open probability o_s and the theoretical equilibrium probability given by

$$o = \frac{1}{1 + \frac{k_{oc}}{k_{co}}}. \tag{13.10}$$

In both plots, we see that the mean values computed in the simulations are quite close to the theoretical values. If we increase the simulation time T, these graphs converge toward the same value.

13.2.2 The Closed to Open Rate k_{co} Does Not Affect the Mean Open Time

We have seen that, theoretically, according to (13.9), the mean open time τ_o is independent of the closed to open rate k_{co}, but the open probability is affected as stated in (13.10). This is illustrated in Fig. 13.3, where we use $k_{oc} = 1$ ms^{-1} and $k_{co} = 1/m$ ms^{-1} and plot the mean open time (left panel) and the open probability (right panel) as functions of m.

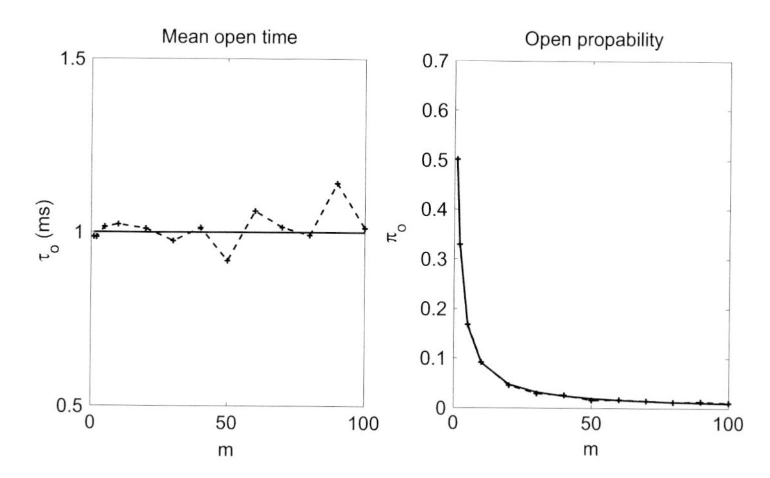

Fig. 13.3 Mean open time (*left*) and open probability (*right*) with $k_{co} = 1/m$ ms^{-1} and $k_{oc} = 1$ ms^{-1}. The mean open time is not affected by changes in k_{co}. The sample values correspond well to the theoretical values

13.2.3 The Mean Open Time in the Presence of Two Open States

In Fig. 13.4, we show the sample mean open time and the theoretical mean open time given by

$$\tau_o = \frac{1}{K} = \frac{k_{ul} + k_{lu}}{k^u_{oc} k_{lu} + k^l_{oc} k_{ul}} \tag{13.11}$$

for the Markov model in Fig. 13.1. In the computations, we have used $k^l_{oc} = 1\,\text{ms}^{-1}$, $k^u_{oc} = 10\,\text{ms}^{-1}$, and $k_{lu} = 0.001\,\text{ms}^{-1}$ and k_{ul} varies. The other parameters of the model do not affect the result, as long as detailed balance holds.

13.2.4 Changing the Mean Open Time Affects the Dynamics of the Transmembrane Potential

We consider the stochastic model of the transmembrane potential given by

$$v_t = g_K(V_K - v) + \gamma g_{Na}(V_{Na} - v), \tag{13.12}$$

where γ is a stochastic variable governed by the two-state Markov model

$$C \underset{k_{co}}{\overset{k_{oc}}{\leftrightarrows}} O.$$

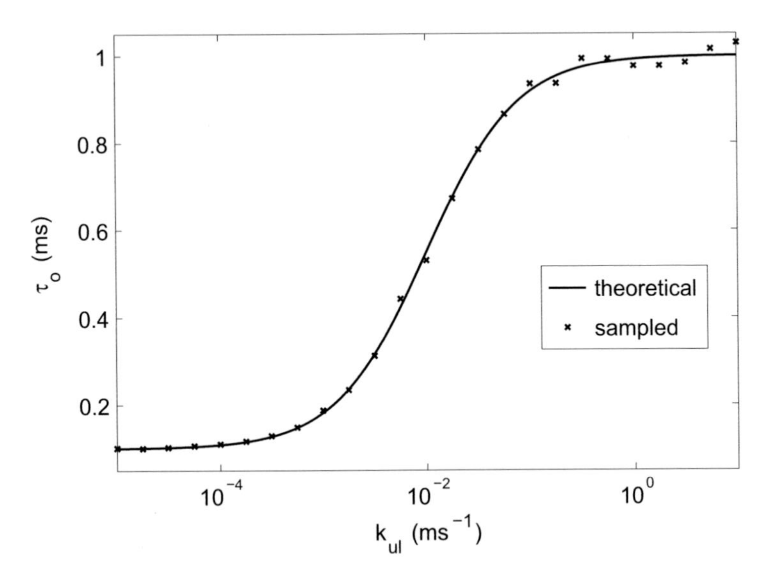

Fig. 13.4 Mean open time for a Markov model with two open states

We use the parameters

$$g_K = \frac{1}{10}\ \text{ms}^{-1},\ g_{Na} = 1\ \text{ms}^{-1}, \tag{13.13}$$
$$V_K = -85\ \text{mV},\ V_{Na} = 45\ \text{mV},$$

and compute solutions using the standard scheme

$$v_{n+1} = v_n - \Delta t\,(g_K\,(v_n - V_K) + \gamma_n g_{Na}(v_n - V_{Na})), \tag{13.14}$$

where the time step is assumed to satisfy the condition

$$\Delta t < \frac{1}{g_K + g_{Na}}. \tag{13.15}$$

Under this condition, we have seen above that, for solutions computed by (13.12), an invariant region is given by

$$\Omega = (V_K, V_+)\,, \tag{13.16}$$

where

$$V_+ = \frac{g_K V_K + g_{Na} V_{Na}}{g_K + g_{Na}}.$$

In Fig. 13.5, we show numerical solutions of (13.12) for

$$k_{oc} = k_{co} = 0.1 \text{ ms}^{-1}, 1 \text{ ms}^{-1}, 10 \text{ ms}^{-1}, 100 \text{ ms}^{-1}.$$

According to the considerations above, the equilibrium open probability is given by

$$o = \frac{1}{1 + \frac{k_{oc}}{k_{co}}},$$

which is constant for the four parameter sets used in Fig. 13.5. The mean open time, however, varies with k_{oc} as

$$\tau_o = \frac{1}{k_{oc}}.$$

For the cases studied in Fig. 13.5, the mean open times are 10, 1, 1/10, and 1/100 ms and we observe that the reduced mean open time greatly reduces the variations of the transmembrane potential.

13.3 Changing the Mean Open Time Affects the Probability Density Functions

The stationary version of the probability density system governing the states of the Markov model

$$C \underset{k_{co}}{\overset{k_{oc}}{\leftrightarrows}} O$$

is given by

$$\frac{\partial}{\partial v}(a_o\rho_o) = k_{co}\rho_c - k_{oc}\rho_o, \tag{13.17}$$
$$\frac{\partial}{\partial v}(a_c\rho_c) = k_{oc}\rho_o - k_{co}\rho_c,$$

where

$$a_o = g_K(V_K - v) + g_{Na}(V_{Na} - v), \tag{13.18}$$
$$a_c = g_K(V_K - v).$$

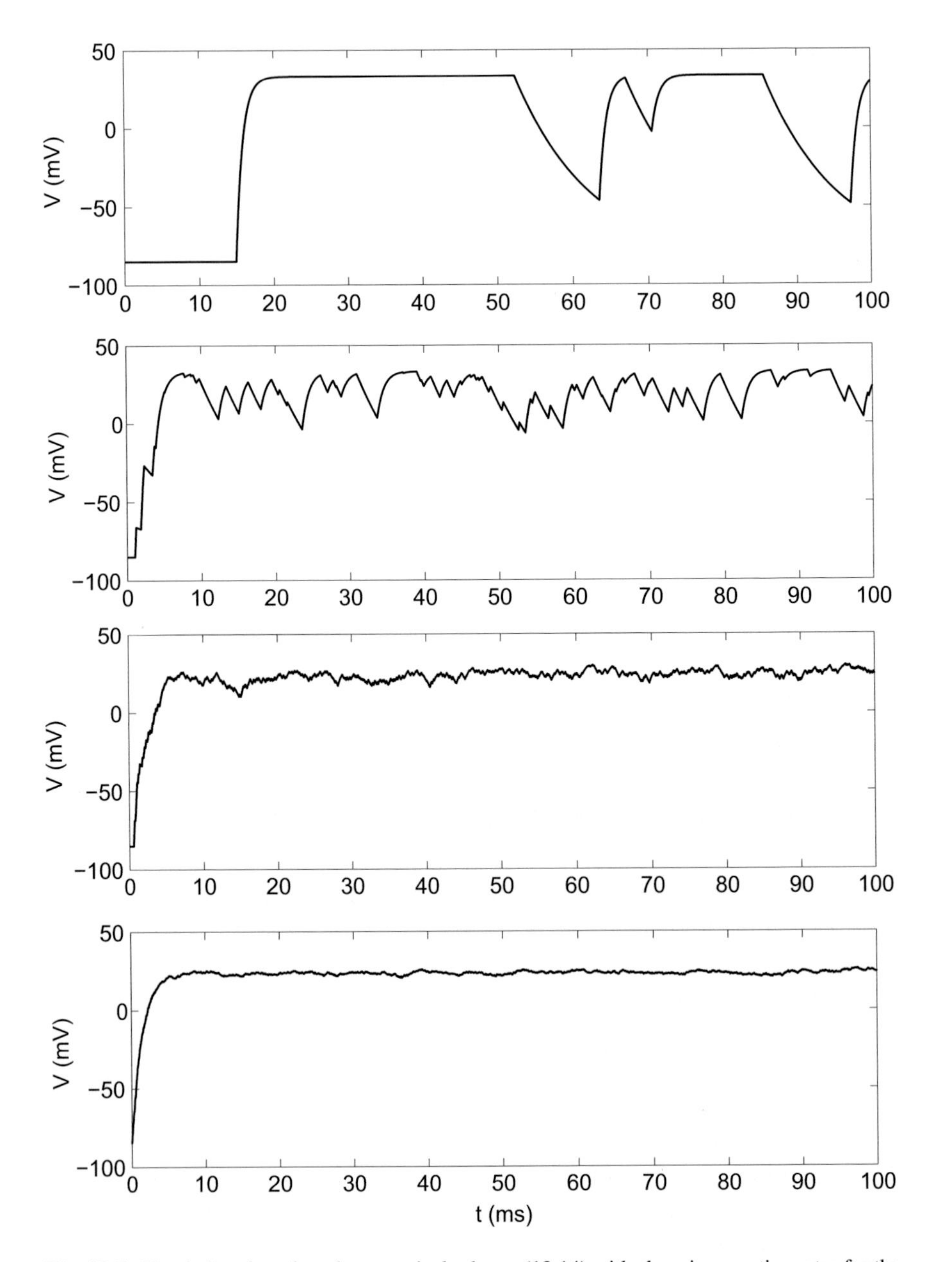

Fig. 13.5 Simulations based on the numerical scheme (13.14) with changing reaction rates for the Markov model. From top to bottom, $k_{oc} = k_{co} = 0.1$, 1, 10, and 100 ms^{-1}. Since $k_{oc} = k_{co}$ for all values, the open probability is kept constant but the mean open time given by $1/k_{oc}$ is decreasing from top to bottom

The analytical solution of this problem is given by

$$\rho_o(v) = Kg_K(V_+ - v)^{\frac{k_{oc}}{g}-1}(v - V_K)^{\frac{k_{co}}{g_K}},$$

$$\rho_c(v) = Kg(V_+ - v)^{\frac{k_{oc}}{g}}(v - V_K)^{\frac{k_{co}}{g_K}-1},$$

where

$$g = g_{Na} + g_K,\ V_+ = \frac{g_{Na}V_{Na} + g_K V_K}{g_{Na} + g_K}$$

and K is chosen such that

$$\int_{V_K}^{V_+} \rho_o + \rho_c = 1,$$

which is given by

$$1/K = \frac{k_{co} + k_{oc}}{a + b}(V_+ - V_K)^{(a+b)}B(a, b),$$

with $a = k_{co}/g_K, b = k_{oc}/g$, and $B(a, b) = \Gamma(a)\Gamma(b)/\Gamma(a + b)$.

In Fig. 13.6, we show the open probability density function for the data given in (13.13) with

$$k_{oc} = k_{co} = 0.1\ \text{ms}^{-1}, 1\ \text{ms}^{-1}, 10\ \text{ms}^{-1}, 100\ \text{ms}^{-1}.$$

Again, we recall that as k_{oc} increases, the mean open time decreases and we observe in the figure that the probability density function becomes narrower.

13.4 Theoretical Drugs for OC-Mutations

We have seen earlier that when mutations increase the open probability by increasing the reaction rate from C to O (k_{co}), the effect of the mutation can be completely repaired by using an optimal closed state blocker. Now we are interested in a mutation that increases the open probability by reducing the reaction rate from O to C (k_{oc}) . Such a mutation increases both the open probability and the mean open time and we will observe that a closed state blocker is unable to repair the effect of such a mutation.

We consider the two-state Markov model

$$C \underset{k_{co}}{\overset{k_{oc}/\mu}{\leftrightarrows}} O, \tag{13.19}$$

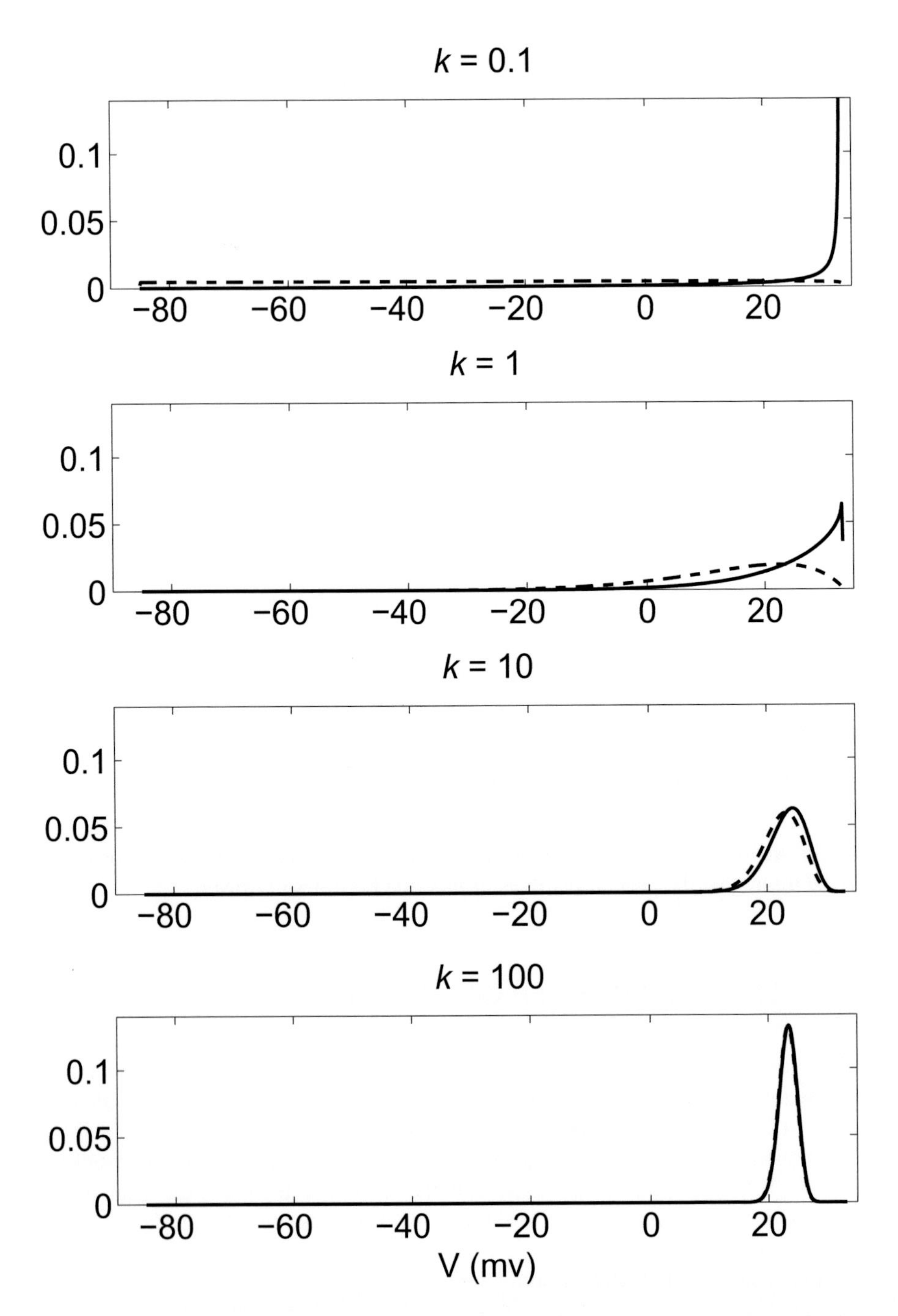

Fig. 13.6 The open probability density function ρ_o (*solid line*) and closed probability density function ρ_c depend on the mean open time given by $1/k_{oc}$. In the figures, we have used $k = k_{oc} = k_{co}$

where $\mu \geqslant 1$ is the mutation severity index; as usual, $\mu = 1$ denotes the wild type. Recall that the equilibrium open probability is given by

$$o = \frac{1}{1 + \frac{k_{oc}}{\mu k_{co}}}$$

and the mean open time is given by

$$\tau_o = \frac{\mu}{k_{oc}},$$

so the mutation clearly increases both the open probability and the mean open time.

13.4.1 The Theoretical Closed State Blocker Does Not Work for the OC-Mutation

Let us start by considering a closed state blocker of the form

$$B \underset{k_{bc}}{\overset{k_{cb}}{\leftrightarrows}} C \underset{k_{co}}{\overset{k_{oc}/\mu}{\leftrightarrows}} O. \tag{13.20}$$

We find that the equilibrium open probability of the mutant in the presence of the closed state blocker is given by

$$o = \frac{1}{1 + \frac{k_{oc}}{k_{co}} \frac{1+\delta_c}{\mu}},$$

where

$$\delta_c = \frac{k_{cb}}{k_{bc}}.$$

Since the wild type equilibrium open probability is given by

$$o = \frac{1}{1 + \frac{k_{oc}}{k_{co}}},$$

the drug will repair the open probability, provided that

$$\frac{1 + \delta_c}{\mu} = 1$$

and therefore the drug must satisfy the usual condition

$$\delta_c = \mu - 1.$$

A drug satisfying this condition will completely repair the equilibrium open probability and that is, of course, good, but it is not enough. Since the mutation represented by (13.19) also affects the mean open time, a drug of the form (13.20) cannot repair that effect of the mutation. To see this, we consider the probability density system defined by

$$\begin{aligned} \frac{\partial}{\partial v}(a_o \rho_o) &= k_{co}\rho_c - \frac{1}{\mu} k_{oc}\rho_o, \\ \frac{\partial}{\partial v}(a_c \rho_c) &= \frac{1}{\mu} k_{oc}\rho_o - (k_{co} + (\mu - 1) k_{bc}) \rho_c + k_{bc}\rho_b, \\ \frac{\partial}{\partial v}(a_c \rho_b) &= (\mu - 1) k_{bc}\rho_c - k_{bc}\rho_b, \end{aligned} \tag{13.21}$$

where, as usual, ρ_o, ρ_c, and ρ_b denote the probability density functions of the open (O), closed (C), and blocked (B) states, respectively, and where the fluxes are defined by (13.18). In Fig. 13.7, we compare the open probability density computed by solving the system (13.21) with the open probability density of the wild type. The

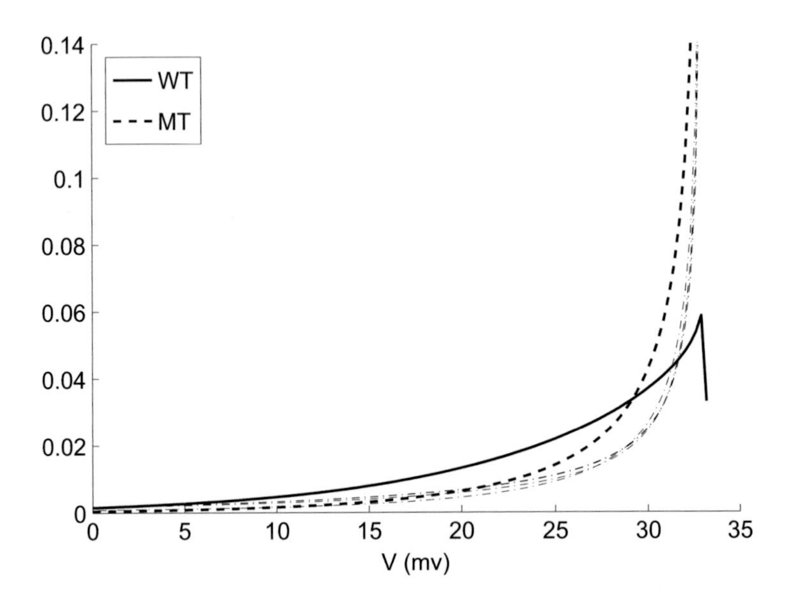

Fig. 13.7 The *solid line* represents the wild type solution and the *dashed line* represents the mutant. Various closed state drugs are applied, but none are able to repair the effect of the mutation

wild type probability density functions are given by

$$\frac{\partial}{\partial v}(a_o\rho_o) = k_{co}\rho_c - k_{oc}\rho_o,$$
$$\frac{\partial}{\partial v}(a_c\rho_c) = k_{oc}\rho_o - k_{co}\rho_c, \tag{13.22}$$

and the probability density functions of the mutant case are given by

$$\frac{\partial}{\partial v}(a_o\rho_o) = k_{co}\rho_c - \frac{1}{\mu}k_{oc}\rho_o,$$
$$\frac{\partial}{\partial v}(a_c\rho_c) = \frac{1}{\mu}k_{oc}\rho_o - k_{co}\rho_c. \tag{13.23}$$

In the computations we have used the parameters given by (13.13) and the rates

$$k_{co} = 1\ \text{ms}^{-1} \text{ and } k_{oc} = 1\ \text{ms}^{-1}.$$

We use three values of the rates k_{bc} and we observe that no parameter is able to repair the open state probability density function of the mutation. In Fig. 13.8, we show the norm of the difference between the open probability density defined by (13.21) and (13.22. The norm is defined by (2.40) on page 46 and we see that no version of the closed state blocker defined by (13.20) is able to repair the effect of the mutations given by (13.19).

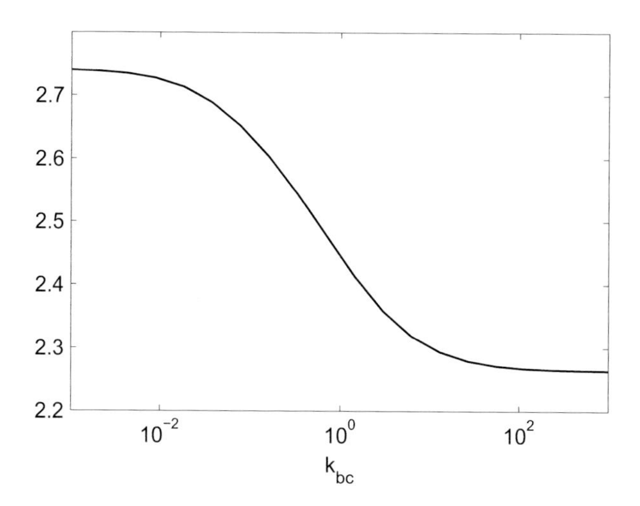

Fig. 13.8 The norm of the difference between the wild type solution and the mutant after the drug is applied. The norm is defined by (2.40) on page 46. We see that no value of the drug parameter k_{bc} for the closed state blocker is able to repair the effect of the mutation

13.4.2 The Theoretical Open State Blocker Repairs the Effect of the OC-Mutation

Next, we consider an open state blocker for the mutation leading to both an increased open probability and an increased mean open time. The theoretical open state blocker can be written in the form

$$C \underset{k_{co}}{\overset{k_{oc}/\mu}{\leftrightarrows}} O \underset{k_{ob}}{\overset{k_{bo}}{\leftrightarrows}} B, \tag{13.24}$$

where the parameters k_{bo} and k_{ob} define the theoretical drug. For this Markov model, the equilibrium open probability is given by

$$o_{\mu} = \frac{1}{1 + \frac{k_{oc}}{\mu k_{co}} + \frac{k_{ob}}{k_{bo}}}$$

and the mean open time is given by

$$\tau_{o,\mu} = \frac{1}{\frac{1}{\mu} k_{oc} + k_{ob}}.$$

Since the associated wild type values are

$$o = \frac{1}{1 + \frac{k_{oc}}{k_{co}}}$$

and

$$\tau_o = \frac{1}{k_{oc}},$$

we want to define the drug such that

$$1 + \frac{k_{oc}}{\mu k_{co}} + \frac{k_{ob}}{k_{bo}} = 1 + \frac{k_{oc}}{k_{co}}$$

and

$$\frac{1}{\mu} k_{oc} + k_{ob} = k_{oc}.$$

To satisfy these two requirements, we find that the drug must be given by

$$\begin{aligned} k_{ob} &= \frac{\mu - 1}{\mu} k_{oc}, \\ k_{bo} &= k_{co}. \end{aligned} \tag{13.25}$$

13.4.3 The Theoretical Open State Blocker Is Optimal

We will show analytically that the open state blocker defined by (13.24) where the parameters are given by (13.25) is an optimal drug, in the sense that the effect of the mutation is completely repaired. We start by observing that the probability density system associated with the Markov model (13.24) is given by

$$\begin{aligned} \frac{\partial}{\partial v}(a_o \rho_o) &= k_{co}\rho_c - (\mu^{-1}k_{oc} + k_{ob})\rho_o + k_{bo}\rho_b, \\ \frac{\partial}{\partial v}(a_c \rho_c) &= \mu^{-1}k_{oc}\rho_o - k_{co}\rho_c, \\ \frac{\partial}{\partial v}(a_c \rho_b) &= k_{ob}\rho_o - k_{bo}\rho_b. \end{aligned} \tag{13.26}$$

If we insert the drug given by (13.25), we obtain the system

$$\begin{aligned} \frac{\partial}{\partial v}(a_o \rho_o) &= k_{co}\rho_c - k_{oc}\rho_o + k_{co}\rho_b, \\ \frac{\partial}{\partial v}(a_c \rho_c) &= \mu^{-1}k_{oc}\rho_o - k_{co}\rho_c, \\ \frac{\partial}{\partial v}(a_c \rho_b) &= \left(1 - \mu^{-1}\right)k_{oc}\rho_o - k_{co}\rho_b. \end{aligned} \tag{13.27}$$

We define

$$\bar{\rho}_c = \rho_c + \rho_b$$

and add the two latter equations of this system to find that ρ_o and $\bar{\rho}_c$ solve the system

$$\begin{aligned} \frac{\partial}{\partial v}(a_o \rho_o) &= k_{co}\bar{\rho}_c - k_{oc}\rho_o, \\ \frac{\partial}{\partial v}(a_c \bar{\rho}_c) &= k_{oc}\rho_o - k_{co}\bar{\rho}_c, \end{aligned} \tag{13.28}$$

which coincides with the system defining the wild type probability density functions (see (13.22) above). We therefore conclude that the open state blocker defined by

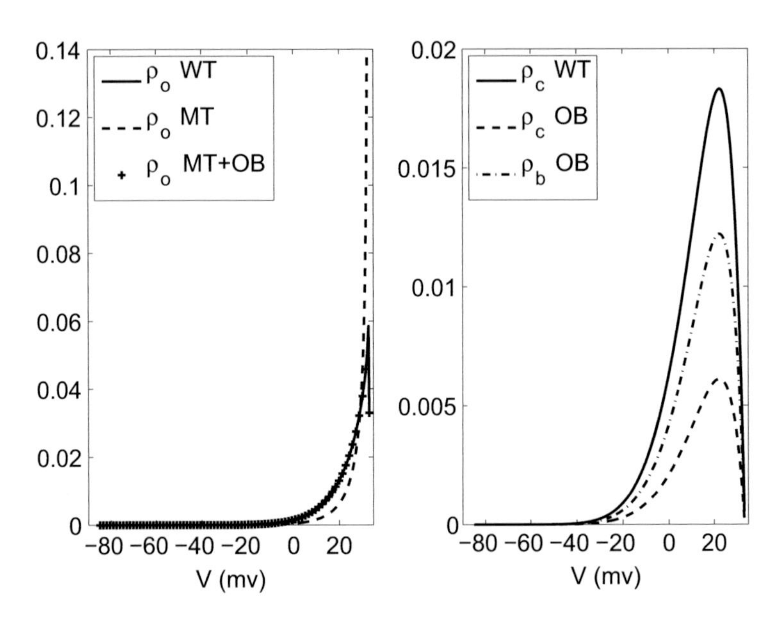

Fig. 13.9 Probability density functions of the wild type, mutant, and mutant in the presence of the open blocker. The open blocker completely repairs the open probability density function of the mutant

the parameters (13.25) completely repairs the probability density functions of the mutant for any value of the mutation severity index.

13.4.3.1 The Probability Density Function of the Blocked State Is Proportional to the Probability Density Function of the Wild Type Closed State

In Fig. 13.9, we show the open probability density functions of the wild type (defined by system (13.22), the mutant (defined by system (13.23) with $\mu = 3$), and the mutant including the optimal drug (defined by system (13.27)). As expected, the open probability is completely repaired by the theoretical drug.

In the right panel of the figure, we show the graph of ρ_c for the wild type (solid line) and for the mutant case in the presence of the open blocker. We show both ρ_c and ρ_b. We note that these graphs seem to have the same shape and we will show that they indeed differ only by a constant.

We start by making the ansatz that for the solution of system (13.27) we have

$$\rho_b = (\mu - 1)\, \rho_c. \tag{13.29}$$

If we insert this into system (13.27), we find that the two latter equations become identical and the system is therefore reduced to the following 2×2 system:

$$\frac{\partial}{\partial v}(a_o \rho_o) = \mu k_{co} \rho_c - k_{oc} \rho_o,$$
$$\frac{\partial}{\partial v}(a_c \rho_c) = \mu^{-1} k_{oc} \rho_o - k_{co} \rho_c. \qquad (13.30)$$

Therefore, we can define

$$\rho_c^* = \mu \rho_c$$

and find that ρ_o and ρ_c^* solve system

$$\frac{\partial}{\partial v}(a_o \rho_o) = k_{co} \rho_c^* - k_{oc} \rho_o,$$
$$\frac{\partial}{\partial v}\left(a_c \rho_c^*\right) = k_{oc} \rho_o - k_{co} \rho_c^*, \qquad (13.31)$$

which is exactly the wild type system. We therefore conclude that

$$\rho_b = (\mu - 1)\, \rho_c = \frac{\mu - 1}{\mu} \rho_c^*, \qquad (13.32)$$

where (ρ_o, ρ_c, ρ_b) solves the system (13.27) and where (ρ_o^*, ρ_c^*) solves the wild type system

$$\frac{\partial}{\partial v}\left(a_o \rho_o^*\right) = k_{co} \rho_c^* - k_{oc} \rho_o^*,$$
$$\frac{\partial}{\partial v}\left(a_c \rho_c^*\right) = k_{oc} \rho_o^* - k_{co} \rho_c^*.$$

13.4.4 Stochastic Simulations Using the Optimal Open State Blocker

In Fig. 13.10, we show the results of numerical simulations using scheme (13.14). We show the result for the wild type model (upper panel), the mutant model (middle panel), and the model of the mutant where the drug defined by (13.25) is used (lower panel).

The graphs show that the effect of the mutation is repaired using the drug (13.25); the solutions are not identical and this is reasonable, since a random number generator is involved in updating the state of the Markov model and therefore two computed solutions will not be identical (not even two wild type solutions).

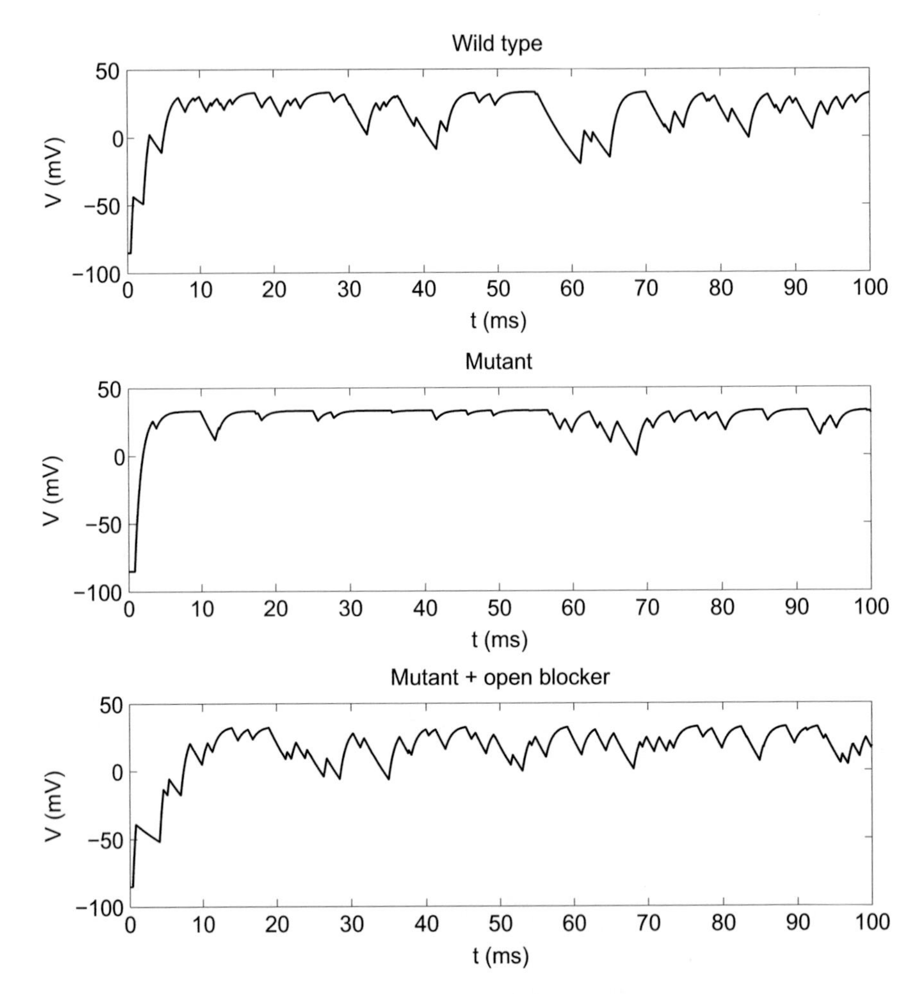

Fig. 13.10 Numerical simulations using scheme (13.14) for wild type data (*upper panel*), mutant data (*center panel*), and mutant data where the drug defined by (13.25) is used (*lower panel*). Observe the long open periods in the middle panel and that these are repaired by the drug (*lower panel*)

However, we note that the qualitative properties of the upper and lower solutions are similar, whereas the mutant case is different due to the increased open probability and prolonged mean open time.

13.5 Inactivated States and Mean Open Time

In Chap. 11, we studied a Markov model including the open state (O), closed state (C), and inactivated state (I). The prototypical Markov model is repeated in Fig. 13.11. As usual, we assumed that the principle of detailed balance holds and therefore the parameters of the Markov model satisfy the equation

$$k_{io}k_{oc}k_{ci} = k_{oi}k_{co}k_{ic}. \tag{13.33}$$

We also introduced a mutation that increased the rates k_{io} and k_{ic} and thus reduced the probability of being in the inactivated state. From what we have just seen, we readily observe that such a mutation does not influence the mean open time; however, if data show that the mean open time is affected, the effect of the mutation must be modeled differently. Another way to model the reduced equilibrium probability of being in the inactivated state is to reduce the rates toward the inactivated state. Such a mutation takes the form

$$\begin{aligned} \bar{k}_{ci} &= k_{ci}/\mu, \\ \bar{k}_{oi} &= k_{oi}/\mu, \end{aligned} \tag{13.34}$$

where $\mu \geqslant 1$ and, as usual, $\mu = 1$ represents the wild type. It follows from (13.33) that the principle of detailed balance also holds for the mutant model:

$$k_{io}k_{oc}\frac{k_{ci}}{\mu} = \frac{k_{oi}}{\mu}k_{co}k_{ic}. \tag{13.35}$$

If we repeat the argument above, we find that the mean open time of the model presented in Fig. 13.11 is given by

$$\tau_o = \frac{1}{k_{oc} + k_{oi}}$$

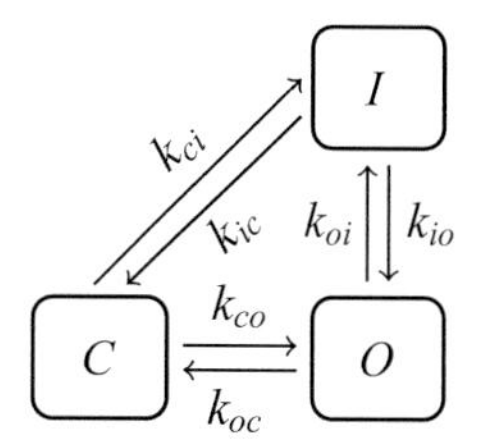

Fig. 13.11 Three-state Markov model. In the mutant case, we replace the rates k_{ci} and k_{oi} by k_{ci}/μ and k_{oi}/μ, respectively, where μ denotes the mutation severity index

for wild type data and

$$\tau_{o,\mu} = \frac{1}{k_{oc} + k_{oi}/\mu}$$

for the mutant case. We note that the mean open time increases as the mutation severity index μ increases. Following the usual steps, we find that the equilibrium probabilities are given by

$$o = \frac{1}{1 + \frac{k_{oc}}{k_{co}} + \frac{k_{oi}}{\mu k_{io}}},$$

$$c = \frac{\frac{k_{oc}}{k_{co}}}{1 + \frac{k_{oc}}{k_{co}} + \frac{k_{oi}}{\mu k_{io}}},$$

$$i = \frac{\frac{k_{oi}}{k_{io}}}{\mu\left(1 + \frac{k_{oc}}{k_{co}}\right) + \frac{k_{oi}}{k_{io}}}.$$

We observe that the equilibrium probability of being in the open and closed states increases as a consequence of the mutation and the equilibrium probability of being in the inactivated state is reduced under the mutation.

13.5.1 A Theoretical Open State Blocker

We observed above that to repair the effect of changes in the mean open time, it is necessary to use an open state blocker. The reason for this is that neither a closed blocker nor an inactivated blocker has any effect on the mean open time and, therefore, it is inconceivable that such blockers can repair the effect of a mutation on the mean open time. An open state blocker directly affects the mean open time and the drug must be tuned to repair the effect of the mutation.

A Markov model that includes an open state blocker is shown in Fig. 13.12. We have already computed formulas for the equilibrium probabilities of a Markov model of this form (see page 170). The inverse ($p = 1/o$) open probability in equilibrium is given by

$$p_{\mu} = 1 + \frac{k_{oc}}{k_{co}} + \frac{1}{\mu}\frac{k_{oi}}{k_{io}}$$

and thus the wild type inverse open probability is given by

$$p = 1 + \frac{k_{oc}}{k_{co}} + \frac{k_{oi}}{k_{io}}.$$

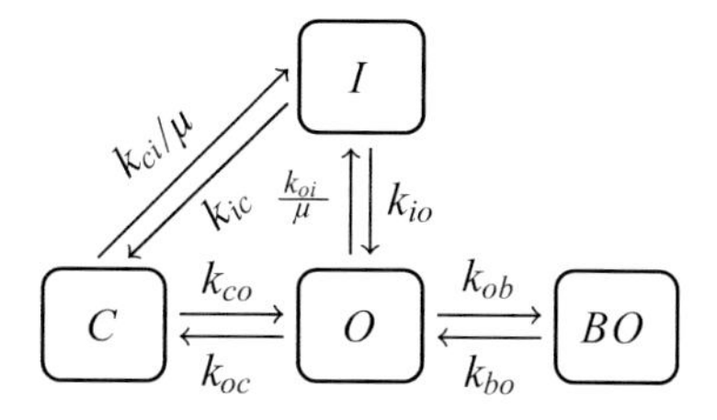

Fig. 13.12 The model represented in Fig. 13.11 is extended to account for the blocker (BO) associated with the open state

Similarly, the inverse open probability in the presence of the open state blocker is given by

$$p_{b,\mu} = 1 + \frac{k_{oc}}{k_{co}} + \frac{1}{\mu}\frac{k_{oi}}{k_{io}} + \frac{k_{ob}}{k_{bo}}.$$

Furthermore, the mean open time of wild type is given by

$$\tau_o = \frac{1}{k_{oi} + k_{oc}}$$

and, when the theoretical drug is included in the mutant case, the mean open time is given by

$$\tau_{o,b,\mu} = \frac{1}{\frac{1}{\mu}k_{oi} + k_{oc} + k_{ob}}.$$

We are now looking for a drug that will repair the equilibrium probability and the mean open time. More precisely, we want to find the parameters k_{bo} and k_{ob} such that $p_{b,\mu} = p$ and $\tau_{o,b,\mu} = \tau_o$. More explicitly, we require that

$$1 + \frac{k_{oc}}{k_{co}} + \frac{1}{\mu}\frac{k_{oi}}{k_{io}} + \frac{k_{ob}}{k_{bo}} = 1 + \frac{k_{oc}}{k_{co}} + \frac{k_{oi}}{k_{io}}$$

and

$$\frac{1}{\mu}k_{oi} + k_{oc} + k_{ob} = k_{oi} + k_{oc}.$$

This is a 2×2 system of equations in the unknowns k_{ob} and k_{bo} and the solution is given by

$$k_{ob} = \left(1 - \mu^{-1}\right) k_{oi} \text{ and } k_{bo} = k_{io}. \tag{13.36}$$

We will see in numerical experiments below that the open state blocker illustrated in Fig. 13.12 where the parameters of the drug are given by (13.36) repairs the effect of the mutation.

13.5.2 *Probability Density Functions Using the Open State Blocker*

We have found a theoretical drug (see (13.36)) for the mutation affecting the rates from O to I and from C to I and we want to assess the drug's usefulness by considering the open probability density functions. For the wild type case, the probability density functions of the states present in the Markov model of Fig. 13.11 are governed by the system

$$
\begin{aligned}
\frac{\partial}{\partial v}(a_o\rho_o) &= k_{co}\rho_c - (k_{oc} + k_{oi})\,\rho_o + k_{io}\rho_i,\\
\frac{\partial}{\partial v}(a_c\rho_c) &= k_{oc}\rho_o - (k_{co} + k_{ci})\,\rho_c + k_{ic}\rho_i,\\
\frac{\partial}{\partial v}(a_c\rho_i) &= k_{oi}\rho_o - (k_{io} + k_{ic})\rho_i + k_{ci}\rho_c.
\end{aligned}
\tag{13.37}
$$

In the mutant case, when the open state blocker is added as indicated in Fig. 13.12, the probability density system is

$$
\begin{aligned}
\frac{\partial}{\partial v}(a_o\rho_o) &= k_{co}\rho_c - \left(k_{oc} + \frac{1}{\mu}k_{oi} + k_{ob}\right)\rho_o + k_{io}\rho_i + k_{bo}\rho_b,\\
\frac{\partial}{\partial v}(a_c\rho_c) &= k_{oc}\rho_o - \left(k_{co} + \frac{1}{\mu}k_{ci}\right)\rho_c + k_{ic}\rho_i,\\
\frac{\partial}{\partial v}(a_c\rho_i) &= \frac{1}{\mu}k_{oi}\rho_o - (k_{io} + k_{ic})\rho_i + \frac{1}{\mu}k_{ci}\rho_c,\\
\frac{\partial}{\partial v}(a_c\rho_b) &= k_{ob}\rho_o - k_{bo}\rho_b.
\end{aligned}
\tag{13.38}
$$

As usual, ρ_o, ρ_c, ρ_i, and ρ_b denote the probability density functions of the open, closed, inactivated, and blocked states, respectively, and the functions of the flux are given by (13.18). By introducing the drug given by (13.36), we obtain the system

$$
\begin{aligned}
\frac{\partial}{\partial v}(a_o\rho_o) &= k_{co}\rho_c - (k_{oc} + k_{oi})\,\rho_o + k_{io}\rho_i + k_{io}\rho_b,\\
\frac{\partial}{\partial v}(a_c\rho_c) &= k_{oc}\rho_o - \left(k_{co} + \frac{1}{\mu}k_{ci}\right)\rho_c + k_{ic}\rho_i,\\
\frac{\partial}{\partial v}(a_c\rho_i) &= \frac{1}{\mu}k_{oi}\rho_o - (k_{io} + k_{ic})\rho_i + \frac{1}{\mu}k_{ci}\rho_c,\\
\frac{\partial}{\partial v}(a_c\rho_b) &= \left(1 - \mu^{-1}\right)k_{oi}\rho_o - k_{io}\rho_b.
\end{aligned}
\tag{13.39}
$$

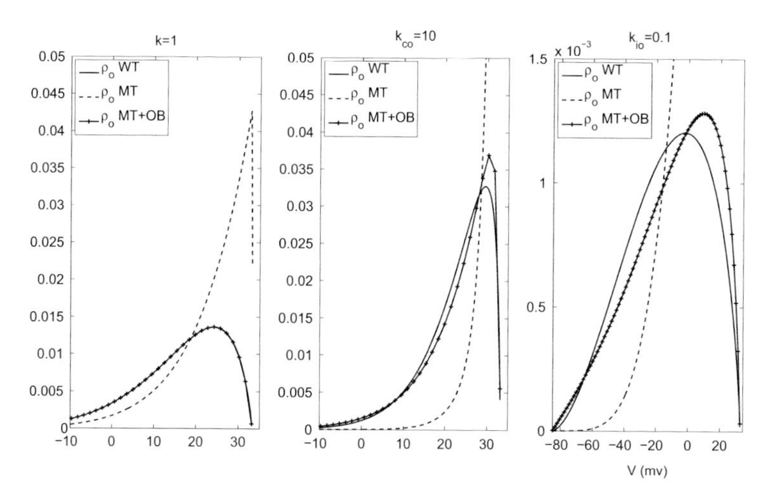

Fig. 13.13 *Left panel*: All rates equal one. The theoretical drug restores ρ_o. *Middle panel*: As in the left panel, except $k_{co} = 10\ \text{ms}^{-1}$. *Right panel*: As in the left panel, except $k_{io} = 0.1\ \text{ms}^{-1}$. For all three cases, $\mu = 10$

In Fig. 13.13, we show solutions of the wild type system (13.37), the mutant system, and the mutant system where the drug is added (13.39). Note that the mutant system is equal to the wild type system, except for the change of the rates k_{ci} and k_{oi} given by

$$\bar{k}_{ci} = k_{ci}/\mu, \tag{13.40}$$
$$\bar{k}_{oi} = k_{oi}/\mu.$$

In Fig. 13.13, we compare the open probability density functions of the three models for three different sets of parameters. In the left panel of Fig. 13.13, we show the open probability of the wild type (solid line), the mutant ($\mu = 10$), and the mutant in the presence of the theoretical open blocker. We see that the effect of the mutation is completely repaired by the drug. Other cases are shown in the center and right panels. The effect of the drug is still good but the effect of the mutation is not completely repaired. These observations are confirmed in Table 13.1. Furthermore, we have tested a large variety of parameters and the results we show here (center and right panels) represent the most difficult cases we could find in experiments. Therefore, we conclude that the theoretical open state blocker illustrated in Fig. 13.12 works very well.

Table 13.1 Statistical properties of ρ_o for the cases shown in Fig. 13.13

	$k = 1$		$k_{co} = 10$		$k_{io} = 0.1$	
	π_o	E_o	π_o	E_o	π_o	E_o
WT	0.333	16.366	0.476	22.995	0.083	−12.867
MT	0.476	23.272	0.833	31.074	0.333	17.702
MT+OB	0.333	16.366	0.476	23.169	0.083	−9.225

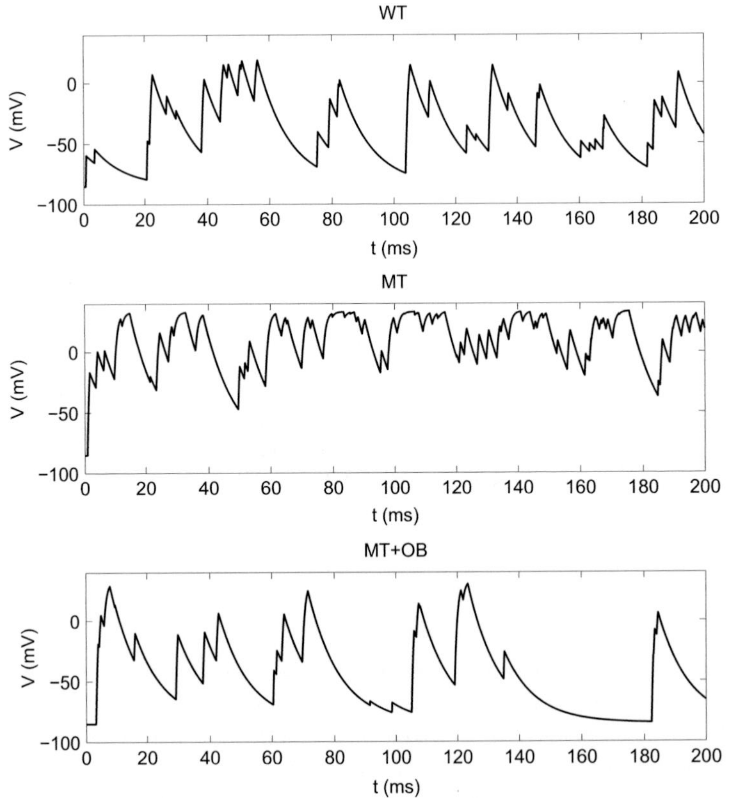

Fig. 13.14 Monte Carlo runs of the case shown in the right panel of Fig. 13.13

13.5.3 Stochastic Simulations Using the Open State Blocker

In Fig. 13.14, we show simulations using the numerical scheme

$$v_{n+1} = v_n - \Delta t\,(g_K\,(v_n - V_K) + \gamma_n g_{Na}(v_n - V_{Na})), \tag{13.41}$$

where the value of the variable γ_n is determined by the Markov model given in Fig. 13.11. For the wild type case, the rates k_{ci} and k_{oi} are used and, in the mutant case, the rates k_{ci}/μ and k_{oi}/μ are used. Furthermore, when the drug is applied in the mutant case, the Markov model is as illustrated in Fig. 13.12, where the rates of the drug are given by (13.36). We observe that, in the mutant case, the channel does not inactivate and therefore more action potentials are generated. When the drug is applied, this effect seems to be removed and the channel again acts more or less as in the wild type case. However, as mentioned above it is not straightforward to compare solutions based on the stochastic model and therefore we emphasis the use of probability density functions.

13.6 Notes

1. The derivation of the formula for the mean open time given by (13.4) can be found in many places (e.g., Keener and Sneyd [42] or Smith [85]).

Chapter 14
The Burst Mode of the Mutant Sodium Channel

We observed above that the effect of the ΔKPQ mutation of the SCN5A gene leading to a delayed sodium current can be modeled by increasing the reaction rates from the inactivated state to the open state and to the permissible state C_0. The model gave results at least qualitatively similar to the experimental data (see Fig. 12.4).

A better-established way of modeling the effect of the mutation is to introduce a so-called burst mode. A simple Markov model including a burst mode is illustrated in Fig. 14.1, where the states of the burst mode are indicated by $*$. Note that when the channel is in the burst mode, there is no inactivated state and therefore the burst mode can be used to model the effect of impaired inactivation. The reaction rates going from the burst mode to the normal mode are given by k^u (where u stands for up) and the reaction rates from the normal mode to the burst mode are given by k^d (where d stands for down). We assume $k^d << k^u$, which means that, for the wild type, the probability of being in the burst mode is very small. The probability of being in the burst mode increases with the mutation severity index μ. As usual, $\mu = 1$ represents the wild type. In the wild type, a channel is basically never in the burst mode and therefore the channel inactivates as it should and no late sodium current is observed. In the mutant case, however, the probability of being in the burst mode is increased. Since there is no inactivated state in the burst mode, the channel fails to inactivate and therefore the probability of being in the open state is increased and therefore we observe a non-negligible late current. This will be illustrated in the numerical computations below.

A. Tveito, G.T. Lines, *Computing Characterizations of Drugs for Ion Channels and Receptors Using Markov Models*, Lecture Notes in Computational Science and Engineering 111, DOI 10.1007/978-3-319-30030-6_14

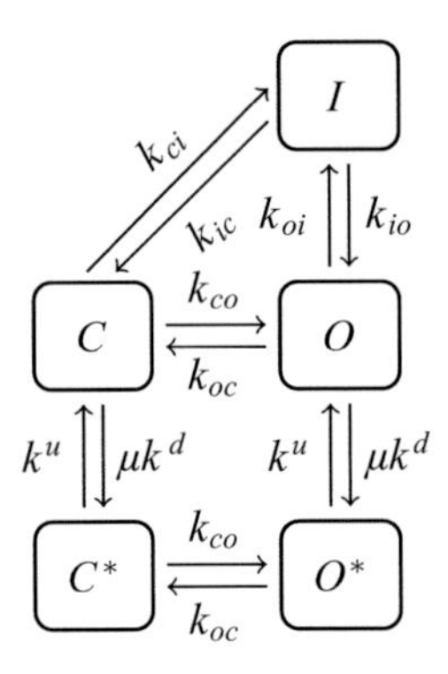

Fig. 14.1 Prototypical model of a sodium channel including a burst mode. The model consists of the states O, I, and C of the normal mode and O^* and C^* of the burst mode (*lower part*)

14.1 Equilibrium Probabilities

We will start by considering the equilibrium states of the prototypical model illustrated in Fig. 14.1. By following the usual steps (see, e.g., page 187) we find the equilibrium probabilities given by

$$o = \frac{1}{1 + \frac{k_{oi}}{k_{io}} + \frac{k_{oc}}{k_{co}} + \frac{\mu k^d}{k^u}\frac{k_{oc}}{k_{co}} + \frac{\mu k^d}{k^u}}, \tag{14.1}$$

$$i = \frac{\frac{k_{oi}}{k_{io}}}{1 + \frac{k_{oi}}{k_{io}} + \frac{k_{oc}}{k_{co}} + \frac{\mu k^d}{k^u}\frac{k_{oc}}{k_{co}} + \frac{\mu k^d}{k^u}}, \tag{14.2}$$

$$c = \frac{\frac{k_{oc}}{k_{co}}}{1 + \frac{k_{oi}}{k_{io}} + \frac{k_{oc}}{k_{co}} + \frac{\mu k^d}{k^u}\frac{k_{oc}}{k_{co}} + \frac{\mu k^d}{k^u}}, \tag{14.3}$$

$$c^* = \frac{\frac{k_{oc}}{k_{co}}\frac{\mu k^d}{k^u}}{1 + \frac{k_{oi}}{k_{io}} + \frac{k_{oc}}{k_{co}} + \frac{\mu k^d}{k^u}\frac{k_{oc}}{k_{co}} + \frac{\mu k^d}{k^u}}, \tag{14.4}$$

$$o^* = \frac{\frac{\mu k^d}{k^u}}{1 + \frac{k_{oi}}{k_{io}} + \frac{k_{oc}}{k_{co}} + \frac{\mu k^d}{k^u}\frac{k_{oc}}{k_{co}} + \frac{\mu k^d}{k^u}}. \tag{14.5}$$

Here, we observe that the equilibrium probability of being in the inactivated state is clearly reduced as the mutation severity index is increased. This is the effect we wanted, since inactivation is impaired in the mutation and the effect is modeled by introducing a burst mode that lacks the inactivated state. Second, we observe that the sum of the open probabilities given by

$$o + o^* = \frac{1 + \mu\frac{k^d}{k^u}}{1 + \frac{k_{oi}}{k_{io}} + \frac{k_{oc}}{k_{co}} + \mu\frac{k^d}{k^u}\frac{k_{oc}}{k_{co}} + \mu\frac{k^d}{k^u}} \tag{14.6}$$

is an increasing function of μ; in fact,

$$\frac{d}{d\mu}\left(o+o^*\right)=\frac{\frac{k^d}{k^u}\frac{k_{oi}}{k_{io}}}{\left(1+\frac{k_{oc}}{k_{co}}+\frac{k_{oi}}{k_{io}}+\mu\frac{k^d}{k^u}\frac{k_{oc}}{k_{co}}+\mu\frac{k^d}{k^u}\right)^2}>0. \tag{14.7}$$

So the model has the two main properties we seek: The equilibrium probability of being in the inactivated state is reduced and the open probability is increased.

14.2 The Mean Open Time

We observed above (see page 196) that the formula for the mean open time can also be derived in the presence of several open states. If we generalize the argument to also take into account the inactivated state, we find that the mean open time of the Markov model illustrated in Fig. 14.1 is given by

$$\tau_{o,\mu}=\frac{\mu k^d+k^u}{\mu k^d k_{oc}+k^u\left(k_{oc}+k_{oi}\right)} \tag{14.8}$$

and, since

$$\frac{d\tau_{o,\mu}}{d\mu}=\frac{k_{oi}k^d k^u}{\left(k^u k_{oc}+k^u k_{oi}+\mu k_{oc}k^d\right)^2}, \tag{14.9}$$

the mean open time increases as a function of the mutation severity index.

14.3 An Optimal Theoretical Open State Blocker

Our aim is now to define an open state drug that can repair both the equilibrium open probability and the mean open time. The structure of the open state blocker is given in Fig. 14.2 and the equilibrium total open probability is now given by

$$\left(o+o^*\right)_{\mu,d}=\frac{1+\mu\frac{k^d}{k^u}}{1+\frac{k_{oi}}{k_{io}}+\frac{k_{oc}}{k_{co}}+\mu\frac{k^d}{k^u}\frac{k_{oc}}{k_{co}}+\mu\frac{k^d}{k^u}+\frac{k_{ob}}{k_{bo}}\left(1+\frac{\mu k^d}{k^u}\right)}. \tag{14.10}$$

Furthermore, the mean open time is now given by

$$\tau_{o,\mu,d}=\frac{\mu k^d+k^u}{\mu k^d\left(k_{oc}+k_{ob}\right)+k^u\left(k_{oc}+k_{oi}+k_{ob}\right)}, \tag{14.11}$$

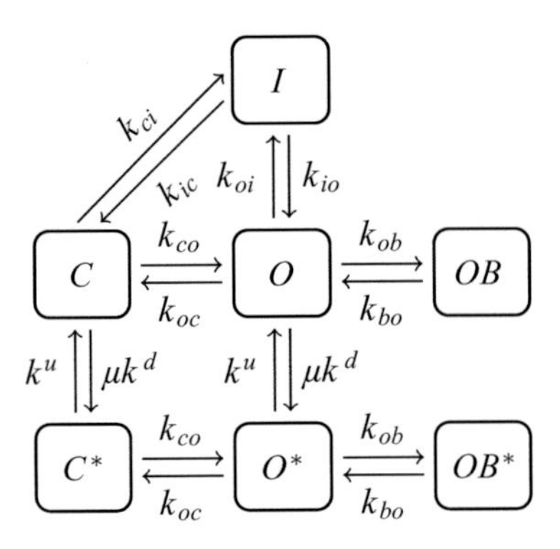

Fig. 14.2 Prototypical model of a sodium channel including a burst mode and an open state blocker. The model consists of the states O, I, C, and OB of the normal mode and O^*, C^*, and OB^* of the burst mode (*lower part*). The states OB and OB^* represent the open blocker and we assume that the rates characterizing the blocker are the same in the normal and burst modes

where the subscript d is used to remind us that this concerns the case where the theoretical drug has been applied.

The task at hand is now to tune the drug such that the equilibrium open probability and the mean open time given by (14.10) and (14.11), respectively, are as close as possible to the equilibrium open probability and the mean open time of the wild type. We regard the parameters k_{ob} and k_{bo} as the unknowns and we want to solve the following 2×2 system of equations:

$$\frac{1+\mu\frac{k^d}{k^u}}{1+\frac{k_{oi}}{k_{io}}+\frac{k_{oc}}{k_{co}}+\mu\frac{k^d}{k^u}\frac{k_{oc}}{k_{co}}+\mu\frac{k^d}{k^u}+\frac{k_{ob}}{k_{bo}}\left(1+\mu\frac{k^d}{k^u}\right)} = \frac{1+\frac{k^d}{k^u}}{1+\frac{k_{oi}}{k_{io}}+\frac{k_{oc}}{k_{co}}+\frac{k^d}{k^u}\frac{k_{oc}}{k_{co}}+\frac{k^d}{k^u}}, \tag{14.12}$$

$$\frac{\mu k^d + k^u}{\mu k^d\left(k_{oc}+k_{ob}\right)+k^u\left(k_{oc}+k_{oi}+k_{ob}\right)} = \frac{k^d+k^u}{k^d k_{oc}+k^u\left(k_{oc}+k_{oi}\right)}, \tag{14.13}$$

where the latter equation determines the on rate, k_{ob}, of the drug,

$$k_{ob} = (\mu - 1)\frac{k^d k^u k_{oi}}{\left(k^u+\mu k^d\right)\left(k^u+k^d\right)}, \tag{14.14}$$

and we note that, in the case of $\mu = 1$, the drug is completely turned off, which is reasonable. Since k_{ob} is known, the off rate of the drug can be computed by solving (14.12). If we define

$$A = \frac{k_{ob}}{k_{bo}}, \tag{14.15}$$

we find from (14.12)

$$A = (\mu - 1)\frac{k_{oi}}{k_{io}} \frac{k^u k^d}{(\mu k^d + k^u)(k^d + k^u)} \tag{14.16}$$

and then the off rate of the drug is given by

$$k_{bo} = A^{-1} k_{ob} = k_{io} \tag{14.17}$$

which is the same as we have in the prototypical model given in Fig. 13.12; see (13.36) on page 217.

14.4 Numerical Experiments

The purpose of this section is to show how the burst mode can be used to represent impaired inactivation and how the theoretical drug derived above works.

14.4.1 Representation of the Late Sodium Current Using the Burst Mode Model

As discussed in Chap. 12, impaired inactivation leads to a late sodium current (see Fig. 12.4). Here, we will see that this effect can also be obtained using a Markov model of the form indicated in Fig. 14.1. In Fig. 14.3, we repeat the computations reported in Fig. 12.4, using the Markov model of Fig. 14.1. The parameters used in this computation are given in Table 14.1. We observe from Fig. 14.3 that $\mu = 20$ seems to represent the late current of Fig. 12.4 fairly well.

14.4.2 The Open State Blocker Repairs the Effect of the Mutation

In Fig. 14.3, we show the late current for the wild type, the mutant $\mu = 20$, and the drug using the optimal open state blocker defined by (14.14) and (14.17). We observe that the late current induced by the mutation is repaired by the open state blocker. The statistics of the open probability density function (for the wild type, the mutant ($\mu = 20$), and the mutant where the drug has been applied) are given in Table 14.2 and the corresponding probability density functions are shown in Fig. 14.4. Again we note that the open blocker repairs the main features of the solution.

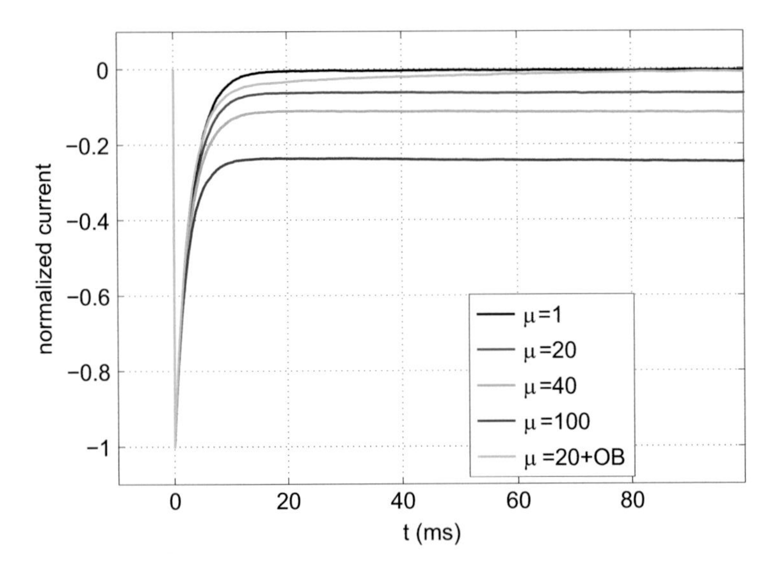

Fig. 14.3 Currents computed using the Markov model illustrated in Fig. 14.2. The simulations are based on averages of 10,000 runs. As expected, the open blocker asymptotically repairs the late current

Table 14.1 Values of the parameters used in the model in Fig. 14.2. The remaining rates are as in Table 12.2

μ	20
k_u	0.0001 ms^{-1}
k_d	0.001 ms^{-1}
k_{ob}	0.0286 ms^{-1}
k_{bo}	0.000824 ms^{-1}

Table 14.2 Statistics of the stationary probability density functions computed using the Markov model illustrated in Fig. 14.2. The subscript o refers to open states and the subscript n refers to non-conducting states

μ	π_o	π_n	E_o	E_n
1	0.59	0.41	31.2	−54.2
20	0.96	0.04	33.1	−52.8
50	0.98	0.02	33.1	−51.3
100	0.99	0.01	33.2	−49.8
20+OB	0.46	0.54	30.2	−57.9

14.5 A More Sophisticated Markov Model

The Markov model presented in Fig. 14.1 above has a structure that is a bit simpler than the Markov model commonly used to model the sodium channel. A more common structure is given in Fig. 14.5. This is the model we studied in Chap. 12. When a burst mode is added to it, the Markov model obtains the form illustrated in Fig. 14.6.

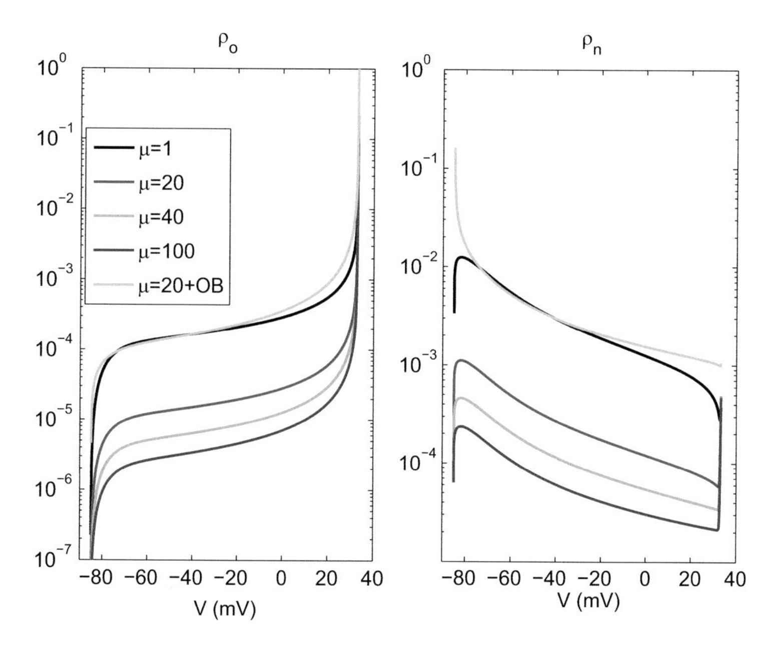

Fig. 14.4 Stationary probability density functions computed using the Markov model illustrated in Fig. 14.2. The open probability density function is given in the left panel and the probability density function of the sum of non-conducting states is given in the right panel. We observe that the open blocker repairs most parts of the probability density functions

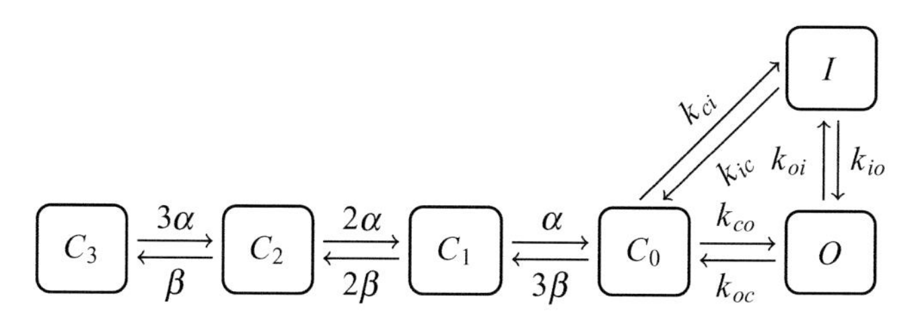

Fig. 14.5 Typical Markov model of a wild type sodium channel consisting of an open state (O), an inactivated state (I), and four closed states (C_0, C_1, C_2, and C_3). This model was analyzed in Chap. 12

To understand how the burst mode changes the properties of the model, it is of interest to compute the equilibrium probabilities. The equilibrium state of the model presented in Fig. 14.6 is characterized by the following system of equations:

$$
\begin{aligned}
&k_{ci}c_0 = k_{ic}i, \quad k_{oi}o = k_{io}i, \quad k_{co}c_0 = k_{oc}o, \\
&3\beta c_0 = \alpha c_1, \;\; 2\alpha c_2 = 2\beta c_1, \;\; 3\alpha c_3 = \beta c_2, \\
&k^u o^* = \mu k^d o, \; k^u c_0^* = \mu k^d c_0, \; k^u c_1^* = \mu k^d c_1, \\
&k^u c_2^* = \mu k^d c_2, \; k^u c_3^* = \mu k^d c_3.
\end{aligned}
\tag{14.18}
$$

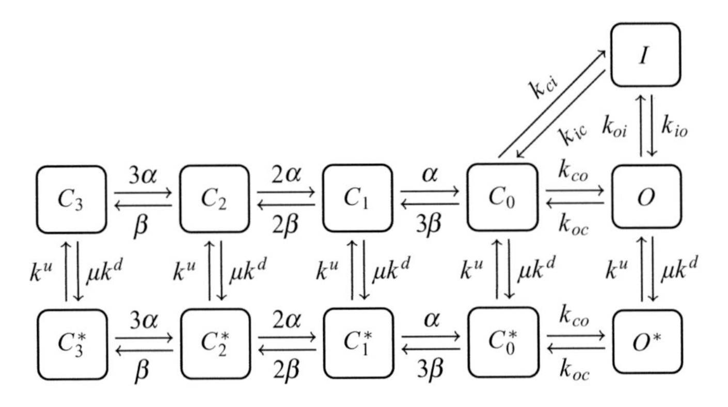

Fig. 14.6 Markov model of the sodium channel. The model consists of the states O, I, C_0, C_1, C_2, and C_3 of the normal mode and O^*, C_0^*, C_1^*, C_2^*, and C_3^* of the burst mode (*lower part*). Note that there is no inactivated state in the burst mode and that μ denotes the mutation severity index. A larger value of μ increases the probability of moving from the normal (*upper*) mode to the burst (*lower*) mode

It follows that

$$i = \frac{k_{oi}}{k_{io}} o, \; c_0 = \frac{k_{oc}}{k_{co}} o,$$

$$c_1 = \frac{3\beta}{\alpha} \frac{k_{oc}}{k_{co}} o, \; c_2 = \frac{3\beta^2}{\alpha^2} \frac{k_{oc}}{k_{co}} o, \; c_3 = \frac{\beta^3}{\alpha^3} \frac{k_{oc}}{k_{co}} o,$$

$$o^* = \mu \frac{k^d}{k^u} o, c_0^* = \mu \frac{k^d}{k^u} \frac{k_{oc}}{k_{co}} o, c_1^* = \mu \frac{3\beta}{\alpha} \frac{k^d}{k^u} \frac{k_{oc}}{k_{co}} o,$$

$$c_2^* = \mu \frac{3\beta^2}{\alpha^2} \frac{k^d}{k^u} \frac{k_{oc}}{k_{co}} o, c_3^* = \mu \frac{\beta^3}{\alpha^3} \frac{k^d}{k^u} \frac{k_{oc}}{k_{co}} o$$

and, since the sum of the probabilities equals one, we have

$$o(\mu) = \frac{1}{\frac{k_{oi}}{k_{io}} + \left(1 + \mu \frac{k^d}{k^u}\right)\left(1 + \frac{k_{oc}}{k_{co}} (1 + \beta/\alpha)^3\right)}$$

and

$$o(\mu) + o^*(\mu) = \frac{1 + \mu \frac{k^d}{k^u}}{\frac{k_{oi}}{k_{io}} + \left(1 + \mu \frac{k^d}{k^u}\right)\left(1 + \frac{k_{oc}}{k_{co}} (1 + \beta/\alpha)^3\right)}.$$

Therefore,

$$\frac{d}{d\mu}\left(o\left(\mu\right)+o^{*}\left(\mu\right)\right)=\frac{\frac{k_{oi}}{k_{io}}\frac{k^{d}}{k^{u}}}{\left(\frac{k_{oi}}{k_{io}}+\left(1+\frac{k_{oc}}{k_{co}}\left(1+\beta/\alpha\right)^{3}\right)\left(1+\mu\frac{k^{d}}{k^{u}}\right)\right)^{2}}>0,$$

so the total open probability increases as the mutation severity index μ increases. This will lead to a sustained sodium current characteristic of the mutation under consideration.

It is also interesting to see how the mutation severity index changes the probability of being in the normal or burst mode. To understand this, we define b and b^{*} as the sum of the probabilities in the normal and burst modes, respectively. By using the equilibrium probabilities derived above, we obtain

$$\frac{b^{*}}{b}=\frac{o^{*}+c_{0}^{*}+c_{1}^{*}+c_{2}^{*}+c_{3}^{*}}{o+c_{0}+c_{1}+c_{2}+c_{3}+i}=\mu\frac{k^{d}}{k^{u}}\frac{1+\frac{k_{oc}}{k_{co}}\left(1+\beta/\alpha\right)^{3}}{\frac{k_{oi}}{k_{io}}+1+\frac{k_{oc}}{k_{co}}\left(1+\beta/\alpha\right)^{3}}$$

and thus the probability of being in the burst mode increases as the mutation severity index increases.

14.6 Numerical Experiments Illustrating the Effect of the Burst Mode

The effect of increasing the mutation severity index of the Markov model given in Fig. 14.6 is shown in Fig. 14.7 using the parameters given in Table 14.3. The associated currents are shown in Fig. 14.8 and we note that when the mutation severity index increases, there is a significant late sodium current (Table 14.4).

14.7 A Theoretical Drug for the Mutation Represented by the Burst Mode

In the simplified Markov model presented in Fig. 14.1 above, we saw that an open blocker was able to repair the effect of the mutation. Now the Markov model is extended (see Fig. 14.6), but it is reasonable to believe that an open blocker is still the best alternative, since both the open probability and the mean open time are affected by the mutation. We consider the Markov model given in Fig. 14.9, where

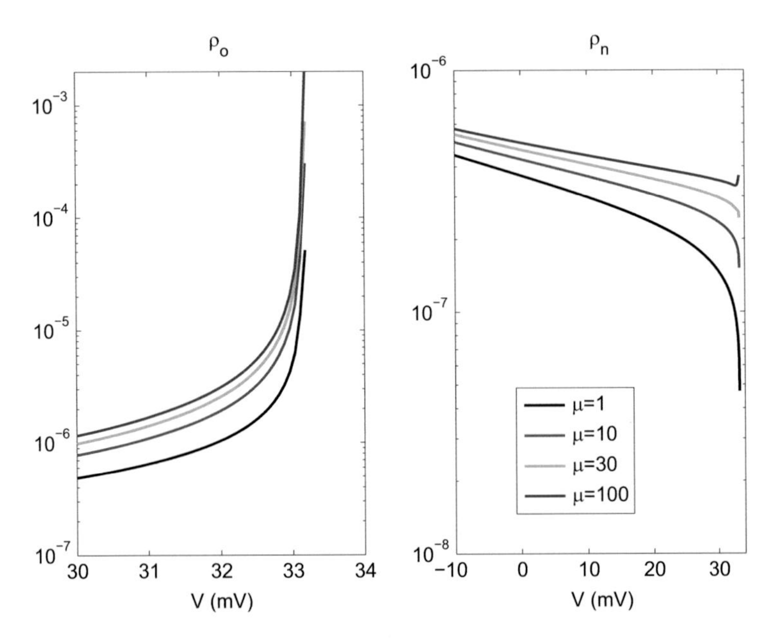

Fig. 14.7 The probability density functions of the open, closed, and inactivated states for the burst mode model. The mutation severity index is given by $\mu = 10, 30$, and 100 and the *black line* represents the wild type. Note that we only show solutions for the values of the transmembrane potential where the solutions differ as a result of the mutations

Table 14.3 Values of the parameters used in the model in Fig. 14.6. The remaining rates are as in Table 12.2 on page 184

μ	1,10,30,100
k_u	0.1 ms^{-1}
k_d	0.01 ms^{-1}

an open blocker is added to both the open states of the Markov model given in Fig. 14.6. By following our usual procedure, we find that

$$\left(o+o^*\right)_{\mu,d} = \frac{1+\mu\frac{k^d}{k^u}}{\frac{k_{ob}}{k_{bo}}\left(1+\mu\frac{k^d}{k^u}\right)+\frac{k_{oi}}{k_{io}}+\left(1+\mu\frac{k^d}{k^u}\right)\left(1+\frac{k_{oc}}{k_{co}}\left(1+\beta/\alpha\right)^3\right)}.$$

The associated mean open time is given by

$$\tau_{o,\mu,d} = \frac{\mu k^d + k^u}{\mu k^d\left(k_{oc}+k_{ob}\right)+k^u\left(k_{oc}+k_{oi}+k_{ob}\right)}. \tag{14.19}$$

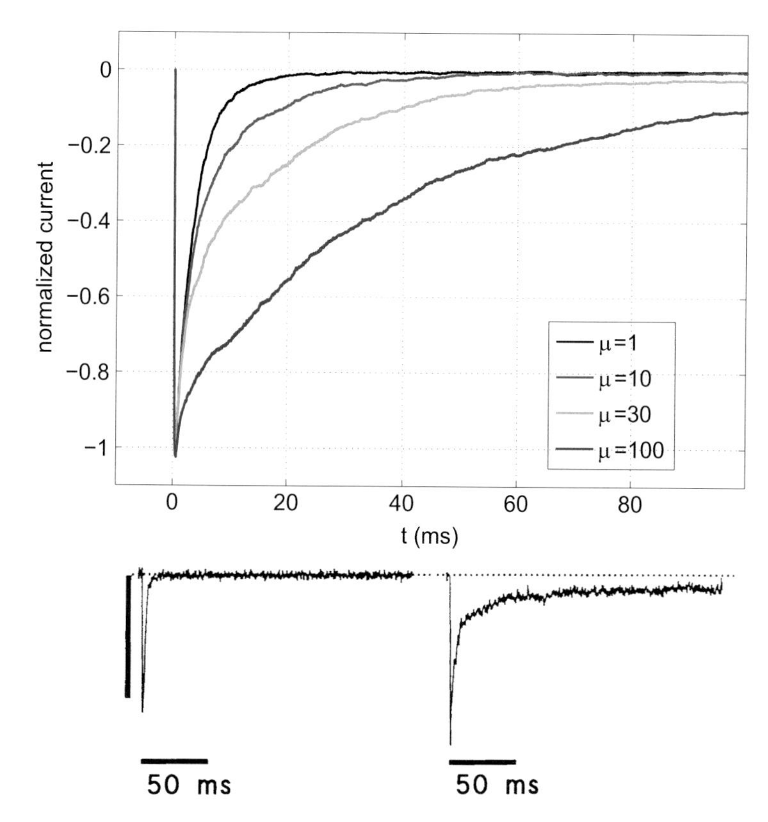

Fig. 14.8 Currents computed using the Markov model including the burst mode (see Fig. 14.6). *Top panel*: Current for $\mu = 1,\ 10,\ 30,\ 100$. Each trace is an average of 10,000 Monte Carlo runs and the current is computed by $I = g_{Na}P_o(v - V_{Na})$, with the transmembrane potential at $v = 0\,\text{mV}$. The currents are normalized so that the wild type current peaks at -1. Here $V_{Na} = 45\,\text{mV}$ and $g_{Na} = 1\,\text{mS/cm}^2$. The lower figures are from Bennett et al. [2]

Table 14.4 Probabilities and expected values of the transmembrane potential for open and non-conducting states for increasing values of the mutation severity index μ

μ	$1000 \times \pi_o$	π_n	E_o	E_c
1	0.05738	0.99994	−53.2	−84.9
10	0.08435	0.99992	−26.1	−84.9
30	0.12109	0.99983	−8.3	−84.9
100	0.22305	0.99978	10.5	−84.9
30+OB	0.05490	0.99995	−57.0	−84.9

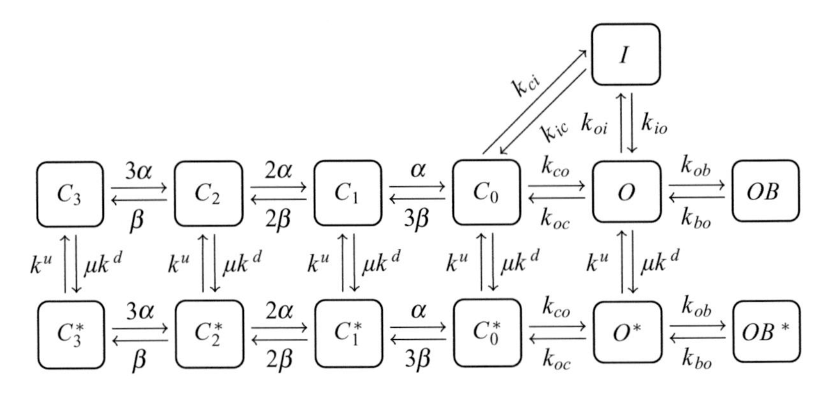

Fig. 14.9 Markov model of the mutant sodium channel with a blocker associated with the open states. The model consists of the states O, I, OB, C_0, C_1, C_2, and C_3 of the normal mode and $OB^*, O^*, C_0^*, C_1^*, C_2^*$, and C_3^* of the burst mode (*lower part*). The drug is characterized by the two parameters k_{bo} and k_{ob}

We now want to tune the drug characterized by the two parameters k_{ob} and k_{bo} such that

$$\left(o + o^*\right)_{\mu,d} \approx \left(o + o^*\right)_{wt}$$

and

$$\tau_{o,\mu,d} \approx \tau_{o,wt},$$

where the subscript *wt* denotes wild type values. As above, we have two equations for the two unknowns k_{ob} and k_{bo} and the solution is given by

$$k_{ob} = (\mu - 1)\frac{k^d k^u k_{oi}}{(k^u + \mu k^d)(k^u + k^d)} \tag{14.20}$$

and

$$k_{bo} = A^{-1} k_{ob}, \tag{14.21}$$

where

$$A = \frac{k_{oi}}{k_{io}} k^u k^d \frac{\mu - 1}{(\mu k^d + k^u)(k^d + k^u)}. \tag{14.22}$$

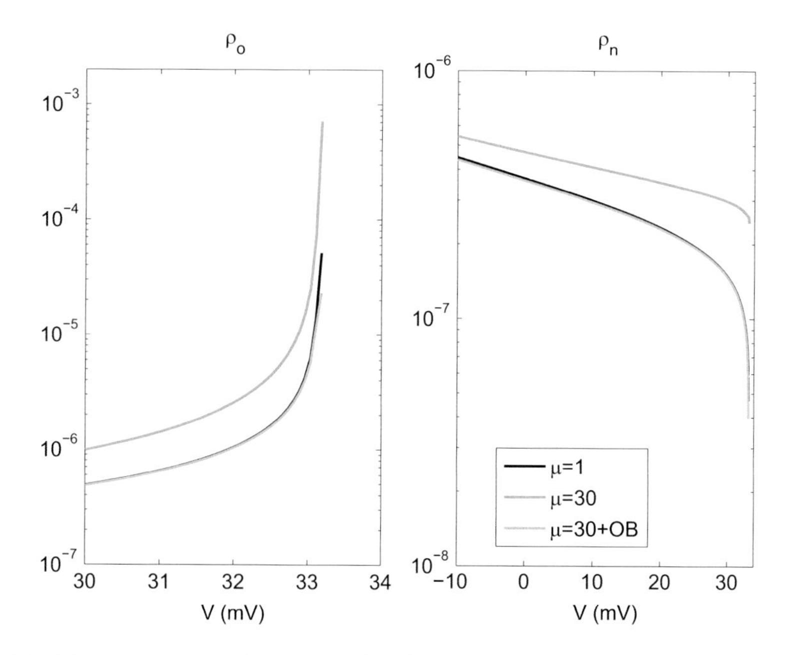

Fig. 14.10 Probability density functions for the wild type, the mutant ($\mu = 30$), and the mutant in the presence of the open blocker. The subscripts o and n refer to open and non-conduction states, respectively, where the states are shown in Fig. 14.9

So we obtain

$$k_{bo} = k_{io}. \tag{14.23}$$

We note that the formulas for the optimal open blocker for the Markov model given in Fig. 14.9 are exactly the same as for the open blocker of the prototype Markov model given in Fig. 14.2.

In Fig. 14.10, we show the probability density functions of the wild type, the mutant (using $\mu = 30$), and the mutant case where the optimal open blocker is applied. The blocker repairs the effect of the mutation and the same effect is seen in Fig. 14.11 where the currents are given; the open blocker removes the late sodium current.

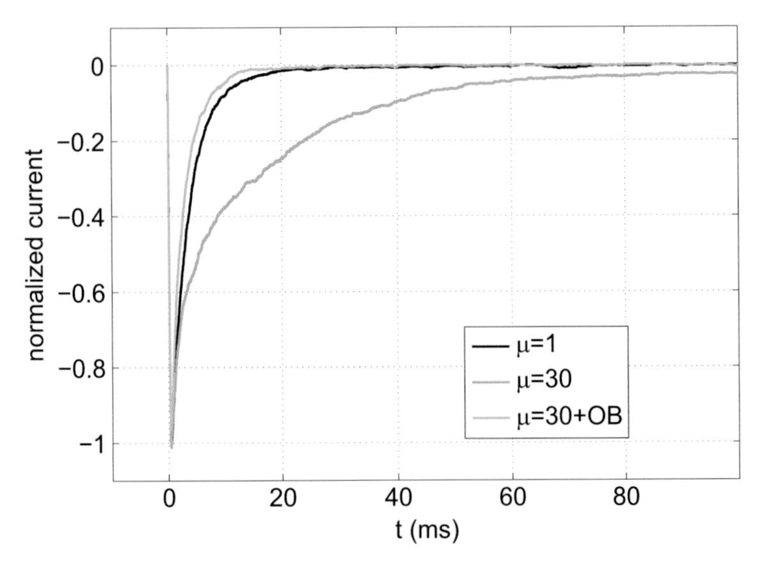

Fig. 14.11 Currents computed using the Markov model given in Fig. 14.9 for the wild type, the mutant ($\mu = 30$), and the mutant in the presence of the open blocker

14.8 Notes

1. The burst mode is discussed by Bennett et al. [2] and modeled in the paper by Clancy and Rudy [14].
2. The form of the model illustrated in Fig. 14.6 is taken from Clancy and Rudy [14], but the functions and parameters of the model are not taken from their paper.
3. As mentioned above, the introduction of a burst mode is a convenient way of modeling the effect of certain mutations. The notion that gating may enter various modes has been considerably extended and studied in the papers by Chakrapani et al. [10–12] and by Ionescu et al. [37]. In the recent paper by Siekmann et al [83] the concept of modal gating is studied and a method for detecting mode changes based on single channel data is developed.

Chapter 15
Action Potentials: Summing Up the Effect of Loads of Ion Channels

In this final chapter we will use the theoretical drugs developed in various chapters above for whole cell simulations. So far we have studied very small parts of a cell. We started by studying the dynamics going on in a single dyad; see Fig. 2.1. The size of one dyad is less than 1/1,000 μm^3[3] and we have been concerned with the concentration of calcium ions in this small volume. We have also studied the voltage dynamics in the vicinity of a single ion channel. The size of a single channel is about 1 nm. Now we address what is going on in a whole cell and it is important to realize that, compared to the single dyad and the single ion channel, the whole cell is huge; a normal ventricular cell is about 30,000 μm^3 [3], or on the order of 30 million times larger than the single dyad.

In the analysis of single channels, we have regarded the state of a channel as a stochastic variable. In the whole cell, however, the effect of a huge number of channels is added and the sum can be modeled using deterministic equations. We will still use the same Markov model formalism in terms of reaction schemes to formulate the models, but now we will use the associated master equations (see page 5) to define the open probability of the channel. Thus we need to solve deterministic systems of ordinary differential equations to find the open probability as a function of time.

Since the state of the channels will be represented using Markov model reaction schemes, we can study mutations in the same manner as we did for the single channel case. Therefore, we can use the results we derived above regarding optimal theoretical drugs for the single channel case for the whole cell case as well. The reasoning behind this was indicated earlier: If a mathematical model of a cell is constructed by using models of a huge number of single channels and we can repair the function of each single channel, the whole cell will be repaired.

In this chapter we will start by introducing a model of the action potential of the whole cell. We will focus on a simplified model that will merely represent the action potential in a qualitatively relevant manner; it will not represent any particular

A. Tveito, G.T. Lines, *Computing Characterizations of Drugs for Ion Channels and Receptors Using Markov Models*, Lecture Notes in Computational Science and Engineering 111, DOI 10.1007/978-3-319-30030-6_15

action potential in a quantitatively correct manner. Using numerical experiments, we will show that the model provides reasonable results for both wild type and various mutations. Finally, we will use the optimal theoretical drugs derived above and see that the effect of various mutations can be repaired using the theoretical drugs.

15.1 Whole Cell Action Potential Model

Our aim is now to introduce a reasonably simple action potential model for a whole cell. We will use the building blocks developed above and add some new features in order to get an action potential that is qualitatively reasonable.

The model consists of six main variables: v, c_e, c_c, c_d, c_j, and c_n. Here v, as usual, denotes the transmembrane potential given in mV. All the other variables are concentrations given in μM; c_e is the extracellular calcium concentration, c_c is the cytosolic concentration, c_d is the concentration of the dyad, c_j is the concentration of the JSR, and finally c_n is the concentration of the NSR; see Fig. 15.1. In addition to these six main variables, we will have variables associated with various Markov models; all these variables are between zero and one; they also denote probabilities and they have no unit. The transmembrane potential is governed by the equation

$$Cv' = -(I_{Na} + I_{Ca} + I_K + I_0) \tag{15.1}$$

where the minus sign is according to convention in the field. Here C denotes the capacitance and is simply a constant that will be specified below. The current I_0 represents a stimulus of the cell and we will use it below to initiate action potentials.

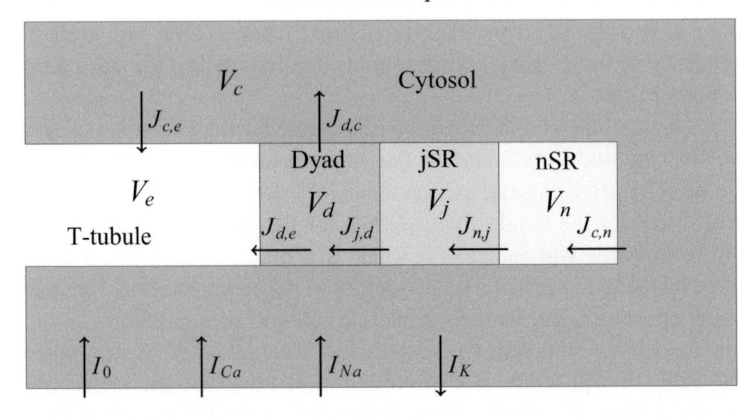

Fig. 15.1 Sketch of the calcium dynamics and the fluxes and pumps involved. The volumes of the cytosol, the dyad, the junctional sarcoplasmic reticulum (JSR) and the network sarcoplasmic reticulum (NSR) are V_c, V_d, V_j, and V_n, respectively

The sodium current I_{Na}, the calcium current I_{Ca}, and the potassium current I_K need some attention and will be handled separately.

In addition to the transmembrane potential, we need to keep track of all five calcium concentrations. By considering Fig. 15.1, we see that the cytosolic concentration can change in three ways[1]: (1) Calcium may diffuse into the cytosolic space from the dyad,[2] leading to an increase in the cytosolic concentrations; (2) it can be pumped from the cytosol into the NSR and thereby reduce the cytosolic concentration; or, finally, (3) it can be pumped out to the extracellular space, thereby reducing the cytosolic concentration. The calcium concentration of the NSR, c_n, will be increased as calcium is pumped into this space from the cytosol and reduced by diffusion into its neighboring space, the JSR. In the JSR the calcium concentration will increase through diffusion from the NSR and be reduced when calcium is released through the ryanodine receptor (RyR) into the dyadic space. Finally, the concentration in the dyad will increase when calcium is released from the JSR to the dyad; it will be reduced as calcium diffuses out to the cytosol and finally it will be increased when calcium is released into the dyad through the L-type calcium channels (LCCs). In mathematical terms, we get the following system of equations:

$$V_c c_c' = J_{d,c} - J_{c,n} - J_{c,e}, \tag{15.2}$$

$$V_n c_n' = J_{c,n} - J_{n,j}, \tag{15.3}$$

$$V_j c_j' = J_{n,j} - J_{j,d}, \tag{15.4}$$

$$V_d c_d' = J_{j,d} - J_{d,c} - J_{d,e}. \tag{15.5}$$

$$V_e c_e' = J_{c,e} + J_{d,e}. \tag{15.6}$$

Here the notation $J_{x,y}$ denotes a flux of calcium from space x to space y. So $J_{d,c}$ denotes the flux of calcium from the dyad (d) to the cytosol (c) and, similarly, $J_{d,e}$ denotes the flux of calcium from the dyad (d) to the extracellular (e) space. Here V_x denotes the volume fraction occupied by the space x (see Table 15.1). The total amount of calcium in the system is given by

$$c = V_c c_c + V_n c_n + V_j c_j + V_d c_d + V_e c_e. \tag{15.7}$$

[1]This is a major simplification; many other things can happen to calcium but this rough description is sufficient for our purposes.

[2]It is important to recall here that when we talk about the dyad now, we really refer to a space representing the sum of all the dyads of the cell. So what used to be a very tiny place is not so tiny anymore.

15.1.1 Conservation of Calcium

It follows from the system (15.2)–(15.6) that

$$c' = 0, \tag{15.8}$$

so the total amount of calcium is conserved no matter how the calcium dynamics of the cell are organized.

15.1.2 Definition of Calcium-Related Fluxes

We need to define all the fluxes entering the system (15.2)–(15.6) and we start with the simple diffusion fluxes. Some of them have been used in earlier chapters, but we need a little more notation here, so we redefine all the terms.

15.1.2.1 Flux $J_{d,c}$ from the Dyad to the Cytosol

We assume that the pure diffusion flux from the dyad to the cytosol can be written as

$$J_{d,c} = k_{d,c}\left(c_d - c_c\right). \tag{15.9}$$

Here we assume that $k_{d,c}$ is a constant and the value used in our computations is given in Table 15.2.

15.1.2.2 Flux $J_{n,j}$ from the NSR to the JSR

Similarly, we assume that the diffusion flux from the NSR to the JSR can be written as

$$J_{n,j} = k_{n,j}\left(c_n - c_j\right), \tag{15.10}$$

where $k_{n,j}$ is assumed to be a constant (see Table 15.2).

Table 15.1 The table shows the relative size of the intracellular spaces. Note that the volume fractions of the intracellular space add up to 100 %. In addition, V_e represents 100 % of the extracellular space. We assume that both the extracellular space and the total intracellular space are 30.4 pL

V_d	0.1 %
V_j	0.3 %
V_n	1 %
V_c	98.6 %

Table 15.2 Constants used to define the fluxes between the different spaces. The constants are in units of 1/ms

$k_{c,n}$	0.01
$k_{j,d}$	0.01
$k_{d,c}$	0.001
$k_{d,e}$	0.0001
$k_{n,j}$	0.0001
$k_{c,e}$	0.00001

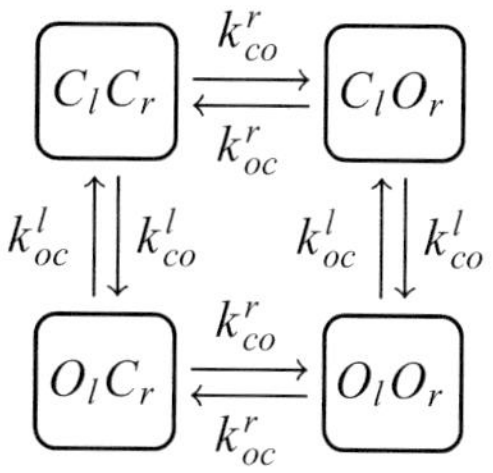

Fig. 15.2 Markov model including four possible states: C_lC_r (both closed), C_lO_r (LCC closed, RyR open), O_lO_r (both open), and O_lC_r (LCC open, RyR closed)

Table 15.3 Reaction rates used in the Markov model illustrated in Fig. 15.2. As usual, $\mu \geq 1$ denotes the mutation severity index of the RyR and $\eta \geq 1$ denotes the mutation severity index of the LCC

RyR	LCC
$k_{co}^r(c_d, c_j) = \mu \frac{c_d^4}{K(c_j)^4 + c_d^4}$ ms^{-1}	$k_{co}^l(v) = \eta\, l_\infty(v)/\tau_l$
$k_{oc}^r = 1$ ms^{-1}	$k_{oc}^l(v) = (1 - l_\infty(v))/\tau_l$
$K(c_j) = 20 + 1000(\frac{1000-c_j}{600})^2$	$l_\infty(v) = \exp(-(\frac{v-55}{10})^2)$
	$\tau_l = 1$ ms

15.1.2.3 RyR Flux $J_{j,d}$ from the JSR to the Dyad

The flux from the JSR to the dyad can be written in the form

$$J_{j,d} = o_{j,d} k_{j,d} \left(c_j - c_d\right), \tag{15.11}$$

where, as usual, $o_{j,d}$ is governed by a Markov model and $k_{j,d}$ is a constant giving the speed of diffusion when the RyR channel (situated between the JSR and the dyad) is open.

The variable $o_{j,d}$ is governed by the Markov model used in Chap. 8. For convenience the Markov model is repeated here in Fig. 15.2 and the functions used in the model are given in Table 15.3. Note that $o_{j,d}$ is the probability of being in the state C_lO_r or the state O_lO_r of the Markov model given in Fig. 15.2.

Table 15.4 Parameters in (15.12)

F	96485.3 C mol^{-1}
R	8.3145 J mol^{-1}K^{-1}
T	310 K
v_0	13.357 mV

15.1.2.4 Flux from the Extracellular Space to the Dyad: $J_{d,e}$

This flux was introduced above (see page 128) and referred to as the Goldman-Hodgkin-Katz (GHK) flux. In the present notation, we write

$$J_{d,e} = o_{d,e} k_{d,e} \frac{c_d - c_e e^{-\frac{v}{v_0}}}{1 - e^{-\frac{v}{v_0}}} \frac{v}{v_0}. \tag{15.12}$$

Here F is Faraday's constant, R is the gas constant, and T is the absolute temperature and we have defined

$$v_0 = \frac{RT}{2F}.$$

The parameters involved in defining the $J_{d,e}$ flux are given in Table 15.4. Furthermore, $o_{d,e}$ is governed by the Markov model given in Fig. 15.2. Here $o_{d,e}$ is the probability of being in the state $O_l C_r$ or the state $O_l O_r$ of the Markov model in Fig. 15.2.

15.1.3 Definition of Calcium Pumps

The terms $J_{c,e}$ and $J_{c,n}$ remain to be defined. These terms are active fluxes, or pumps, that continuously remove calcium from the cytosol and out to the extracellular domain ($J_{c,e}$) and into the NSR ($J_{c,n}$). These pumps transport calcium against a considerable concentration gradient and the operation therefore requires energy. In our model we do not track the energy consumption and we simply introduce the pumps:

$$J_{c,e} = k_{c,e}(c_c - c_e/18000) \tag{15.13}$$

and

$$J_{c,n} = k_{c,n}(c_c - c_n/10000). \tag{15.14}$$

15.1.4 *Definition of the Currents*

The currents I_{Na}, I_K and I_{Ca} of (15.1) remain to be defined. Each current will be written in the form

$$I_x = o_x g_x (v - v_x),$$

where o_x is the open probability of the channel given by the continuous version of a Markov model, g_x is the maximum conductance of the channel, and v_x is the resting potential.

15.1.4.1 Sodium Current I_{Na}

The sodium current has been studied above; see Chaps. 12 and 14. The model takes the form

$$I_{Na} = o_{Na} g_{Na} (v - v_{Na}), \tag{15.15}$$

where the open probability o_{Na} is the sum of the probability of being in the O or the O^* state of the Markov model of Fig. 15.3.

15.1.4.2 Potassium Current I_K

The potassium current is written in the form

$$I_K = (o_K g_K(v) + g_{K1}(v))(v - v_K), \tag{15.16}$$

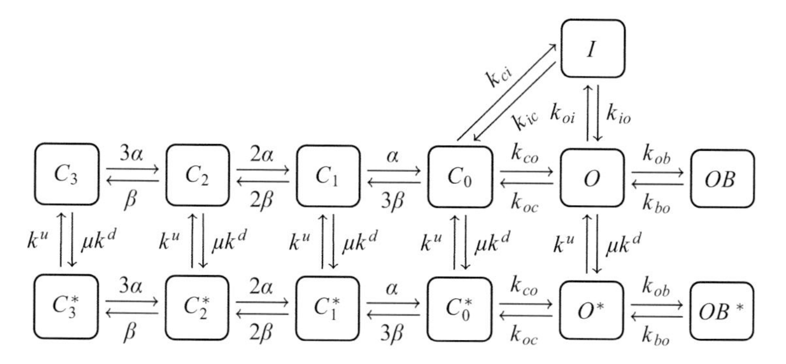

Fig. 15.3 This figure is a copy of Fig. 14.9 and it illustrates a Markov model of the mutant sodium channel. The model consists of the states O, I, OB, C_0, C_1, C_2, and C_3 of the normal mode and $OB^*, O^*, C_0^*, C_1^*, C_2^*$, and C_3^* of the burst mode (*lower part*)

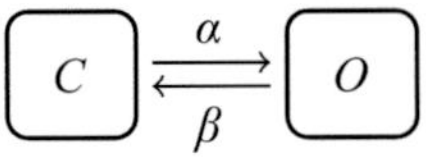

$$C \underset{\beta}{\overset{\alpha}{\rightleftarrows}} O$$

Fig. 15.4 Markov model of a potassium channel consisting of one closed and one open state

where the open probability o_K is given by the Markov model of Fig. 15.4 with rates

$$\alpha(v) = e^{-7+0.03v},$$
$$\beta(v) = e^{-8-0.03v}.$$

The voltage-dependent conductances are given by

$$g_K(v) = 0.1e^{-0.03v},$$
$$g_{K1}(v) = \frac{1}{1+e^{0.1v+10}}.$$

15.1.4.3 Calcium Current I_{Ca}

The calcium current is given by the calcium flux $J_{d,e}$ from the dyad to the extracellular space plus the flux $J_{c,e}$ from the cytosol to the extracellular space. In order to use these fluxes in the equation governing the transmembrane potential, we need convert to current density,

$$I_{Ca} = 2F\frac{V}{A}(-J_{d,e} - J_{c,e}). \tag{15.17}$$

Here $V = 30.4$ pL is the cell volume and $A = 1.4 \cdot 10^{-4}$ cm^2 is the cell area.

15.1.5 Markov Models in Terms of Systems of Differential Equations

The model of the action potential for a whole cell is a system of ordinary differential equations. For parts of the system this is clear from the equations, but for the Markov models, this may seem unclear. In Sect. 1.3 we explained how to formulate a system of ordinary differential equation associated with the reaction scheme defining a Markov model. Since the Markov models considered in the present chapter are considerably more complex, we will give one more example of this transition in order to clarify matters. To this end, consider the Markov model presented in Fig. 15.5. The associated system of ordinary differential equations governing the

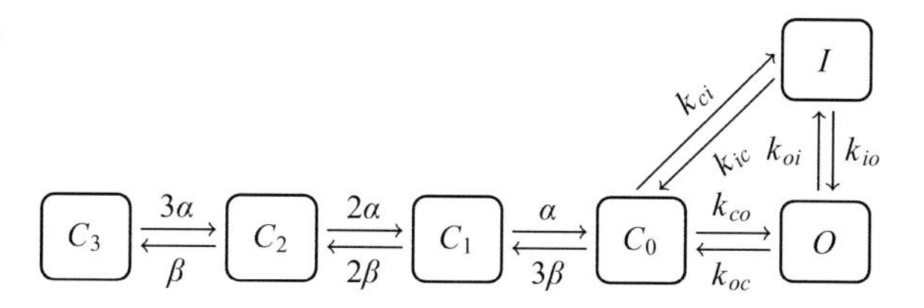

Fig. 15.5 Markov model of a wild type sodium channel consisting of an open state (O), an inactivated state (I), and four closed states (C_0, C_1, C_2, and C_3)

probabilities is given by

$$
\begin{aligned}
o' &= k_{io}i + k_{co}c_0 - (k_{oc} + k_{oi})\, o, \\
i' &= k_{oi}o + k_{ci}c_0 - (k_{io} + k_{ic})\, i, \\
c_0' &= k_{oc}o + k_{ic}i + \alpha c_1 - (k_{co} + k_{ci} + 3\beta)\, c_0, \\
c_1' &= 3\beta c_0 + 2\alpha c_2 - (2\beta + \alpha)\, c_1, \\
c_2' &= 2\beta c_1 + 3\alpha c_3 - (2\alpha + \beta)\, c_2, \\
c_3' &= \beta c_2 - 3\alpha c_3.
\end{aligned}
$$

Here, o denotes the open probability of the sodium channel, c_0 is the probability of the C_0 state, and so forth. Ideally, we would write o_{Na} for o, $c_{0,Na}$ for c_0, and so forth, but it becomes clumsy. Since these variables represent probabilities, they sum to one (for all time) and we can therefore reduce the number of unknowns in the system by one.

Based on this example, it should be straightforward to formulate the system of ordinary differential equations associated with the more complex Markov model given in Fig. 15.3.

15.2 Numerical Simulations Using the Action Potential Model for Wild Type Markov Models

The complete version of the model presented above can be written in the compact form

$$Cv' = -\left(I_{Na} + I_{Ca} + I_K + I_0\right), \qquad (15.18)$$

$$u' = F(v, u), \qquad (15.19)$$

where v is the transmembrane potential and all other variables are gathered in the vector u. The initial conditions used in the simulations are given in Table 15.5. In addition, we need to specify the applied current I_0. This current will be zero most of the time, but it will be turned on every 500 ms in order to mimic periodic stimulation

Table 15.5 Initial conditions. The Markov models for the LCC and RyR were initially set to closed and the Markov model for sodium channel was set to be in the state C_3. Starting with these conditions, the code is run for 1,000 cycles in order to generate the initial conditions used in generating the figures below. The exact numbers obtained depend upon the chosen cycle length

v	-85 mV
c_d	0.1 μM
c_c	0.1 μM
c_j	1,000 μM
c_n	1,000 μM
c_e	1,800 μM

of the cell. More specifically, we hold $I_0 = -6$ mV/ms for 5 ms at the start of each cycle.

15.2.1 Single Action Potential

In Fig. 15.6 we show the transmembrane potential and all the calcium concentration for a single action potential. There are a number of interesting effects acting together to generate the action potential. Let us consider some of them in some detail.

In Fig. 15.7 we show the first 20 ms of the computation. In the left panel we show the transmembrane potential v (upper left panel), the open probability o_{Na} (middle left panel), and the sodium current I_{Na} (lower left panel). Observe that when the cell is stimulated by the applied current I_0, the transmembrane potential increases. This increase leads to an increased open probability of the sodium channel. When the sodium channel opens, the sodium current becomes large (or very negative, to be precise), which leads to a fast increase of the transmembrane potential. As the transmembrane potential reaches its peak value (at about 15 ms), the open probability starts to decline, since the channel inactivates. In the three right panels, we show the calcium concentration of the dyad c_d (upper right panel), the calcium flux $J_{d,e}$ (middle right panel), and the open probability of the RyR channel (lower right panel). We see that when the transmembrane potential starts increasing, the calcium flux $J_{d,e}$ increases and the calcium concentration of the dyad increases. This increase leads to the increased open probability (lower right panel) of the RyR channel and therefore the dyad concentration increases rapidly.

In Fig. 15.8, we show the return to the stable equilibrium solution. In the left panel, we show the transmembrane (upper left panel), the open probability of the LCC (middle left panel), and the open probability of the gated potassium channel. After the sodium channel has switched off (see Fig. 15.7), the calcium current contributes to a continued depolarized state. However, after about 20 ms the transmembrane potential starts declining because of a substantial (positive) potassium current.

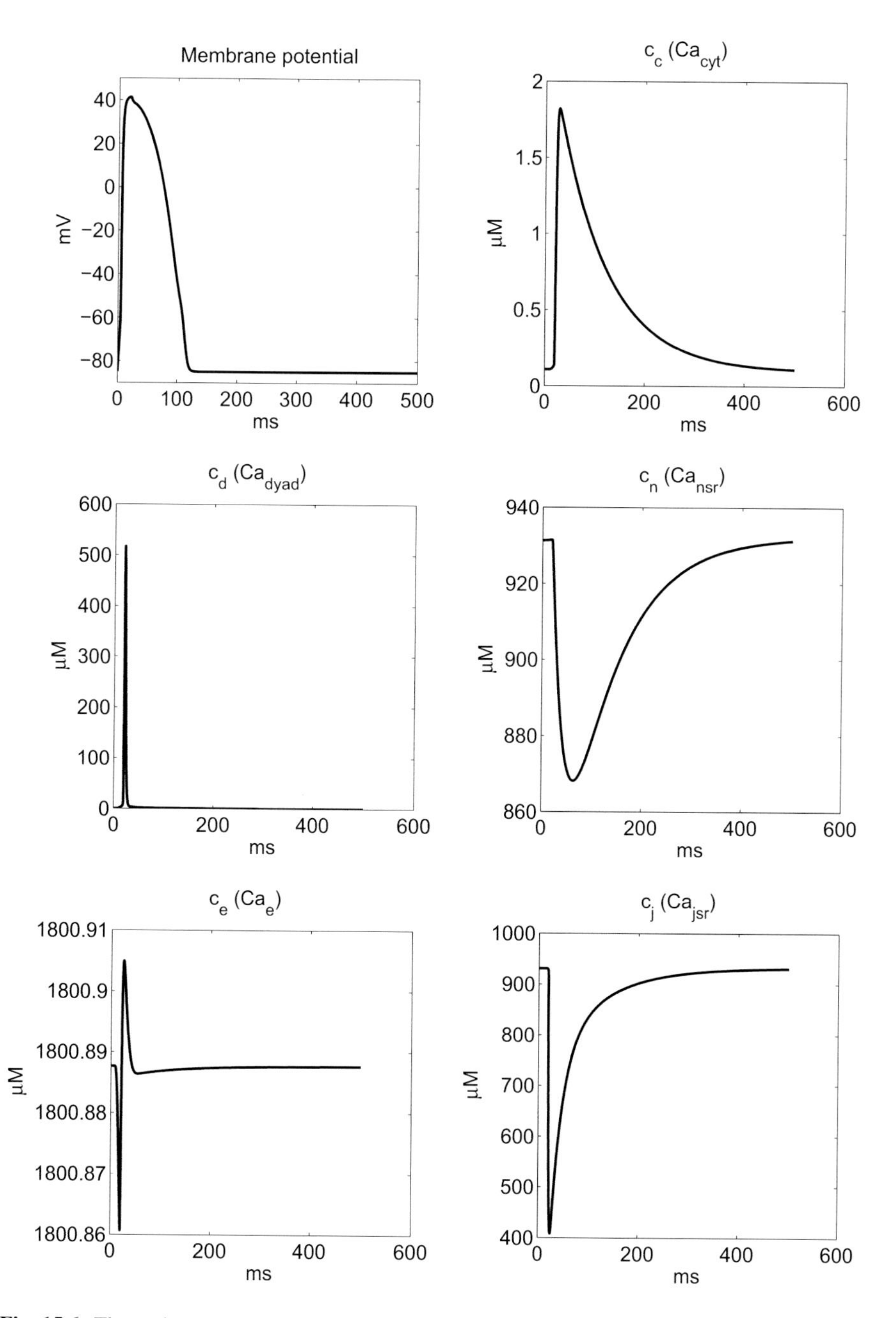

Fig. 15.6 The action potential of the model described in the present chapter. The membrane potential (*upper left*) and the dynamics of the five calcium concentrations are shown for 500 ms. The action potential is initiated by holding $I_0 = -6$ mV/ms for 5 ms. All variables return to their resting values after about 500 ms

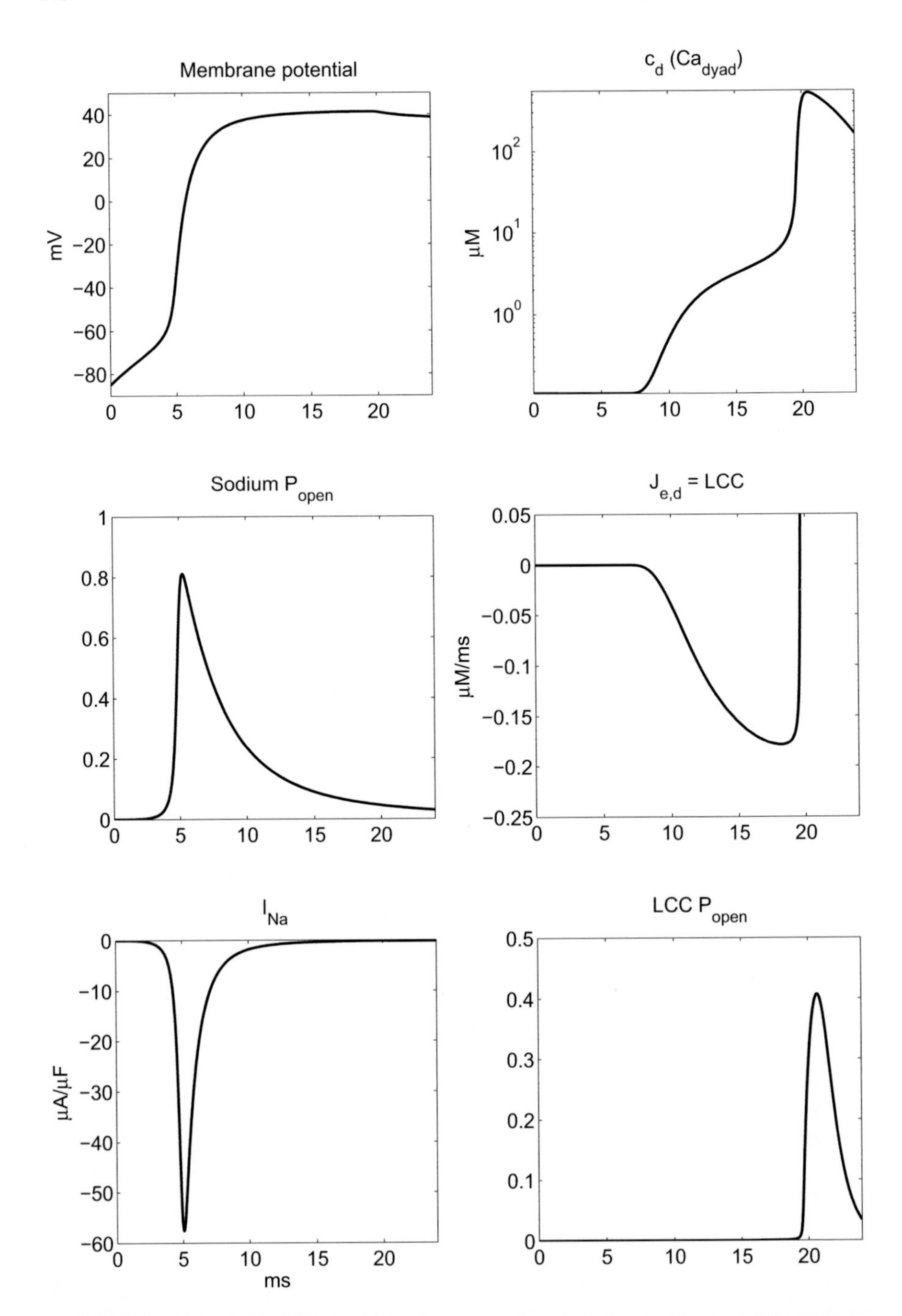

Fig. 15.7 The first 20 ms of the simulation shown in Fig. 15.6. Note the log scale in the *upper right panel*. There we see a slow rise due to the LCC opening, followed by a fast rise due to the RyR opening

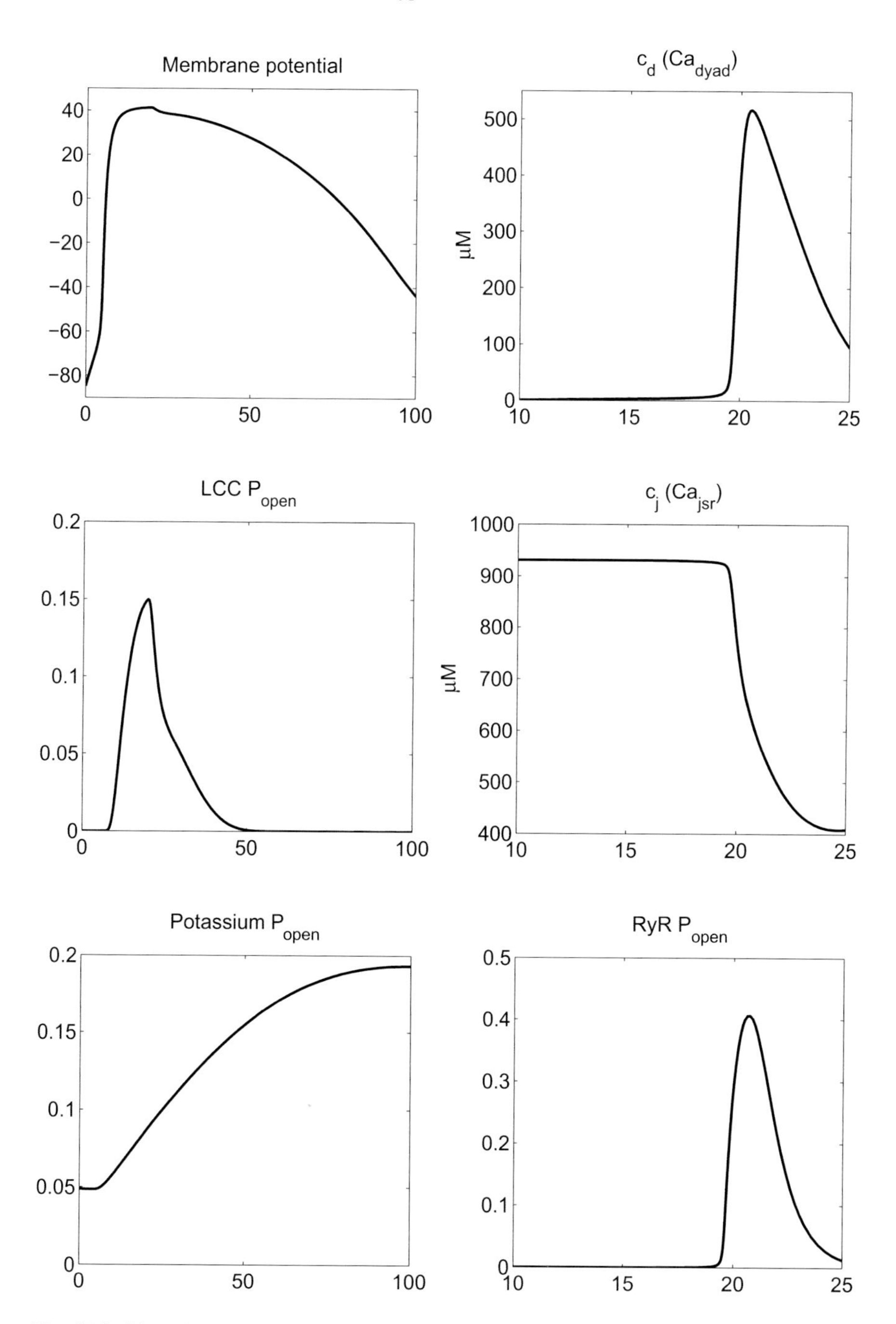

Fig. 15.8 After about 15 ms, the transmembrane potential (*upper left*) reaches its peak value and enters the plateau phase before it starts to decline toward the stable equilibrium solution

In the right panels, we follow the development of the calcium concentration of the dyad c_d (upper right panel), the calcium concentration c_j of the JSR, (middle right panel), and the open probability of the RyR channel, denoted $o_{j,d}$ (lower right panel).

15.2.2 *Many Action Potentials*

In Fig. 15.9, we show the action potential for a simulation running for 25,000 ms. The left panel shows the transmembrane potential v (upper left panel), the calcium concentration c_d of the dyad (middle left panel), and the extracellular calcium concentration c_e (lower left panel). From top to bottom in the right panels, we show the cytosolic calcium concentration c_c, the NSR calcium concentration c_n, and finally the JSR calcium concentration c_j. All variables return to their initial values and the rhythm seems to be perfect.

15.3 Changing the Mean Open Time of the Sodium Channel While Keeping the Equilibrium Probability Fixed Changes the Action Potential

We consider a case where we multiply all rates of the Markov model (see Fig. 15.3) of the sodium channel by the same factor. Here we use the wild type case ($\mu = 1$) and the drug parameters (k_{ob}, k_{bo}) are set to zero. This will change the mean open time, but not the equilibrium probabilities. The results are given in Fig. 15.10, where the blue line illustrates the results using default parameters, the red line represents the solution when all the rates are multiplied by 1.3, and finally the green line represents the solution when all the rates are multiplied by 0.7. We observe that the action potential changes substantially when the rates are changed (and the mean open time is changed), even though the equilibrium probabilities are kept unchanged.

15.4 Numerical Simulations Using the Action Potential Model When the Cell Is Affected by a Mutation

We will use the model of the action potential for the whole cell introduced above to study the effect of mutations. We have studied many different theoretical models of mutations earlier, but here we will limit ourselves to study the effect of one theoretical model of a sodium channel mutation, one model of a RyR mutation, and

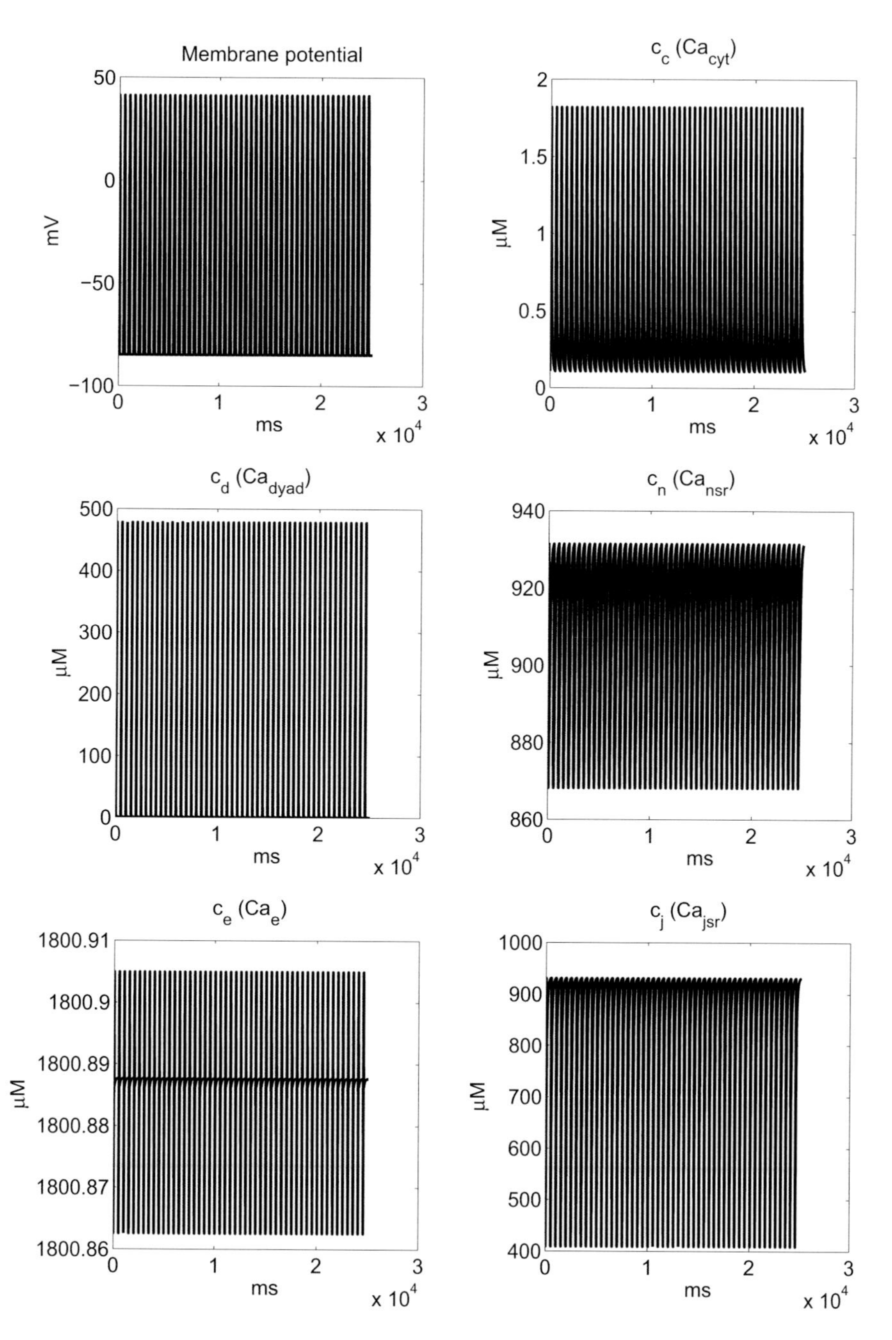

Fig. 15.9 The action potential running for 25,000 ms (50 beats). All variables return to their equilibrium values before a new action potential is initiated (every 500 ms)

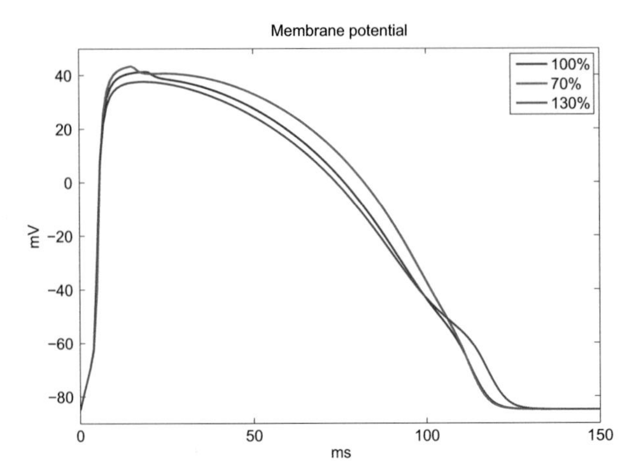

Fig. 15.10 Slower dynamics (*green*) lead to later inactivation, yielding a higher plateau. Quicker dynamics (*red*) lead to faster recovery from inactivation, allowing a stronger late current

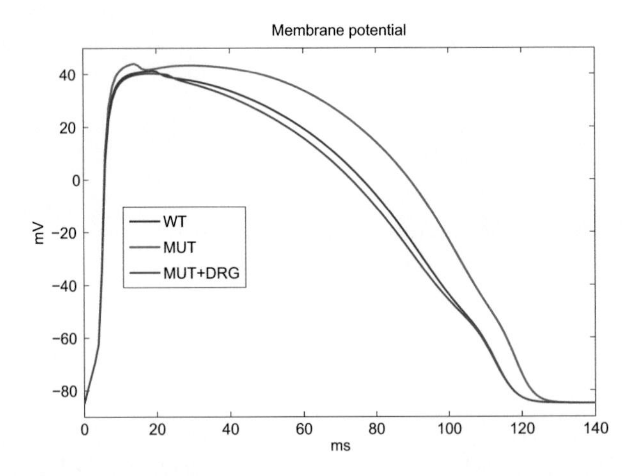

Fig. 15.11 The figure shows the action potential of the wild type (*blue*), the mutant (*green*), and the mutant after the application of the drug (*red*)

one model of an LCC mutation. We will also see how the theoretical drugs derived above handle these mutations.

15.4.1 Mutation of the Sodium Channel

We consider a mutation of the sodium channel of the form presented in Fig. 15.3. In Fig. 15.11 we show simulation results comparing the wild type ($\mu = 1$, blue), the mutant ($\mu = 10$, green), and a simulation (red) where a drug is applied to the mutant case. The Markov model describing the open state drug is given in Fig. 15.3, where we have used drug parameters given by

$$k_{bo} = k_{io}, \text{ and } k_{ob} = (\mu - 1) \frac{k^d k^u k_{oi}}{(k^u + \mu k^d)(k^u + k^d)};$$

see (14.20) and (14.23). As in the single channel case, we observe that the theoretical drug is able to repair the effect of the mutation.

15.4.2 *Mutation of the RyR*

In Fig. 15.12 we have simulated mutation in the RyR using the Markov model given in Fig. 15.2. The figure shows the wild type (blue, $\mu = 1$), the mutant (green, $\mu = 3$), and the mutant where the drug has been applied (red). We have used a closed state drug computed as described in (3.5) and (3.9) and we observe that the theoretical drug is able to repair the effect of the mutation.

15.4.3 *Mutation of the LCC*

In Fig. 15.13 we have simulated mutation in the LCC channel, using $\eta = 3$. We model the mutation and the drug as defined in (3.5) and (3.9). As usual, k_{bc} is a free

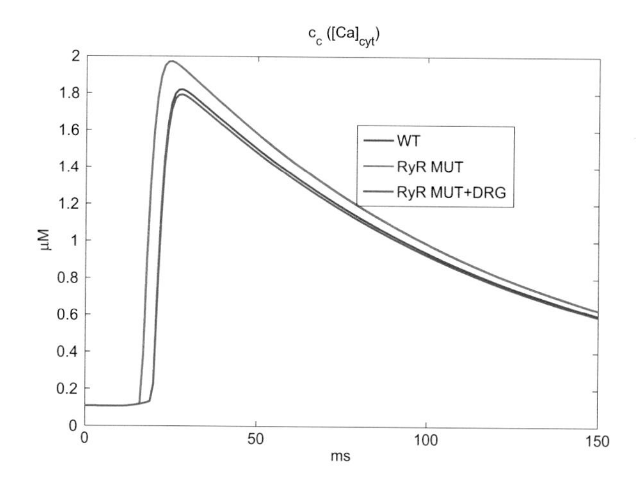

Fig. 15.12 The cytosolic calcium concentration for wild type (*blue*, $\mu = 1$), the mutant (*green*, $\mu = 3$), and the mutant after the application of the drug (*red*). We have used a closed state drug as defined in (3.5) with $k_{bc} = 0.5 \text{ ms}^{-1}$ and $k_{cb} = (\mu - 1)k_{bc}$; see (3.9)

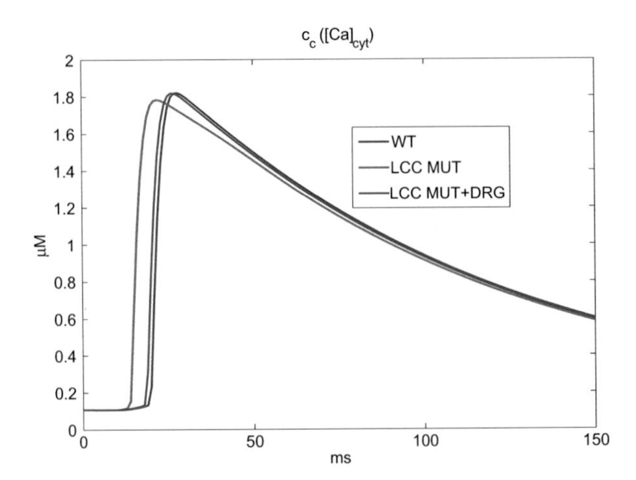

Fig. 15.13 LCC mutation. The cytosolic calcium concentration for the wild type (*blue*, $\eta = 1$), the mutant (*green*, $\eta = 3$), and the mutant case where the theoretical drug is applied (*red*). In the computations we have used $k_{bc} = 0.05\ \text{ms}^{-1}$; for larger values of k_{bc} the results overlap with the wild type case

parameter that must be chosen sufficiently large. Again, we note that the theoretical drug repairs the effect of the mutation.

15.5 Notes

1. The action potential model discussed in Sect. 15.1 and used throughout this chapter is only of qualitative relevance; no effort is made to mimic the properties of one particular cell. The field of models for the action potential is huge and growing. A great collection of models is provided by the Auckland Bioengineering Institute at the University of Auckland and their collaborators; see CellML.org. Recent models tend to be increasingly complex and hard to deal with from a mathematical perspective, but clearly the models become more and more realistic in terms of mimicking the properties of the actual action potential. As mentioned earlier, there are comprehensive introductions to the cardiac action potential, such as Rudy [74] and Rudy and Silva [75].
2. In these notes we have used Matlab as the computational platform for all our simulations. For solving ordinary differential equations we have used the ODE15s function. However, solving the ordinary differential equations modeling the single cell action potential has received a great deal of attention and numerical methods suited for this problem have been developed. An early alternative was developed by Rush and Larsen [76]; the method was improved to second by Sundnes et al. [92] and comparisons of several methods were provided by Marsh et al. [56] and Campos et al. [8]; see also Stary and Biktashev [88]. From

a programming perspective, the explicit Euler scheme is always an attractive alternative, but for stiff problems the stability requirement often excludes that method. For instance, if we use the explicit Euler method with a fixed time step to compute the solutions shown in Fig. 15.6, we need about 26,000 time-steps, whereas the ODE15s method needs 335 time steps.

Bibliography

1. F.G. Ball, Y. Cai, J.B. Kadane, A. O'hagan, Bayesian inference for ion–channel gating mechanisms directly from single–channel recordings, using markov chain monte carlo. Proc. R. Soc. Lond. A Math. Phys. Eng. Sci. **455**(1988), 2879–2932 (1999)
2. P.B. Bennett, K. Yazawa, N. Makita, A.L. George Jr., Molecular mechanism for an inherited cardiac arrhythmia. Nature **376**, 683–685 (1995)
3. D.M. Bers, *Excitation-Contraction Coupling and Cardiac Contractile Force* (Kluwert Academic, Dordrecht, 2001)
4. D.M. Bers, Cardiac excitation–contraction coupling. Nature **415**(6868), 198–205 (2002)
5. D.M. Bers, Calcium cycling and signaling in cardiac myocytes. Ann. Rev. Physiol. **70**, 23–49 (2008)
6. P.C. Bressloff, *Stochastic Processes in Cell Biology*, vol. 41. Interdisciplinary Applied Mathematics (Springer International Publishing, New York, 2014)
7. P.C. Bressloff, *Waves in Neural Media*. Lecture Notes on Mathematical Modelling in the Life Sciences (Springer, New York, 2014)
8. R.S. Campos, F.O. Campos, J.M. Gomes, C. de Barros Barbosa, M. Lobosco, R.W. Dos Santos, Comparing high performance techniques for the automatic generation of efficient solvers of cardiac cell models. Computing **95**(1), 639–660 (2013)
9. J. Chai, J. Hake, N. Wu, M. Wen, X. Cai, G.T. Lines, J. Yang, H. Su, C. Zhang, X. Liao, Towards simulation of subcellular calcium dynamics at nanometre resolution. Int. J. High Perform. Comput. Appl. **29**(1), 51–63 (2013)
10. S. Chakrapani, J.F. Cordero-Morales, V. Jogini, A.C. Pan, D. Marien Cortes, B. Roux, E. Perozo, On the structural basis of modal gating behavior in K+ channels. Nature Struct. Mole. Biol. **18**(1), 67–74 (2011)
11. S. Chakrapani, J.F. Cordero-Morales, E. Perozo, A quantitative description of KcsA gating I: Macroscopic currents. J. General Physiol. **130**(5), 465–478 (2007)
12. S. Chakrapani, J.F. Cordero-Morales, E. Perozo, A quantitative description of KcsA gating II: Single-channel currents. J. General Physiol. **130**(5), 479–496 (2007)
13. R. Chandra, C. Frank Starmer, A.O. Grant, Multiple effects of KPQ deletion mutation on gating of human cardiac Na^+ channels expressed in mammalian cells. AJP Heart Circulatory Physiol. **274**(5), H1643–H1654 (1998)
14. C.E. Clancy, Y. Rudy, Linking a genetic defect to its cellular phenotype in a cardiac arrhythmia. Nature **400**, 566–569 (1999)

A. Tveito, G.T. Lines, *Computing Characterizations of Drugs for Ion Channels and Receptors Using Markov Models*, Lecture Notes in Computational Science and Engineering 111, DOI 10.1007/978-3-319-30030-6

15. C.E. Clancy, Y. Rudy, Na^+ channel mutation that causes both Brugada and long-QT syndrome phenotypes: A simulation study of mechanism. Circulation **105**(10), 1208–1213 (2002)
16. C.E. Clancy, Z.I. Zhu, Y. Rudy, Pharmacogenetics and anti-arrhythmic drug therapy: A theoretical investigation. AJP Heart Circulatory Physiol. **292**(1), H66–H75 (2007)
17. D. Colquhoun, A.G. Hawkes, K. Srodzinski, Joint distributions of apparent open and shut times of single-ion channels and maximum likelihood fitting of mechanisms. Phil. Trans. R. Soc. Lond. A Math. Phys. Eng. Sci. **354**(1718), 2555–2590 (1996)
18. D. Colquhoun, K.A. Dowsland, M. Beato, A.J.R. Plested, How to impose microscopic reversibility in complex reaction mechanisms. Biophys. J. **86**(6), 3510–3518 (2004)
19. D. Colquhoun, A.G. Hawkes, Relaxation and fluctuations of membrane currents that flow through drug-operated channels. Proc. R. Soc. Lond. B Biol. Sci. **199**(1135), 23–262 (1977)
20. D. Colquhoun, A.G. Hawkes, On the stochastic properties of single ion channels. Proc. R. Soc. Lond. B Biol. Sci. **211**(1183), 205–235 (1981)
21. D. Colquhoun, A.G. Hawkes, On the stochastic properties of bursts of single ion channel openings and of clusters of bursts. Phil. Trans. R. Soc. B Biol. Sci. **300**, 1–59 (1982)
22. P. Dayan, L.F. Abbott, *Theoretical Neuroscience*, vol. 806 (MIT Press, Cambridge, 2001)
23. G.B. Ermentrout, D.H. Terman, *Mathematical Foundations of Neuroscience*, vol. 35 (Springer, New York, 2010)
24. M. Fink, D. Noble, Markov models for ion channels: Versatility versus identifiability and speed. Phil. Trans. R. Soc. A Math. Phys. Eng. Sci. **367**(1896), 2161–2179 (2009)
25. P.C. Franzone, L.F. Pavarino, S. Scacchi, *Mathematical Cardiac Electrophysiology*, vol. 13 (Springer International Publishing, New York, 2014)
26. D.T. Gillespie, Exact stochastic simulation of coupled chemical reactions. J. Phys. Chem. **81**(25), 2340–2361 (1977)
27. E. Gin, M. Falcke, L.E. Wagner, D.I. Yule, J. Sneyd, Markov chain Monte Carlo fitting of single-channel data from inositol trisphosphate receptors. J. Theor. Biol. **257**(3), 460–474 (2009)
28. L. Glass, P. Hunter, A. McCulloch, *Theory of Heart: Biomechanics, Biophysics, and Nonlinear Dynamics of Cardiac Function* (Springer, New York, 2012)
29. E. Grandi, F.S. Pasqualini, D.M. Bers, A novel computational model of the human ventricular action potential and Ca transient. J. Mol. Cell. Cardiol. **48**(1), 112–121 (2010)
30. J. Hake, A.G. Edwards, Z. Yu, P.M. Kekenes-Huskey, A.P. Michailova, J. Andrew McCammon, M.J. Holst, M. Hoshijima, A.D. McCulloch, Modelling cardiac calcium sparks in a three-dimensional reconstruction of a calcium release unit. J. Physiol. **590**(18), 4403–4422 (2012)
31. B. Hille, Local anesthetics: hydrophilic and hydrophobic pathways for the drug-receptor reaction. J. General Physiol. **69**(4), 497–515 (1977)
32. B. Hille, *Ion Channels of Excitable Membranes*, vol. 507 (Sinauer Sunderland, MA, 2001)
33. A.L. Hodgkin, A.F. Huxley, A quantitative description of membrane current and its application to conduction and excitation in nerve. J. Physiol. **117**(4), 500–544 (1952)
34. L.M. Hondeghem, B.G. Katzung, Time- and voltage-dependent interactions of antiarrhythmic drugs with cardiac sodium channels. Biochimica et Biophysica Acta **472**(3–4), 373–398 (1977)
35. M.A. Huertas, G.D. Smith, The dynamics of luminal depletion and the stochastic gating of Ca^{2+}-activated Ca^{2+} channels and release sites. J. Theor. Biol. **246**(2), 332–354 (2007)
36. M.A. Huertas, G.D. Smith, S. Györke, Ca^{2+} alternans in a cardiac myocyte model that uses moment equations to represent heterogeneous junctional SR Ca^{2+}. Biophys. J. **99**, 377–387 (2010)
37. L. Ionescu, C. White, K.-H. Cheung, J. Shuai, I. Parker, J.E. Pearson, J. Kevin Foskett, D.-O. Daniel Mak, Mode switching is the major mechanism of ligand regulation of $InsP_3$ receptor calcium release channels. J. General Physiol. **130**(6), 631–645 (2007)
38. E.M. Izhikevich, *Dynamical Systems in Neuroscience* (MIT Press, Cambridge, 2007)

39. K. Jacobs, *Stochastic Processes for Physicists: Understanding Noisy Systems* (Cambridge University Press, Cambridge, 2010)
40. N. Jost, K. Acsai, B. Horváth, T. Bányász, I. Baczkó, M. Bitay, G. Bogáts, P.P. Nánási, Contribution of I_{Kr} and I_{K1} to ventricular repolarization in canine and human myocytes: Is there any influence of action potential duration? Basic Res. Cardiol. **104**, 33–41 (2009)
41. A.M. Katz, *Physiology of the Heart* (Lippincott Williams & Wilkins, Baltimore, 2010)
42. J. Keener, J. Sneyd, *Mathematical Physiology* (Springer, New York, 2009)
43. J. Keener, J. Sneyd, *Mathematical Physiology: I: Cellular Physiology* (Springer, New York, 2010)
44. J. Keener, J. Sneyd, *Mathematical Physiology II: Systems Physiology* (Springer, New York, 2010)
45. J.P. Keener, K. Bogar, A numerical method for the solution of the bidomain equations in cardiac tissue. Chaos Interdiscip. J. Nonlinear Sci. **8**(1), 234–241 (1998)
46. J.C. Lagarias, J.A. Reeds, M.H. Wright, P.E. Wright, Convergence properties of the Nelder–Mead simplex method in low dimensions. SIAM J. Optim. **9**(1), 112–147 (1998)
47. E.G. Lakatta, D. DiFrancesco, What keeps us ticking: A funny current, a calcium clock, or both? J. Mole. Cell. Cardiol. **47**(2), 157–170 (2009)
48. R.J. LeVeque, *Finite Volume Methods for Hyperbolic Problems* (Cambridge Texts in Applied Mathematics, Cambridge, 2002)
49. P. Li, A.V. Holden, Intracellular Ca^{2+} nonlinear wave behaviours in a three dimensional ventricular cell model. Phys. D Nonlinear Phenomena **238**(11), 992–999 (2009)
50. P. Li, G.T. Lines, M.M. Maleckar, A. Tveito, Mathematical models of cardiac pacemaking function. Frontiers Comput. Phys. **1**(20), 1–25 (2013)
51. P. Li, W. Wei, X. Cai, C. Soeller, M.B. Cannell, A.V. Holden, Computational modelling of the initiation and development of spontaneous intracellular Ca^{2+} waves in ventricular myocytes. Phil. Trans. R. Soc. Lond. A Math. Phys. Eng. Sci. **368**(1925), 3953–3965 (2010)
52. R. Loaiza, N.A. Benkusky, P.P. Powers, T. Hacker, S. Noujaim, M.J. Ackerman, J. Jalife, H.H. Valdivia, Heterogeneity of ryanodine receptor dysfunction in a mouse model of catecholaminergic polymorphic ventricular tachycardia. Circ. Res. **112**(2), 298–308 (2013)
53. D. Logan, *Applied Partial Differential Equations* (Springer, New York, 2014)
54. W.E. Louch, J.T. Koivumäki, P. Tavi, Calcium signalling in developing cardiomyocytes: Implications for model systems and disease. J. Physiol. **593**(5), 1047–1063 (2015)
55. W.E. Louch, O.M. Sejersted, F. Swift, There goes the neighborhood: Pathological alterations in T-tubule morphology and consequences for cardiomyocyte handling. J. Biomed. Biotechnol. **2010**, 17 (2010). Article ID: 503906. doi:10.1155/2010/503906
56. M.E. Marsh, S.T. Ziaratgahi, R.J. Spiteri, The secrets to the success of the Rush–Larsen method and its generalizations. IEEE Trans. Biomed. Eng. **59**(9), 2506–2515 (2012)
57. B. Mazzag, C.J. Tignanelli, G.D. Smith, The effect of residual Ca^{2+} on the stochastic gating of Ca^{2+} -regulated Ca^{2+} channel models. J. Theor. Biol. **235**(1), 121–150 (2005)
58. J.A. Nelder, R. Mead, A simplex method for function minimization. Comput. J. **7**(4), 308–313 (1965)
59. C. Nicolai, F. Sachs, Solving ion channel kinetics with the QuB software. Biophys. Rev. Lett. **8**(03n04), 191–211 (2013)
60. M. Nivala, E. de Lange, R. Rovetti, Z. Qu, Computational modeling and numerical methods for spatiotemporal calcium cycling in ventricular myocytes. Frontiers Physiol. **3**(114), (2012)
61. D. Noble, Cardiac action and pacemaker potentials based on the Hodgkin–Huxley equations. Nature **188**, 495–497 (1960)
62. D. Noble, A modification of the Hodgkin–Huxley equations applicable to Purkinje fibre action and pacemaker potentials. J. Physiol. **160**, 317–352 (1962)
63. D.Q. Nykamp, D. Tranchina, A population density approach that facilitates large-scale modeling of neural networks: Analysis and an application to orientation tuning. J. Comput. Neurosci. **8**(1), 19–50 (2000)
64. T. O'Hara, L. Virág, A. Varró, Y. Rudy, Simulation of the undiseased human cardiac ventricular action potential: Model formulation and experimental validation. PLoS Comput. Biol. **7**(5), e1002061 (2011)

65. J. Patlak, Molecular kinetics of voltage-dependent Na^{+} channels. Physiol. Rev. **71**(4), 1047–1080 (1991)
66. R. Plonsey, R.C. Barr, *Bioelectricity, A Quantitative Approach* (Springer, New York, 2007)
67. A.J. Pullan, L.K. Cheng, M.L. Buist, *Mathematically Modelling the Electrical Activity of the Heart: From Cell to Body Surface and Back Again* (World Scientific, Singapore, 2005)
68. F. Qin, A. Auerbach, F. Sachs, Estimating single-channel kinetic parameters from idealized patch-clamp data containing missed events. Biophys. J. **70**, 264–280 (1996)
69. F. Qin, A. Auerbach, F. Sachs, A direct optimization approach to hidden Markov modeling for single channel kinetics. Biophys. J. **79**, 1915–1927 (2000)
70. Z. Qu, A. Garfinkel, An advanced algorithm for solving partial differential equation in cardiac conduction. IEEE Trans. Biomed. Eng. **46**(9), 1166–1168 (1999)
71. Z. Qu, G. Hu, A. Garfinkel, J.N. Weiss, Nonlinear and stochastic dynamics in the heart. Phys. Rep. **543**(2), 61–162 (2014)
72. R. Rosales, J.A. Stark, W.J Fitzgerald, S.B. Hladky, Bayesian restoration of ion channel records using hidden markov models. Biophys. J. **80**(3), 1088–1103 (2001)
73. R.A. Rosales, Mcmc for hidden markov models incorporating aggregation of states and filtering. Bull. Math. Biol. **66**(5), 1173–1199 (2004)
74. Y. Rudy, From genes and molecules to organs and organisms: Heart. Comprehensive Biophys. **9**, 268–327 (2012)
75. Y. Rudy, J.R. Silva, Computational biology in the study of cardiac ion channels and cell electrophysiology. Q. Rev. Biophys. **39**(1), 57–116 (2006)
76. S. Rush, H. Larsen, A practical algorithm for solving dynamic membrane equations. IEEE Trans. Biomed. Eng. **BME-25**(4), 389–392 (1978)
77. B. Sakmann, E. Neher, Patch clamp techniques for studying ionic channels in excitable membranes. Ann. Rev. Phys. **46**(1), 455–472 (1984)
78. B. Sakmann, E. Neher (eds.), *Single-Channel Recording* (Springer, New York, 1995)
79. M. Santillán, *Chemical Kinetics, Stochastic Processes, and Irreversible Thermodynamics* (Springer International Publishing, New York, 2014)
80. H.J. Schroll, G.T. Lines, A. Tveito, On the accuracy of operator splitting for the monodomain model of electrophysiology. Int. J. Comput. Math. **84**(6), 871–885 (2007)
81. D. Shaya, M. Kreir, R.A. Robbins, S. Wong, J. Hammon, A. Brüggemann, D.L. Minor Jr., Voltage-gated sodium channel (Na_V) protein dissection creates a set of functional pore-only proteins. Proc. Natl. Acad. Sci. **108**(30), 12313–12318 (2011)
82. I. Siekmann, J. Sneyd, E.J. Crampin, MCMC can detect nonidentifiable models. Biophys. J. **103**(11), 2275–2286 (2012)
83. I. Siekmann, J. Sneyd, E.J. Crampin, Statistical analysis of modal gating in ion channels. Proc. R. Soc. Lond. A Math. Phys. Eng. Sci. **470**(2166), 20140030 (2014)
84. I. Siekmann, L.E. Wagner II, D. Yule, C. Fox, D. Bryant, E.J. Crampin, J. Sneyd, MCMC Estimation of Markov models for ion channels. Biophys. J. **100**(8), 1919–1929 (2011)
85. G.D. Smith, Modeling the stochastic gating of ion channels. In *Computational Cell Biology*, vol. 20 of *Interdisciplinary Applied Mathematics*, chapter 11, pp. 285–319, ed. by C.P. Fall, E.S. Marland, J.M. Wagner, J.J. Tyson (Springer, New York, 2002)
86. L. Song, K.L. Magleby, Testing for microscopic reversibility in the gating of maxi k+ channels using two-dimensional dwell-time distributions. Biophys. J. **67**(1), 91 (1994)
87. C.F. Starmer, How antiarrhythmic drugs increase the rate of sudden cardiac death. Int. J. Bifurcat. Chaos **12**(9), 1953–1968 (2002)
88. T. Stary, V.N. Biktashev, Exponential integrators for a Markov chain model of the fast sodium channel of cardiomyocytes. IEEE Trans. Biomed. Eng. **62**(4), 1070–1076 (2015)
89. M.D. Stern, L.-S. Song, H. Cheng, J.S.K. Sham, H.T. Yang, K.R. Boheler, E. Ríos, Local control models of cardiac excitation-contraction coupling. A possible role for allosteric interactions between ryanodine receptors. J. General Physiol. **113**(3), 469–489 (1999)
90. D. Sterratt, B. Graham, A. Gillies, D. Willshaw, *Principles of Computational Modelling in Neuroscience* (Cambridge University Press, Cambridge, 2011)
91. W.A. Strauss, *Partial Differential Equations, An Introduction* (Wiley, New York, 2008)

92. J. Sundnes, R. Artebrant, O. Skavhaug, A. Tveito, A second order algorithm for solving dynamic cell membrane equations. IEEE Trans. Biomed. Eng. **56**(10), 2546–2548 (2009)
93. J. Sundnes, G.T. Lines, X. Cai, B.F. Nielsen, K.-A. Mardal, A. Tveito, *Computing the Electrical Activity in the Heart*, vol. 1 (Springer, Berlin, Heidelberg, 2007)
94. J. Sundnes, G.T. Lines, A. Tveito, An operator splitting method for solving the bidomain equations coupled to a volume conductor model for the torso. Math. Biosci. **194**(2), 233–248 (2005)
95. P. Swietach, K.W. Spitzer, R.D. Vaughan-Jones, Ca^{2+}-mobility in the sarcoplasmic reticulum of ventricular myocytes is low. Biophys. J. **95**(3), 1412–1427 (2008)
96. A. Tveito, H.P. Langtangen, B.F. Nielsen, X. Cai, *Elements of Scientific Computing*, vol. 7 (Springer, Berlin, Heidelberg, 2010)
97. A. Tveito, G.T. Lines, A note on a method for determining advantageous properties of an anti-arrhythmic drug based on a mathematical model of cardiac cells. Math. Biosci. **217**(2), 167–173 (2009)
98. A. Tveito, G.T. Lines, J. Hake, A.G. Edwards, Instabilities of the resting state in a mathematical model of calcium handling in cardiac myocytes. Math. Biosci. **236**(2), 97–107 (2012)
99. A. Tveito, G.T. Lines, P. Li, A. McCulloch, Defining candidate drug characteristics for Long-QT (LQT3) syndrome. Math. Biosci. Eng. **8**(3), 861–873 (2011)
100. A. Tveito, R. Winther, *Introduction to Partial Differential Equations: A Computational Approach*, vol. 29 (Springer, Berlin, Heidelberg, 2005)
101. G. Ullah, D.-O. Daniel Mak, J.E Pearson, A data-driven model of a modal gated ion channel: The inositol 1, 4, 5-trisphosphate receptor in insect sf9 cells. J. General Physiol. **140**(2), 159–173 (2012)
102. G.S.B. Williams, M.A. Huertas, E.A. Sobie, M. Saleet Jafri, G.D. Smith, A probability density approach to modeling local control of calcium-induced calcium release in cardiac myocytes. Biophys. J. **92**, 2311–2328 (2007)
103. G.S.B. Williams, M.A. Huertas, E.A. Sobie, M. Saleet Jafri, G.D. Smith, Moment closure for local control models of calcium-induced calcium release in cardiac myocytes. Biophys. J. **95**, 1689–1703 (2008)
104. R.L. Winslow, J.L. Greenstein, Cardiac myocytes and local signaling in nano-domains. Prog. Biophys. Mole. Biol. **107**, 48–59 (2011)
105. R.L. Winslow, A. Tanskanen, M. Chen, J.L. Greenstein, Multiscale modeling of calcium signaling in the cardiac dyad. Ann. New York Acad. Sci. **1080**, 362–375 (2006)

Editorial Policy

1. Volumes in the following three categories will be published in LNCSE:

i) Research monographs
ii) Tutorials
iii) Conference proceedings

Those considering a book which might be suitable for the series are strongly advised to contact the publisher or the series editors at an early stage.

2. Categories i) and ii). Tutorials are lecture notes typically arising via summer schools or similar events, which are used to teach graduate students. These categories will be emphasized by Lecture Notes in Computational Science and Engineering. **Submissions by interdisciplinary teams of authors are encouraged.** The goal is to report new developments – quickly, informally, and in a way that will make them accessible to non-specialists. In the evaluation of submissions timeliness of the work is an important criterion. Texts should be well-rounded, well-written and reasonably self-contained. In most cases the work will contain results of others as well as those of the author(s). In each case the author(s) should provide sufficient motivation, examples, and applications. In this respect, Ph.D. theses will usually be deemed unsuitable for the Lecture Notes series. Proposals for volumes in these categories should be submitted either to one of the series editors or to Springer-Verlag, Heidelberg, and will be refereed. A provisional judgement on the acceptability of a project can be based on partial information about the work: a detailed outline describing the contents of each chapter, the estimated length, a bibliography, and one or two sample chapters – or a first draft. A final decision whether to accept will rest on an evaluation of the completed work which should include

- at least 100 pages of text;
- a table of contents;
- an informative introduction perhaps with some historical remarks which should be accessible to readers unfamiliar with the topic treated;
- a subject index.

3. Category iii). Conference proceedings will be considered for publication provided that they are both of exceptional interest and devoted to a single topic. One (or more) expert participants will act as the scientific editor(s) of the volume. They select the papers which are suitable for inclusion and have them individually refereed as for a journal. Papers not closely related to the central topic are to be excluded. Organizers should contact the Editor for CSE at Springer at the planning stage, see *Addresses* below.

In exceptional cases some other multi-author-volumes may be considered in this category.

4. Only works in English will be considered. For evaluation purposes, manuscripts may be submitted in print or electronic form, in the latter case, preferably as pdf- or zipped ps-files. Authors are requested to use the LaTeX style files available from Springer at http://www.springer.com/gp/authors-editors/book-authors-editors/manuscript-preparation/5636 (Click on LaTeX Template → monographs or contributed books).

For categories ii) and iii) we strongly recommend that all contributions in a volume be written in the same LaTeX version, preferably LaTeX2e. Electronic material can be included if appropriate. Please contact the publisher.

Careful preparation of the manuscripts will help keep production time short besides ensuring satisfactory appearance of the finished book in print and online.

5. The following terms and conditions hold. Categories i), ii) and iii):

Authors receive 50 free copies of their book. No royalty is paid.
Volume editors receive a total of 50 free copies of their volume to be shared with authors, but no royalties.

Authors and volume editors are entitled to a discount of 33.3 % on the price of Springer books purchased for their personal use, if ordering directly from Springer.

6. Springer secures the copyright for each volume.

Addresses:

Timothy J. Barth
NASA Ames Research Center
NAS Division
Moffett Field, CA 94035, USA
barth@nas.nasa.gov

Michael Griebel
Institut für Numerische Simulation
der Universität Bonn
Wegelerstr. 6
53115 Bonn, Germany
griebel@ins.uni-bonn.de

David E. Keyes
Mathematical and Computer Sciences
and Engineering
King Abdullah University of Science
and Technology
P.O. Box 55455
Jeddah 21534, Saudi Arabia
david.keyes@kaust.edu.sa

and

Department of Applied Physics
and Applied Mathematics
Columbia University
500 W. 120 th Street
New York, NY 10027, USA
kd2112@columbia.edu

Risto M. Nieminen
Department of Applied Physics
Aalto University School of Science
and Technology
00076 Aalto, Finland
risto.nieminen@aalto.fi

Dirk Roose
Department of Computer Science
Katholieke Universiteit Leuven
Celestijnenlaan 200A
3001 Leuven-Heverlee, Belgium
dirk.roose@cs.kuleuven.be

Tamar Schlick
Department of Chemistry
and Courant Institute
of Mathematical Sciences
New York University
251 Mercer Street
New York, NY 10012, USA
schlick@nyu.edu

Editor for Computational Science
and Engineering at Springer:
Martin Peters
Springer-Verlag
Mathematics Editorial IV
Tiergartenstrasse 17
69121 Heidelberg, Germany
martin.peters@springer.com

Lecture Notes in Computational Science and Engineering

1. D. Funaro, *Spectral Elements for Transport-Dominated Equations.*
2. H.P. Langtangen, *Computational Partial Differential Equations.* Numerical Methods and Diffpack Programming.
3. W. Hackbusch, G. Wittum (eds.), *Multigrid Methods V.*
4. P. Deuflhard, J. Hermans, B. Leimkuhler, A.E. Mark, S. Reich, R.D. Skeel (eds.), *Computational Molecular Dynamics: Challenges, Methods, Ideas.*
5. D. Kröner, M. Ohlberger, C. Rohde (eds.), *An Introduction to Recent Developments in Theory and Numerics for Conservation Laws.*
6. S. Turek, *Efficient Solvers for Incompressible Flow Problems.* An Algorithmic and Computational Approach.
7. R. von Schwerin, *Multi Body System SIMulation.* Numerical Methods, Algorithms, and Software.
8. H.-J. Bungartz, F. Durst, C. Zenger (eds.), *High Performance Scientific and Engineering Computing.*
9. T.J. Barth, H. Deconinck (eds.), *High-Order Methods for Computational Physics.*
10. H.P. Langtangen, A.M. Bruaset, E. Quak (eds.), *Advances in Software Tools for Scientific Computing.*
11. B. Cockburn, G.E. Karniadakis, C.-W. Shu (eds.), *Discontinuous Galerkin Methods.* Theory, Computation and Applications.
12. U. van Rienen, *Numerical Methods in Computational Electrodynamics.* Linear Systems in Practical Applications.
13. B. Engquist, L. Johnsson, M. Hammill, F. Short (eds.), *Simulation and Visualization on the Grid.*
14. E. Dick, K. Riemslagh, J. Vierendeels (eds.), *Multigrid Methods VI.*
15. A. Frommer, T. Lippert, B. Medeke, K. Schilling (eds.), *Numerical Challenges in Lattice Quantum Chromodynamics.*
16. J. Lang, *Adaptive Multilevel Solution of Nonlinear Parabolic PDE Systems.* Theory, Algorithm, and Applications.
17. B.I. Wohlmuth, *Discretization Methods and Iterative Solvers Based on Domain Decomposition.*
18. U. van Rienen, M. Günther, D. Hecht (eds.), *Scientific Computing in Electrical Engineering.*
19. I. Babuška, P.G. Ciarlet, T. Miyoshi (eds.), *Mathematical Modeling and Numerical Simulation in Continuum Mechanics.*
20. T.J. Barth, T. Chan, R. Haimes (eds.), *Multiscale and Multiresolution Methods.* Theory and Applications.
21. M. Breuer, F. Durst, C. Zenger (eds.), *High Performance Scientific and Engineering Computing.*
22. K. Urban, *Wavelets in Numerical Simulation.* Problem Adapted Construction and Applications.
23. L.F. Pavarino, A. Toselli (eds.), *Recent Developments in Domain Decomposition Methods.*

24. T. Schlick, H.H. Gan (eds.), *Computational Methods for Macromolecules: Challenges and Applications.*
25. T.J. Barth, H. Deconinck (eds.), *Error Estimation and Adaptive Discretization Methods in Computational Fluid Dynamics.*
26. M. Griebel, M.A. Schweitzer (eds.), *Meshfree Methods for Partial Differential Equations.*
27. S. Müller, *Adaptive Multiscale Schemes for Conservation Laws.*
28. C. Carstensen, S. Funken, W. Hackbusch, R.H.W. Hoppe, P. Monk (eds.), *Computational Electromagnetics.*
29. M.A. Schweitzer, *A Parallel Multilevel Partition of Unity Method for Elliptic Partial Differential Equations.*
30. T. Biegler, O. Ghattas, M. Heinkenschloss, B. van Bloemen Waanders (eds.), *Large-Scale PDE-Constrained Optimization.*
31. M. Ainsworth, P. Davies, D. Duncan, P. Martin, B. Rynne (eds.), *Topics in Computational Wave Propagation.* Direct and Inverse Problems.
32. H. Emmerich, B. Nestler, M. Schreckenberg (eds.), *Interface and Transport Dynamics.* Computational Modelling.
33. H.P. Langtangen, A. Tveito (eds.), *Advanced Topics in Computational Partial Differential Equations.* Numerical Methods and Diffpack Programming.
34. V. John, *Large Eddy Simulation of Turbulent Incompressible Flows.* Analytical and Numerical Results for a Class of LES Models.
35. E. Bänsch (ed.), *Challenges in Scientific Computing - CISC 2002.*
36. B.N. Khoromskij, G. Wittum, *Numerical Solution of Elliptic Differential Equations by Reduction to the Interface.*
37. A. Iske, *Multiresolution Methods in Scattered Data Modelling.*
38. S.-I. Niculescu, K. Gu (eds.), *Advances in Time-Delay Systems.*
39. S. Attinger, P. Koumoutsakos (eds.), *Multiscale Modelling and Simulation.*
40. R. Kornhuber, R. Hoppe, J. Périaux, O. Pironneau, O. Wildlund, J. Xu (eds.), *Domain Decomposition Methods in Science and Engineering.*
41. T. Plewa, T. Linde, V.G. Weirs (eds.), *Adaptive Mesh Refinement – Theory and Applications.*
42. A. Schmidt, K.G. Siebert, *Design of Adaptive Finite Element Software.* The Finite Element Toolbox ALBERTA.
43. M. Griebel, M.A. Schweitzer (eds.), *Meshfree Methods for Partial Differential Equations II.*
44. B. Engquist, P. Lötstedt, O. Runborg (eds.), *Multiscale Methods in Science and Engineering.*
45. P. Benner, V. Mehrmann, D.C. Sorensen (eds.), *Dimension Reduction of Large-Scale Systems.*
46. D. Kressner, *Numerical Methods for General and Structured Eigenvalue Problems.*
47. A. Boriçi, A. Frommer, B. Joó, A. Kennedy, B. Pendleton (eds.), *QCD and Numerical Analysis III.*
48. F. Graziani (ed.), *Computational Methods in Transport.*
49. B. Leimkuhler, C. Chipot, R. Elber, A. Laaksonen, A. Mark, T. Schlick, C. Schütte, R. Skeel (eds.), *New Algorithms for Macromolecular Simulation.*

50. M. Bücker, G. Corliss, P. Hovland, U. Naumann, B. Norris (eds.), *Automatic Differentiation: Applications, Theory, and Implementations.*
51. A.M. Bruaset, A. Tveito (eds.), *Numerical Solution of Partial Differential Equations on Parallel Computers.*
52. K.H. Hoffmann, A. Meyer (eds.), *Parallel Algorithms and Cluster Computing.*
53. H.-J. Bungartz, M. Schäfer (eds.), *Fluid-Structure Interaction.*
54. J. Behrens, *Adaptive Atmospheric Modeling.*
55. O. Widlund, D. Keyes (eds.), *Domain Decomposition Methods in Science and Engineering XVI.*
56. S. Kassinos, C. Langer, G. Iaccarino, P. Moin (eds.), *Complex Effects in Large Eddy Simulations.*
57. M. Griebel, M.A Schweitzer (eds.), *Meshfree Methods for Partial Differential Equations III.*
58. A.N. Gorban, B. Kégl, D.C. Wunsch, A. Zinovyev (eds.), *Principal Manifolds for Data Visualization and Dimension Reduction.*
59. H. Ammari (ed.), *Modeling and Computations in Electromagnetics: A Volume Dedicated to Jean-Claude Nédélec.*
60. U. Langer, M. Discacciati, D. Keyes, O. Widlund, W. Zulehner (eds.), *Domain Decomposition Methods in Science and Engineering XVII.*
61. T. Mathew, *Domain Decomposition Methods for the Numerical Solution of Partial Differential Equations.*
62. F. Graziani (ed.), *Computational Methods in Transport: Verification and Validation.*
63. M. Bebendorf, *Hierarchical Matrices.* A Means to Efficiently Solve Elliptic Boundary Value Problems.
64. C.H. Bischof, H.M. Bücker, P. Hovland, U. Naumann, J. Utke (eds.), *Advances in Automatic Differentiation.*
65. M. Griebel, M.A. Schweitzer (eds.), *Meshfree Methods for Partial Differential Equations IV.*
66. B. Engquist, P. Lötstedt, O. Runborg (eds.), *Multiscale Modeling and Simulation in Science.*
67. I.H. Tuncer, Ü. Gülcat, D.R. Emerson, K. Matsuno (eds.), *Parallel Computational Fluid Dynamics 2007.*
68. S. Yip, T. Diaz de la Rubia (eds.), *Scientific Modeling and Simulations.*
69. A. Hegarty, N. Kopteva, E. O'Riordan, M. Stynes (eds.), *BAIL* 2008 – *Boundary and Interior Layers.*
70. M. Bercovier, M.J. Gander, R. Kornhuber, O. Widlund (eds.), *Domain Decomposition Methods in Science and Engineering XVIII.*
71. B. Koren, C. Vuik (eds.), *Advanced Computational Methods in Science and Engineering.*
72. M. Peters (ed.), *Computational Fluid Dynamics for Sport Simulation.*
73. H.-J. Bungartz, M. Mehl, M. Schäfer (eds.), *Fluid Structure Interaction II - Modelling, Simulation, Optimization.*
74. D. Tromeur-Dervout, G. Brenner, D.R. Emerson, J. Erhel (eds.), *Parallel Computational Fluid Dynamics 2008.*
75. A.N. Gorban, D. Roose (eds.), *Coping with Complexity: Model Reduction and Data Analysis.*

76. J.S. Hesthaven, E.M. Rønquist (eds.), *Spectral and High Order Methods for Partial Differential Equations.*

77. M. Holtz, *Sparse Grid Quadrature in High Dimensions with Applications in Finance and Insurance.*

78. Y. Huang, R. Kornhuber, O.Widlund, J. Xu (eds.), *Domain Decomposition Methods in Science and Engineering XIX.*

79. M. Griebel, M.A. Schweitzer (eds.), *Meshfree Methods for Partial Differential Equations V.*

80. P.H. Lauritzen, C. Jablonowski, M.A. Taylor, R.D. Nair (eds.), *Numerical Techniques for Global Atmospheric Models.*

81. C. Clavero, J.L. Gracia, F.J. Lisbona (eds.), *BAIL 2010 – Boundary and Interior Layers, Computational and Asymptotic Methods.*

82. B. Engquist, O. Runborg, Y.R. Tsai (eds.), *Numerical Analysis and Multiscale Computations.*

83. I.G. Graham, T.Y. Hou, O. Lakkis, R. Scheichl (eds.), *Numerical Analysis of Multiscale Problems.*

84. A. Logg, K.-A. Mardal, G. Wells (eds.), *Automated Solution of Differential Equations by the Finite Element Method.*

85. J. Blowey, M. Jensen (eds.), *Frontiers in Numerical Analysis - Durham 2010.*

86. O. Kolditz, U.-J. Gorke, H. Shao, W. Wang (eds.), *Thermo-Hydro-Mechanical-Chemical Processes in Fractured Porous Media - Benchmarks and Examples.*

87. S. Forth, P. Hovland, E. Phipps, J. Utke, A. Walther (eds.), *Recent Advances in Algorithmic Differentiation.*

88. J. Garcke, M. Griebel (eds.), *Sparse Grids and Applications.*

89. M. Griebel, M.A. Schweitzer (eds.), *Meshfree Methods for Partial Differential Equations VI.*

90. C. Pechstein, *Finite and Boundary Element Tearing and Interconnecting Solvers for Multiscale Problems.*

91. R. Bank, M. Holst, O. Widlund, J. Xu (eds.), *Domain Decomposition Methods in Science and Engineering XX.*

92. H. Bijl, D. Lucor, S. Mishra, C. Schwab (eds.), *Uncertainty Quantification in Computational Fluid Dynamics.*

93. M. Bader, H.-J. Bungartz, T. Weinzierl (eds.), *Advanced Computing.*

94. M. Ehrhardt, T. Koprucki (eds.), *Advanced Mathematical Models and Numerical Techniques for Multi-Band Effective Mass Approximations.*

95. M. Azaïez, H. El Fekih, J.S. Hesthaven (eds.), *Spectral and High Order Methods for Partial Differential Equations ICOSAHOM 2012.*

96. F. Graziani, M.P. Desjarlais, R. Redmer, S.B. Trickey (eds.), *Frontiers and Challenges in Warm Dense Matter.*

97. J. Garcke, D. Pflüger (eds.), *Sparse Grids and Applications – Munich 2012.*

98. J. Erhel, M. Gander, L. Halpern, G. Pichot, T. Sassi, O. Widlund (eds.), *Domain Decomposition Methods in Science and Engineering XXI.*

99. R. Abgrall, H. Beaugendre, P.M. Congedo, C. Dobrzynski, V. Perrier, M. Ricchiuto (eds.), *High Order Nonlinear Numerical Methods for Evolutionary PDEs - HONOM 2013.*

100. M. Griebel, M.A. Schweitzer (eds.), *Meshfree Methods for Partial Differential Equations VII.*

101. R. Hoppe (ed.), *Optimization with PDE Constraints - OPTPDE 2014.*

102. S. Dahlke, W. Dahmen, M. Griebel, W. Hackbusch, K. Ritter, R. Schneider, C. Schwab, H. Yserentant (eds.), *Extraction of Quantifiable Information from Complex Systems.*

103. A. Abdulle, S. Deparis, D. Kressner, F. Nobile, M. Picasso (eds.), *Numerical Mathematics and Advanced Applications - ENUMATH 2013.*

104. T. Dickopf, M.J. Gander, L. Halpern, R. Krause, L.F. Pavarino (eds.), *Domain Decomposition Methods in Science and Engineering XXII.*

105. M. Mehl, M. Bischoff, M. Schäfer (eds.), *Recent Trends in Computational Engineering - CE2014.* Optimization, Uncertainty, Parallel Algorithms, Coupled and Complex Problems.

106. R.M. Kirby, M. Berzins, J.S. Hesthaven (eds.), *Spectral and High Order Methods for Partial Differential Equations - ICOSAHOM'14.*

107. B. Jüttler, B. Simeon (eds.), *Isogeometric Analysis and Applications 2014.*

108. P. Knobloch (ed.), *Boundary and Interior Layers, Computational and Asymptotic Methods – BAIL 2014.*

109. J. Garcke, D. Pflüger (eds.), *Sparse Grids and Applications – Stuttgart 2014.*

110. H. P. Langtangen, *Finite Difference Computing with Exponential Decay Models.*

111. A. Tveito, G.T. Lines, *Computing Characterizations of Drugs for Ion Channels and Receptors Using Markov Models.*

For further information on these books please have a look at our mathematics catalogue at the following URL: www.springer.com/series/3527

Monographs in Computational Science and Engineering

1. J. Sundnes, G.T. Lines, X. Cai, B.F. Nielsen, K.-A. Mardal, A. Tveito, *Computing the Electrical Activity in the Heart.*

For further information on this book, please have a look at our mathematics catalogue at the following URL: www.springer.com/series/7417

Texts in Computational Science and Engineering

1. H. P. Langtangen, *Computational Partial Differential Equations.* Numerical Methods and Diffpack Programming. 2nd Edition
2. A. Quarteroni, F. Saleri, P. Gervasio, *Scientific Computing with MATLAB and Octave.* 4th Edition
3. H. P. Langtangen, *Python Scripting for Computational Science*. 3rd Edition
4. H. Gardner, G. Manduchi, *Design Patterns for e-Science.*
5. M. Griebel, S. Knapek, G. Zumbusch, *Numerical Simulation in Molecular Dynamics.*
6. H. P. Langtangen, *A Primer on Scientific Programming with Python.* 4th Edition
7. A. Tveito, H. P. Langtangen, B. F. Nielsen, X. Cai, *Elements of Scientific Computing.*
8. B. Gustafsson, *Fundamentals of Scientific Computing.*
9. M. Bader, *Space-Filling Curves.*
10. M. Larson, F. Bengzon, *The Finite Element Method: Theory, Implementation and Applications.*
11. W. Gander, M. Gander, F. Kwok, *Scientific Computing: An Introduction using Maple and MATLAB.*
12. P. Deuflhard, S. Röblitz, *A Guide to Numerical Modelling in Systems Biology.*
13. M. H. Holmes, *Introduction to Scientific Computing and Data Analysis.*
14. S. Linge, H. P. Langtangen, *Programming for Computations* - A Gentle Introduction to Numerical Simulations with MATLAB/Octave.
15. S. Linge, H. P. Langtangen, *Programming for Computations* - A Gentle Introduction to Numerical Simulations with Python.

For further information on these books please have a look at our mathematics catalogue at the following URL: www.springer.com/series/5151

Printed in the United States
By Bookmasters